Pseudoscience in Therapy

When experiencing mental health challenges, we all deserve treatments that actually work. Whether you are a healthcare consumer, student, or mental health professional, this book will help you recognize implausible, ineffective, and even harmful therapy practices while also considering recent controversies. Research-supported approaches are identified in this book and expanded upon in a companion volume. Chapters cover every major mental disorder and are written by experts in their respective fields. *Pseudoscience in Therapy* is of interest to students taking courses in psychotherapy, counseling, clinical psychology, and behavior therapy, as well as practitioners looking for a guide to supported therapeutic techniques.

Stephen Hupp, PhD, is a licenced clinical psychologist and professor at Southern Illinois University Edwardsville, USA, where he has won the Great Teacher Award and the Champion for Diversity Award. His edited books include *Investigating Pop Psychology* (2023), *Pseudoscience in Child and Adolescent Psychotherapy* (2019), and *Child and Adolescent Psychotherapy: Components of Evidence-Based Treatments for Youth and Their Parents* (2018). His coauthored books include *Great Myths of Child Development* (2015), *Great Myths of Adolescence* (2019), and *Thinking Critically about Child Development* (2020). He has also written a skeptical game book for children called *Dr. Huckleberry's True or Malarkey? Superhuman Abilities* (2021).

Cara L. Santa Maria, MS, MA, is a public communicator of science and doctoral candidate in clinical psychology at Fielding Graduate University, USA. She has won several awards for science and public interest journalism, including three Los Angeles Area Emmy Awards, the Knight Foundation Innovation Give Forward Award, a Golden Mic Award, and an LA Press Club Award. She is coauthor of *The Skeptics' Guide to the Universe* (2018), and she hosts numerous podcasts including *The Skeptics' Guide to the Universe*, *Fixed That for You*, and *Talk Nerdy with Cara Santa Maria*, which was once featured as a category on *Jeopardy!* She was a correspondent for National Geographic's *Brain Games* and *Explorer*, as well as Netflix's *Bill Nye Saves the World*.

Other Books in This Series

- *Science-Based Therapy*
- *Child and Adolescent Psychotherapy: Components of Evidence-Based Treatments for Youth and Their Parents*
- *Pseudoscience in Child and Adolescent Psychotherapy: A Skeptical Field Guide*

Other Books by Stephen Hupp

- *Dr. Huckleberry's True or Malarkey? Superhuman Abilities*
- *Investigating Pop Psychology: Pseudoscience, Fringe Science, and Controversies*
- *Great Myths of Child Development*
- *Great Myths of Adolescence*
- *Thinking Critically about Child Development: Examining Myths and Misunderstandings*

Other Book by Cara L. Santa Maria

- *The Skeptics' Guide to the Universe: How to Know What's Really Real in a World Increasingly Full of Fake*

Pseudoscience in Therapy

A Skeptical Field Guide

Edited by

Stephen Hupp
Southern Illinois University Edwardsville

Cara L. Santa Maria
Fielding Graduate University

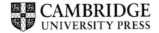

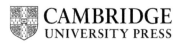
CAMBRIDGE
UNIVERSITY PRESS

Shaftesbury Road, Cambridge CB2 8EA, United Kingdom

One Liberty Plaza, 20th Floor, New York, NY 10006, USA

477 Williamstown Road, Port Melbourne, VIC 3207, Australia

314–321, 3rd Floor, Plot 3, Splendor Forum, Jasola District Centre,
New Delhi – 110025, India

103 Penang Road, #05–06/07, Visioncrest Commercial, Singapore 238467

Cambridge University Press is part of Cambridge University Press & Assessment,
a department of the University of Cambridge.

We share the University's mission to contribute to society through the pursuit of
education, learning and research at the highest international levels of excellence.

www.cambridge.org
Information on this title: www.cambridge.org/9781316519226

DOI: 10.1017/9781009000611

First published 2023

A catalogue record for this publication is available from the British Library.

Library of Congress Cataloging-in-Publication Data
Names: Hupp, Stephen, editor. | Santa Maria, Cara, 1983- editor.
Title: Pseudoscience in therapy : a skeptical field guide / edited by Stephen Hupp,
Southern Illinois University Edwardsville, Cara L. Santa Maria, Fielding
Graduate University.
Description: Cambridge, United Kingdom ; New York, NY : Cambridge University
Press, 2023. | Includes bibliographical references and index.
Identifiers: LCCN 2022054989 | ISBN 9781316519226 (hardback) |
ISBN 9781009005104 (paperback) | ISBN 9781009000611 (ebook)
Subjects: LCSH: Psychotherapy. | Pseudoscience. | Medical misconceptions.
Classification: LCC RC480.5 .P714 2023 | DDC 616.89/14–dc23/eng/20230111
LC record available at https://lccn.loc.gov/2022054989

ISBN 978-1-316-51922-6 Hardback
ISBN 978-1-009-00510-4 Paperback

To my daughter, Vyla Mae Hupp, who has already started changing the world.

(S. H.)

To all those who have supported me on my skeptical journey, I thank you from the bottom of my heart.

(C. L. S. M.)

Contents

Contributors

Damla Aksen, MS, doctoral student of psychology at Binghamton University (SUNY).

Erin F. Alexander, MS, doctoral student of psychology at Binghamton University (SUNY).

Monica Ramirez Basco, PhD, Licensed Clinical Psychologist and Founding Fellow of the Academy of Cognitive Therapy. Author of the book *The Bipolar Workbook, Tools for Controlling Your Mood Swings, Second Edition* (2015).

Jennifer Battles, PhD MS, Primary Care Clinical Psychologist and a member of the Eating Disorder Treatment Team at VA St. Louis Healthcare System.

Brooke L. Bennett, PhD, Postdoctoral Research Fellow at UConn's Rudd Center for Food Policy and Health.

Kirsten Bootes, MA, doctoral student of psychology at the University of Utah.

Emily Braley, MA, doctoral student of psychology at the University of Utah.

Colleen E. Carney, PhD, CPsych, Associate Professor of Psychology at Ryerson University in Canada. Author of the book *Goodnight Mind for Teens: Skills to Help You Quiet Noisy Thoughts and Get the Sleep You Need* (2020).

R. Trent Codd, III, EdS, BCBA, VP of Clinical Services for the Carolinas, Refresh Mental Health. Co-author of the book *Nonlinear Contingency Analysis: Going Beyond Cognition and Behavior in Clinical Practice* (2021).

Olivier Dodier, PhD, Contract Lecturer of Psychology at the University of Nîmes in France.

Claudia Drossel, PhD, Associate Professor of Psychology at Eastern Michigan University. Co-editor of the book *Applications of Behavior Analysis in Healthcare and Beyond* (2021).

Brandon A. Gaudiano, PhD, Professor in the Department of Psychiatry and Human Behavior at the Warren Alpert Medical School of Brown University and in the Department of Behavioral and Social Sciences at the School of Public Health. Editor of the book *Incorporating Acceptance and Mindfulness into the Treatment of Psychosis: Current Trends and Future Directions* (2015).

Harriet Hall, MD, retired family physician. Author of the book *Women Aren't Supposed to Fly: The Memoirs of a Female Flight Surgeon* (2008).

Michael B. Himle, PhD, Associate Professor of Psychology and the Director of Clinical Training at the University of Utah.

David C. Hodgins, PhD, RPsych, FCAHS, Professor of Psychology at the University of Calgary in Canada. Co-editor of the book *Research and Measurement Issues in Gambling Studies* (2007).

Danae L. Hudson, PhD, Professor of Psychology at Missouri State University. Co-author of the book *Revel Psychology* (2019).

Stephen Hupp, PhD, Professor of Psychology at Southern Illinois University Edwardsville. Co-editor of the book *Investigating Pop Psychology: Pseudoscience, Fringe Science, and Controversies* (2023).

Matthew D. Johnson, PhD, Professor of Psychology at Binghamton University. Author of the book *Great Myths of Intimate Relationships: Dating, Sex, and Marriage* (2016).

Hyoun S. Kim, PhD, Assistant Professor of Psychology at Ryerson University in Canada and Director of the Addictions and Mental Health Lab.

Samlau Kutana, BA, graduate student in the Psychology Department at the Memorial University of Newfoundland in Canada.

Parky H. Lau, MA, doctoral student of psychology at Ryerson University in Canada.

Jamie M. Loor, PhD, Postdoctoral Fellow at the University of New Mexico.

Steven Jay Lynn, PhD, Distinguished Professor of Psychology at Binghamton University (SUNY). Co-editor of the book *Evidence-Based Psychotherapy: The State of the Science and Practice* (2018).

Brittany L. Mason, PhD, Scientific Review Officer for the National Institute of Health.

Dean McKay, PhD, Professor of Psychology at Fordham University. Co-editor of the book *Complexities in Obsessive Compulsive and Related Disorders: Advances in Conceptualization and Treatment* (2021).

Harald Merckelbach, PhD, Professor of Psychology at Maastricht University in the Netherlands. Author of the book *Good Stories Are Rarely True* (2020).

Henry Otgaar, PhD, Professor of Psychology at Maastricht University in the Netherlands. Co-editor of the book *Finding the Truth in the Courtroom: Dealing with Deception, Lies, and Memories* (2017).

Jacqueline Pachis, MS, BCBA, doctoral student of psychology at Eastern Michigan University.

Joel Paris, MD, Emeritus Professor of Psychiatry at McGill University in Canada. Author of the book *Treatment of Borderline Personality Disorder: A Guide to Evidence-Based Practice, Second Edition* (2020).

Lawrence Patihis, PhD, Senior Lecturer of Psychology at the University of Plymouth in the United Kingdom. Author of the book *Trauma, Memory, and Law: Enhanced Lectures on Repressed Memories, Memory Distortions, and Trauma* (2022).

Devon L. L. Polaschek, PhD, DipClinPsyc, MNZM, Te Kura Whatu Oho Mauri | School of Psychology and Te Puna Haumaru | New Zealand Institute of Security and Crime Science, University of Waikato. Co-editor of *The Wiley International Handbook of Correctional Psychology* (2019).

Craig P. Polizzi, PhD, completed a doctoral degree in psychology at Binghamton University (SUNY).

Caroline F. Pukall, PhD, Professor of Psychology at Queen's University in Canada. Editor of the book *Human Sexuality: A Contemporary Introduction, Third Edition* (2020).

J. Russell Ramsay, PhD, Professor of Psychology at the University of Pennsylvania Perelman School of Medicine. Author of the book *Rethinking Adult ADHD: Helping Clients Turn Intentions into Actions* (2020).

Gerald M. Rosen, PhD, Clinical Professor Emeritus of Psychology at the University of Washington. Co-editor of the book *Clinician's Guide to Posttraumatic Stress Disorder* (2010).

Cara L. Santa Maria, MS, MA, doctoral candidate in clinical psychology at Fielding Graduate University. Co-author of the book *The Skeptics' Guide to the Universe: How to Know What's Really Real in a World Increasingly Full of Fake* (2018).

Fiona Sleight, MS, doctoral student in psychology at Binghamton University (SUNY).

Jonathan N. Stea, PhD, RPsych, Adjunct Assistant Professor of Psychology at the University of Calgary in Canada. Co-editor of the book *Investigating Clinical Psychology: Pseudoscience, Fringe Science, and Controversies* (in press).

Elizabeth Thompson, PhD, clinical psychologist and Assistant Professor of Psychiatry and Human Behavior at the Warren Alpert Medical School of Brown University and Research Scientist at Rhode Island Hospital.

Jason C. Travers, PhD, BCBA-D, Associate Professor of Teaching and Learning at Temple University. Author of the book *Sexuality Education* (2018).

Katherine Visser, PhD, Staff Psychologist with the Lifespan Physician's Group in Providence, RI.

Brianna Wellen, PhD, doctoral student of psychology at the University of Utah.

Brooke L. Whisenhunt, PhD, Professor of Psychology at Missouri State University. Co-author of the book *Psychological Disorders* 5e (2023).

Igor Yakovenko, PhD, RPsych, Assistant Professor in the Department of Psychology at Dalhousie University in Canada.

Preface

Stephen Hupp

This book is a curated collection of bad ideas. Now you might be thinking, *I don't really need a curated collection of bad ideas.* But before you put this book down, there's something you should know. You've already started collecting bad ideas, and your collection will likely continue to grow.

Fortunately, this book is also a curated collection of good ideas, and you already have a lot of good ideas in your collection, as well. In fact, you might already be effective at distinguishing between the bad and the good; however, you've learned so many ideas that it's sometimes rather tricky to tell the difference. Thus, a field guide can come in handy to help you sort through and evaluate your current collection of ideas while also giving you a quick reference for when you're exposed to new ideas.

Each chapter of this book has a section that identifies *pseudoscience* – or bad ideas – related to therapy. Each chapter also has a section that identifies *research-supported approaches* – or good ideas – related to therapy. Thus, each chapter will distinguish between these two extremes. To be fair, however, some ideas cannot simply be labeled bad or good. That is to say, there's a fuzzy area between the extremes, and because of this challenge, the pseudoscience section of each chapter acknowledges this fuzzy area by discussing questionable ideas and other controversies as well.

Focus and Structure

This book focuses on pseudoscience and questionable ideas related to therapy with adults while another book in this series focuses on youth (i.e., *Pseudoscience in Child and Adolescent Psychotherapy*). Chapter 1 defines broad issues related to understanding pseudoscience and research-supported approaches. All of the other chapters describe conditions that are commonly the focus of clinical attention, and they do so in the same order that they are covered in the *Diagnostic and Statistical*

Manual of Mental Disorders, Fifth Edition, Text Revision. Chapter authors focus on some or all of the following:

- diagnostic controversies
- questionable assessment practices
- myths that influence treatment
- implausible treatments
- ineffective treatments
- potentially harmful treatments
- undermining evidence-based treatments.

Expert Contributors

Book chapters are written by both clinicians and researchers, the majority of whom are licensed psychologists who also engage in university-based research. Additionally, one chapter is from a family physician and another chapter is from a professor of psychiatry. Contributors are from the United States, the United Kingdom, Canada, France, and the Netherlands. Many also regularly engage in science communication activities. Several have published prominent books. Lastly, all of the book's contributors are strong advocates for science-based practices in therapy. In sum, each chapter is a great starting point for helping you distinguish between bad ideas and good ideas about therapy.

Target Audience

The goal of this book is to be a handy reference for all therapists including psychologists, counselors, social workers, psychiatrists, and professionals in related disciplines. Relatedly, it may serve as a supplementary text for graduate courses in psychotherapy and counseling. By covering the same broad topics, it works well in tandem with another book in this series, *Science-Based Therapy*.

Acknowledgments

We are extremely thankful to all of the chapter authors that gave their time to this project. We are equally thankful to everyone at Cambridge University Press who worked to bring this book to life. In particular, Stephen Acerra helped shape all of the books in this series, and Rowan Groat saw this particular book through to completion. Reshma Xavier coordinated the final stages of production, and Sara Brunton was a superb copyeditor. Finally, Scott O. Lilienfeld was a skeptical trailblazer who influenced this book in countless ways.

Thinking Critically about Therapy

Cara L. Santa Maria

As students, researchers, and clinicians, we spend a fair amount of time and effort grappling with the question of how best to approach psychotherapy with our clients. We attempt to focus on what we know works, even if we haven't thought too much about the how and the why behind its efficacy. In my not-so-humble opinion, we should be engaging in honest discussions about not only what works, but also what *doesn't* work.

Truth be told, the mental health field has a long history of dubious claims, quack practitioners, and downright dangerous pseudoscience among its ranks (Fasce, 2018; Lilienfeld et al., 2003). Whether its peddlers are aiming to make an easy dollar or they genuinely believe in the curative properties of their particular brand of snake oil, outcomes are often the same. Therapists have the potential to do great harm to clients if they employ methods that are ineffective, or worse, dangerous to their mental and physical health.

Clinical psychologists, marriage and family therapists, counselors, social workers, psychiatrists, and other mental health practitioners are guided by the ethical principles of their individual disciplines to deliver high-quality treatment to clients in their time of need. In order to do that, we must think critically about therapy. This includes developing a skill dubbed by Carl Sagan (1995) as baloney detection. Sagan described a *baloney detection kit* as including the "tools of skeptical thinking" (p. 210), and this kit can aid in recognizing deception, falsehoods, propaganda, and – you guessed it – pseudoscience.

1.1 Pseudoscience and Questionable Ideas

Pseudoscience is, by definition, fake. Its prefix *pseudo-* is derived from ancient Greek and translates to false, feigned, or deceived. Pseudoscience is something that might look and sound like science – even claiming to be science – but it is incompatible with the scientific method. While it is outside the scope of this book to offer a lengthy philosophical treatise on the tenets of the scientific method, suffice it to say that for something to be accepted as science, it must be testable, reproducible, and verifiable. Pseudoscience lacks one or more of these fundamental qualities.

Especially pernicious is pseudoscience that has managed to infiltrate mainstream psychotherapy practice. Some of the more egregious examples include past-life regression (Pignotti & Thyer, 2019), facilitated communication (Scherr et al., 2019), and conversion therapy (Helms, 2019). These interventions are not only implausible and ineffective, but they are often detrimental.

It is important to remember that pseudoscience can cause harm in several distinct ways. Perhaps most obvious is the capacity for such interventions to induce physical or psychological pain or distress. As mental health practitioners, this is clearly not something we want to do. We are in the business of healing, not hurting. Yet we also don't want to deprive our clients of the time and resources necessary to improve their wellbeing by offering treatments that do not work. If a person is suffering and they spend money and effort on an intervention that won't help them, is this not a type of harm? Finally, when therapists utilize pseudoscience in their practice, they erode trust in the very institutions we ask them to find credible. When clients are burned by their providers, they are less likely to return for treatment, leading to a negative feedback loop of worse and worse outcomes, often for the most vulnerable members of society.

Unfortunately, it is not always easy to differentiate science from pseudoscience. Epistemologists have long contended with the somewhat fuzzy line between science and nonscience. There's even a name for this fuzzy line: the demarcation problem (Pigliucci & Boudry, 2014). Although several prominent philosophers have recommended strategies for dealing with the issue, healthy debate continues to this day (Hansson, 2021).

Yet the ability to sniff out and reject pseudoscience is not just a philosophical one. The demarcation problem has practical implications in areas ranging from public policy to journalism to healthcare. There is no single, foolproof method for baloney detection. In fact, the culmination of our training as scientist-practitioners is only the start. We must be vigilant and maintain a healthy balance between skepticism and open-mindedness. We must practice neuropsychological humility, recognizing cognitive biases and errors of thinking not just in others, but in ourselves. We must critically evaluate the available evidence and make reasonable judgments about claims. And perhaps most importantly, we must continue to ask ourselves the simple question: how do we know what we know?

1.2 Evidence-Informed Practice

I promise I'm not including the following section to confuse you, and I'm definitely not doing it to undermine everything I've said to this point. In fact, its inclusion is a calculated attempt to further refine your baloney detection kit. You see, when we take a deep dive into the outcome literature of various psychotherapeutic interventions, we find that, unfortunately, they don't really work in the same way as pharmacological ones. While many argue that the medical model is sufficient for designing and carrying out psychological research, I assert that the same mechanisms for evaluating the safety and efficacy of a drug don't always translate to testing the effects of psychotherapy.

In fact, it is increasingly safe to say that outcome research in psychotherapy points to its efficacy across several treatment modalities (Barlow, 2010; Wampold & Imel, 2015). Yet *efficacy* and *effectiveness* are two different animals (Baker et al., 2008). Efficacy refers to the outcomes of clinical research under ideal conditions, with little attention paid to applicability. Effectiveness research, on the other hand, involves real-world settings and is considered by many to be a more useful standard than efficacy alone (Hunsley, 2007; Lambert, 2013). For what good is a well-designed, well-controlled study if its outcomes don't translate to actual clients in need?

Psychotherapy's experimental efficacy usually applies whether the treatment offered is theoretically aligned with cognitive-behavioral, humanistic-existential, psychodynamic, or any number of orientations, due to the common factors that underlie all bona fide approaches (Castonguay, 2013). Several decades of high-quality studies support this assertion, yet the beginnings of such investigations were not as promising (Wampold & Imel, 2015).

Famously, Eysenck's (1952) earliest systematic review of the psychotherapy literature raised serious questions about its absolute efficacy. Yet, improvements to study design and statistical technique eventually gave way to the meta-analysis, a standard used to establish outcome measures to this day. After thousands of individual trials and hundreds of meta-analyses, consensus reveals that psychotherapy is not only efficacious but robustly so. In fact, cumulative effect sizes range between .75 and .85, representing a large effect by social science and even medical standards (Barlow, 2010; Wampold & Imel, 2015).

Unfortunately, the vast majority of the research referenced above involves ideal clinical conditions. When reviewing the effectiveness – or real-world – outcome measures for psychotherapy, the picture becomes murkier. An early strategy for determining the practical value of psychotherapy was the clinical representativeness model, in which meta-analyses are performed to determine which factors exert influence when comparing community settings to the laboratory. Smith and Glass (1977) performed such an analysis and found that, unfortunately, laboratory findings did not readily translate to community settings. Since then, more sophisticated techniques like benchmarking have shown some evidence that psychotherapy in practice is effective (Hunsley, 2007).

In addition to legitimate validity concerns about the translation of research to practice, several challenges currently face clinicians, educators, and policymakers who have been tasked with utilizing evidence-based practices (i.e., only those treatments that have robust research literature supporting their efficacy and/or effectiveness). For example, Barlow and colleagues (2013) point out that a paucity of efficacy research on ethnic minority individuals exists in the United States. Combined with concerns about comorbidity – the vast majority of psychological research involves a single complaint or diagnosis – and other types of individual variability, the applicability of outcome research becomes questionable. In addition, Gaudiano and Miller (2013) describe a narrow focus on short-term outcomes that ignores potential downstream benefits. Similarly, Lambert (2013) calls for an increased focus on developing mechanisms for real-time assessment of treatment effectiveness in individual clients, as far too often clinicians rely on lagging research to inform current practice.

This brings us to the crux of the issue at hand, namely, to what extent should practitioners solely utilize evidence-based practice in their clinical work? Isn't it in the best interest of the client to receive care that is held to the highest possible standard? This is a difficult proposition with which to argue, and at its surface, a resounding "of course!" appears to be in order. However, as mentioned in the previous sections of this chapter, the issue at hand is much more complicated than it would seem superficially.

I personally am a staunch supporter of evidence-based practice in medicine and have made a career of debunking pseudoscience in my work as a public science communicator. For one example of my efforts, check out our book *The Skeptics' Guide to the Universe* (Novella, Novella, Santa Maria, Novella, & Bernstein, 2018). As a psychotherapist, I align with the humanistic-existential orientation, a theoretical stance that disavows statistical homogenization of individual clients and even cautions against labeling through diagnosis. It appears to me that a balancing act must be performed by each and every clinician in an effort to provide the highest possible standard of care for their clients. Indeed, utilizing best practices from therapeutic techniques that are known to produce positive outcomes is generally a safe (and beneficent) bet. Yet, doing so at the expense of individualized, authentic, and meaningful care will surely backfire.

I agree with the recommendations made by Baker and colleagues (2008) to set a high standard in scientific education for each and every therapist-in-training. I believe that this will prepare clinicians for the real-world challenges they will face in the clinic, hospital, or private therapy room. Yet I also believe we must remember that therapists, like clients, are unique individuals with rich and complex needs. Because of this, a manualized, one-size-fits-all model is not and will never be the answer. Perhaps instead of describing the ideal psychotherapeutic intervention as evidence-based, a more appropriate term might be evidence-informed. This approach is firmly rooted in a scientific foundation, while still leaving room for adaptability, nuance, and clinical intuition. It does not leave room, however, for pseudoscience. When a treatment has been sufficiently debunked, is based upon dubious claims, or lacks a valid mechanism of action, it has no place in the therapeutic relationship. Pseudoscience is harmful, for the myriad reasons delineated in this volume.

1.3 What Exactly Is Evidence?

As psychological researchers and practitioners, we strive to utilize the best available evidence in making prudent decisions about standards of care. Yet we don't often take the time to think critically about how we define high-quality evidence. Indeed, the randomized controlled trial (RCT) is generally considered to be the gold standard in psychotherapy research. Although it has, in many ways, been a boon to the field, it also introduces legitimate concerns. Below, I will detail some of the methodological issues seen in staunchly evidence-based treatments as well as suggested improvements for translational research.

According to Kazdin (2008), one of the biggest difficulties that RCTs have brought to the surface concerns the deep disconnect often found between research and practice. Although RCTs consistently show that psychotherapy is beneficial when compared to no treatment (absolute efficacy), there is less evidence favoring the relative efficacy of individual treatments, regardless of the clinical orientation of the psychotherapist or the client population (Beutler & Forrester, 2014). Furthermore, effectiveness research is often limited or nonexistent. As opposed to efficacy research, effectiveness studies occur in community settings, offering a better measure of the generalizability of research to practice. This makes them a better indicator of the usefulness of evidence-based treatments (Tolin et al., 2015).

Additionally, the standard methodology of controlling all variables while manipulating only those of interest is incredibly challenging when working with real people (both therapists and clients alike). There are myriad confounds at play, as well as mediating and moderating variables. Fortunately for us and unfortunate for RCTs, human beings are neither mice nor fruit flies. Kazdin (2008) argues that participants in controlled trials generally have less severe psychopathology and fewer comorbid disorders than those in actual clinical treatment. If an intervention is found to be useful for an "ideal" research participant, does it actually offer any real-world benefit to clients in the clinic? RCTs often ignore the rich context of the clinical milieu, leaving out considerations such as typical life stressors, meaning-making, and navigating tough decisions. Instead, clinical trials are laser-focused on diagnosis and symptomatology, representing a less-than-realistic view of typical psychotherapy.

What may then follow are manualized treatments that offer something of a one-size-fits-all approach to intervention. Constructive critics recommend searching for moderating variables outside of the treatment paradigm or diagnosis to improve study design, making it more inclusive and robust (Beutler & Forrester, 2014). In addition, Tolin and colleagues (2015) offer several recommendations, such as moving away from measures of statistical significance and toward effect size estimates (something that is becoming increasingly common in the research literature). In addition, because clinical judgment is often not included as a measured factor in RCTs, an increased focus on mechanisms of change, moderating variables, and qualitative research may fill the void.

It is important to note, however, that RCTs have brought much rigor and benefit to the field of psychotherapy research. Controlled trials move the field as a whole away from clinical anecdotes toward verifiable evidence. They also aid in removing bias and helping to identify confounding variables. Yet in the predominantly cognitive-behavioral RCT model, diagnosis often dominates, and pathology reduction is front and center. By comparison, the humanistic approach places greater emphasis on revealing and encouraging the strengths of the client. Of course, many psychotherapists are adept at finding a healthy balance of multiple approaches. It is important that we remain skeptical even of the gold standards we often utilize in psychotherapy research and practice. They may not translate to real-world settings, especially with clients of color, gender minorities, and those with complex cases involving comorbid diagnoses and biopsychosocial stressors.

1.4 Science-Based Treatments

With all of the above cautions in mind, there's one more major topic to discuss. When considering the evidence base regarding a therapeutic approach, it's helpful to understand what goes into characterizing a treatment as *evidence-based* or even *science-based*. In the 1990s, a task force from the Society of Clinical Psychology (Division 12 of the American Psychological Association) published a set of criteria for identifying *empirically validated treatments* (American Psychological Association Task Force on the Promotion and Disseminating of Psychological Procedures, 1995). Since then, experts have changed the label to *empirically supported treatments* (Chambless & Hollon, 1998) and later, *evidence-based treatments* (American Psychological Association Presidential Task Force on Evidence-Based Practice, 2006). Throughout the evolution of this label, the criteria have remained largely intact. In short, in order for a treatment to qualify for the highest level of the *evidence-based* characterization, it typically needs research support from at least two high-quality RCTs by at least two different teams.

Given the criticisms of this approach (some of which have been identified in previous sections of this chapter), other additions and revisions have been suggested. For example, *plausibility* is often highlighted as an important characteristic (Hupp et al., 2019). Tolin and colleagues (2015) have made several additional suggestions, such as placing a greater emphasis on: (a) systematic reviews, (b) clinical significance, (c) generalization of findings, (d) long-term efficacy, and (e) identification of evidence-based *components* within treatment packages. These factors collectively define *science-based treatments*. A more thorough discussion on this topic can be found in other books in this series – *Science-Based Therapy* (Hupp & Tolin, in press) and *Child and Adolescent Psychotherapy* (Hupp, 2018).

1.5 Conclusion

In the pages that follow, we have invited individuals with expertise in various mental health fields to share their wisdom about the pseudoscience they often encounter. We have asked them to detail implausible, ineffective, and harmful treatments, with a focus on potential outcomes for clients. They also describe diagnostic controversies, questionable assessment practices, and myths that tend to influence treatment. To be clear, not everything in this book can fairly be labeled *pseudoscience*, as there is a fuzzy line filled with many questions, controversies, and otherwise untested ideas. And while we have asked the chapter authors to dedicate the majority of their chapters to highlighting pseudoscience and questionable ideas, they also include brief sections on treatments that are informed by the best available evidence. That is, each chapter will have a Research-Supported Approaches section, meant to be inclusive of the many possible ways of identifying what works in therapy (i.e., authors had the freedom to frame the discussion in terms of evidence-informed treatments, evidence-based treatments, and/or science-based treatments). [It should be noted that the authors were encouraged to focus primarily on therapy for adults as *Pseudoscience in Child and Adolescent Psychotherapy* (Hupp, 2019) is available for additional reference.] We enthusiastically thank the chapter authors for their participation in this book.

Now it's time to start honing that baloney detection kit of yours. Keep an eye out for dubious claims, hyped-up anecdotes, and panaceas. Check your own confirmation bias – that is, the tendency to only seek out evidence that supports your beliefs and dismiss evidence to the contrary. Practice your neuropsychological humility. And above all else, help the mental health field prioritize clients' wellbeing by utilizing assessment, diagnostic, and treatment paradigms that are informed by high-quality evidence. In doing so, you will encourage beneficence and reduce maleficence – the hallmarks of ethical psychotherapy.

Cara L. Santa Maria, M.S., M.A., is a doctoral candidate in clinical psychology at Fielding Graduate University. She is co-author of the book *The Skeptics' Guide to the Universe: How to Know What's Really Real in a World Increasingly Full of Fake* (2018).

References

American Psychological Association Presidential Task Force on Evidence-Based Practice. (2006). Evidence-based practice in psychology. *American Psychologist, 61*, 271–285.

American Psychological Association Task Force on Promotion and Dissemination of Psychological Procedures. (1995). Training in and dissemination of empirically-validated psychological treatments: Report and recommendations. *The Clinical Psychologist, 48*, 3–23.

Baker, T., McFall, R., & Shodham, V. (2008). Current status and future prospects of clinical psychology: Toward a scientifically principled approach to mental and behavioral health care. *Psychological Science in the Public Interest, 9*, 68–103.

Barlow, D. H. (2010). Negative effects from psychological treatments: A perspective. *American Psychologist, 65*(1), 13–20.

Barlow, D. H., Bullis, J. R., Comer, J. S., & Ametaj, A. A. (2013). Evidence-based psychological treatments: An update and a way forward. *Annual Review of Clinical Psychology, 9*, 1–27.

Beutler, L. E., & Forrester, B. (2014). What needs to change: Moving from "research informed" practice to "empirically effective" practice. *Journal of Psychotherapy Integration, 24*(3), 168–177.

Castonguay, L. G. (2013). Psychotherapy outcome: An issue worth re-visiting 50 years later. *Psychotherapy, 50*(1), 52–67.

Chambless, D. L., & Hollon, S. D. (1998). Defining empirically supported therapies. *Journal of Consulting and Clinical Psychology, 66*(1), 7–18.

Eysenck, H. J. (1952). The effects of psychotherapy: An evaluation. *Journal of Consulting Psychology, 16*, 319–324.

Fasce, A. (2018). Divan couches and gurus: The origin and dangers of clinical pseudopsychology. *Mètode Science Studies Journal, 8*, 165–171.

Gaudiano, B. A., & Miller, I. W. (2013). The evidence-based practice of psychotherapy: Facing the challenges that lie ahead. *Clinical Psychology Review, 33*, 813–824.

Hansson, S. O. (2021). Science and pseudo-science, *The Stanford Encyclopedia of Philosophy*. https://plato.stanford.edu/archives/fall2021/entries/pseudo-science/.

Helms, S. W. (2019). What is gay conversion therapy? In S. Hupp (ed.), *Pseudoscience in child and adolescent psychotherapy: A skeptical field guide* (pp. 292–293). Cambridge University Press.

Hunsley, J. (2007). Addressing key challenges in evidence-based practice in psychology. *Professional Psychology: Research and Practice, 38*(2), 113–121.

Hupp, S. (2018). *Child and adolescent psychotherapy: Components of evidence-based treatments for youth and their parents.* Cambridge University Press.

Hupp, S. (2019). *Pseudoscience in child and adolescent psychotherapy: A skeptical field guide.* Cambridge University Press.

Hupp, S., Mercer, J., Thyer, B. A., & Pignotti, M. (2019). Critical thinking about psychotherapy. In S. Hupp (Ed.), *Pseudoscience in child and adolescent psychotherapy: A skeptical field guide.* Cambridge University Press.

Hupp, S., & Tolin, D. (in press). *Science-based therapy.* Cambridge University Press.

Kazdin, A. E. (2008). Evidence-based treatment and practice: New opportunities to bridge clinical research and practice, enhance the knowledge base, and improve care. *American Psychologist, 63*, 146–159.

Lambert, M. J. (2013). Outcome in psychotherapy: The past and important advances. *Psychotherapy*, *50*(1), 42–51.

Lilienfeld, S. O., Lynn, S. J., & Lohr, J. M. (Eds.). (2003). *Science and pseudoscience in clinical psychology*. New York, NY: The Guilford Press.

Novella, S., Novella, B., Santa Maria, C., Novella, J., & Bernstein, E. (2018). *The skeptics' guide to the universe: How to know what's really real in a world increasingly full of fake*. Grand Central Publishing.

Pigliucci, M., & Boudry, M. (2014). *Philosophy of pseudoscience: Reconsidering the demarcation problem*. University of Chicago Press.

Pignotti, M., & Thyer, B., (2019). Obsessions and compulsions. In S. Hupp (Ed.), *Pseudoscience in child and adolescent psychotherapy: A skeptical field guide* (pp. 159–171). Cambridge University Press.

Sagan, C. (1995). *The demon-haunted world: Science as a candle in the dark*. Random House.

Scherr, J. F., Kryszak, E. M., & Mulick, J. A. (2019). Autism spectrum. In S. Hupp (Ed.), *Pseudoscience in child and adolescent psychotherapy: A skeptical field guide* (pp. 28–49). Cambridge University Press.

Smith, M. L., & Glass, G. V. (1977). Meta-analysis of psychotherapy outcome studies. *American Psychologist*, *32*, 752–760.

Tolin, D. F., McKay, D., Forman, E. M., Klonsky, E. D., & Thombs, B. D. (2015). Empirically supported treatment: Recommendations for a new model. *Clinical Psychology: Science and Practice*, *22*, 317–338.

Wampold, B. J., & Imel, Z. E. (2015). *The great psychotherapy debate: The evidence for what makes psychotherapy work*. 2nd edn. Routledge.

Depression

R. Trent Codd, III

Major depressive disorder (American Psychiatric Association [APA], 2022) is characterized by five or more symptoms that have persisted for at least two weeks. One symptom must be depressed mood or diminished interest or pleasure in most activities. Others may include significant changes in weight or appetite disturbance, sleep disturbance, psychomotor agitation or retardation, fatigue, feelings of worthlessness or inappropriate guilt, diminished ability to think or concentrate, indecisiveness, and recurrent thoughts of death, suicidal impulses, or actions. These symptoms must represent a change from previous functioning.

Persistent depressive disorder (previously known as dysthymia; APA, 2022) consists of depressed mood that persists for at least two years in adults, is present most of the time, and is associated with at least two of the following symptoms: appetite disturbance, low energy or fatigue, low self-esteem, sleep disturbance, difficulty concentrating or making decisions, or feelings of hopelessness. The symptoms of major depressive and persistent depressive disorder must cause clinically significant distress or impairment in important areas of functioning. Although the *Diagnostic and Statistical Manual of Mental Disorders, Fifth Edition, Text Revision* (DSM-5-TR) separately categorizes other disorders that contain depressive features, this chapter's focus is primarily limited to the above disorders.

2.1 Pseudoscience and Questionable Ideas

This chapter will address several topics that pertain to controversies and pseudoscience related to depressive disorders. Two primary diagnostic and assessment controversies will be described. Then, several treatments will be critiqued.

2.1.1 Diagnostic and Assessment Controversies

2.1.1.1 Should Grief Be Captured within the Major Depressive Disorder Diagnosis?

A primary area of controversy has pertained to the symptoms of grief being captured by the diagnosis of major depressive disorder in the *Diagnostic and Statistical Manual of Mental Disorders, Fifth Edition* (DSM-5; APA, 2013). Because there is substantial symptom overlap with grief and major depressive disorder, there is concern that mental health clinicians are unable to reliably distinguish between the two. The concern is greater with nonmental health specialty practitioners, such as primary care providers, who have less patient contact time (i.e., less time to fully assess) and less training in psychiatric diagnosing relative to licensed mental health practitioners in specialty settings. This is notable because most patients are seen, and antidepressants prescribed, in primary care settings by these practitioners (Barkil-Oteo, 2013). This combination of factors may result in diagnostic excess, effectively pathologizing normative reactions to interpersonal loss. Previous editions of the DSM addressed this difficulty by making patients ineligible for a diagnosis of major depressive disorder when they had experienced the loss of a loved one within a certain period (e.g., two months in the DSM-IV). Such time-based bereavement exclusions were removed in DSM-5 (Frances, 2013), which permitted major depressive disorder to be diagnosed even when assessors were unable to distinguish the grief symptom picture from the mood disturbance. The DSM-5 supported prudent diagnostic practices around this issue by allowing the use of clinical judgment when attempting to differentiate grief from major depressive disorder. However, many experienced diagnosticians questioned whether accurate discriminations are possible (e.g., Frances, 2013).

The latest edition of the diagnostic manual, the DSM-5-TR (APA, 2022), has recently added a new diagnosis – prolonged grief disorder. This diagnosis can be provided if an adult's persistent grief lasts at least 12 months, causes significant impairment, and meets at least 4 of 10 specific symptoms. However, this diagnosis is housed in the trauma and related stressors section of the manual. Over time, we'll get to see the pros and cons of this addition.

2.1.1.2 Can Imaging Technology Facilitate Diagnosis and Treatment?

Single photon emission computed tomography (SPECT) is a type of imaging technology that uses radioactive isotopes injected into the bloodstream to measure blood flow in the brain (Amen & Easton, 2021). Some clinicians use this imaging technology to facilitate psychiatric diagnosis and treatment, and proponents contend that psychiatry has undervalued the clinical utility of SPECT scans (Amen, 2008). A related website suggests that it is possible to "use brain imaging technology to identify your specific brain type, so we are able to tailor a targeted treatment plan to enhance your quality of life" (Amen Clinics, n.d.a., para. 1). In addition, a depression-specific section of the website suggests that SPECT enhances the ability to determine how patients will respond to treatment, at least in part, through the identification of depression-related brain patterns. According to the website, "there are 7 different brain patterns associated with depression, and knowing your type can be the key to getting the most effective treatment" (Amen Clinics, n.d.b., para. 6).

These claims are controversial in the psychiatric and neurological communities. For example, Robert Burton (2008) refers to SPECT scans as a "brain scam," in the title of a related article. In letters to the editor of the *Journal of Psychiatry* (Adinoff & Devous, 2010a), two psychiatrists assert that claims related to SPECT were not supported by the scientific evidence and that "there is presently no evidence to support neuroimaging techniques to aid, substantiate, or otherwise illuminate the diagnosis and treatment of psychiatric disorders" (Adinoff & Devous, 2010b, p. 1125). Satel and Lilienfeld (2013, p. 24) indicate that there is "near universal agreement among psychiatrists and psychologists that scans cannot presently be used to diagnose mental illness." Whether or not SPECT scans are useful in optimizing patient care is largely an untested question. In a summary of the controversy, Hall (2013) lays out several criticisms of SPECT scans, suggesting that this approach: (a) does not provide accurate diagnosis, (b) has limited research, (c) exposes patients to potentially unnecessary radiation, and (d) is expensive. Further, SPECT scans for depression are not generally covered by insurance (see Farah & Gillihan, 2012, and Bernstein, 2016, for more discussion).

2.1.2 Implausible, Ineffective, and Controversial Treatments

2.1.2.1 Apispuncture

The application of bee stings to one or more specific acupuncture points – apispuncture – has been offered as a treatment for depression (Abd El-Wahab & Eita, 2015). This intervention appears to be based on two problematic assumptions: (1) that acupuncture in general is efficacious in the treatment of depression, and (2) that bee stings enhance the effectiveness of traditional acupuncture. Neither assumption is supported by scientific evidence.

The conclusions articulated in a Cochrane review (Smith et al., 2018) of acupuncture for the treatment of depression did not support the contention that it is clinically efficacious. The authors indicated that the existing empirical evidence is of low or very low quality, advising cautious interpretation. Furthermore, they report that the effects of acupuncture relative to medication and psychotherapy are uncertain. Moreover, randomized controlled research has demonstrated that acupuncture is not effective for depression (Allen et al., 2006). Additionally, it is implausible as a treatment for depression (see Novella, 2010, for additional critique of the research).

Adverse events associated with treatments should always be investigated. However, the frequency of adverse events associated with acupuncture is unknown as most trials examined do not report these data. The authors of the Cochrane review emphasized the need for high-quality randomized trials before conclusions regarding efficacy and effectiveness could be made (Smith et al., 2018). Given that the efficacy of acupuncture for depression is highly questionable, it is problematic to build upon the intervention with live bee stings. One cannot assume the ability to enhance the efficacy of a treatment that has weak evidence of efficacy to begin with.

Only one empirical study of apispuncture – using bee stings – for depression was located after a thorough literature search (Abd El-Wahab & Eita, 2015). Although they reported significant reductions in depression from pre- to post-intervention in their sample, this study contained several methodological weaknesses. Most notably, the intervention was tested on a small convenience sample ($n = 37$) that was not randomly assigned to treatment and control conditions, thus failing to adequately control for threats to validity. Furthermore, the depressive nature of the tested clinical population was unclear. For example, the authors first indicated the purpose of the study was to evaluate "the effectiveness of live bee sting acupuncture on first episode of depression" (Abd El-Wahab & Eita, 2015, p. 21), but later specified that a diagnosis of major depression was an exclusion criterion. *Beck Depression Inventory* (Beck et al., 1961) scores were reported for their sample, however, which revealed moderate (59.5%) and severe (40.5%) levels of depression pre-treatment.

Two additional difficulties with this study involve the discussion of the proposed mechanism of action and the rationale provided for the investigation. For example, the description of acupuncture's mechanism of action was vague and offered in contradictory ways. They suggested acupuncture works by "restoring the proper flow of the patient's life force" (Abd El-Wahab & Eita, 2015, p. 20), at other times suggesting it impacts various biological substances such as neurotransmitters, while also indicating that the precise mechanism of action is unknown. An additional rationale provided was that live bee stings provoke an immune response that causes antidepressant effects. Finally, one of the rationales given for the study was that conventional therapy had significant limitations. Although no existing treatment realizes perfect outcomes, several robust treatments are indeed available for depressive disorders (see more on this in the Research-Supported Approaches section).

2.1.2.2 Other Complementary and Alternative Medicine Approaches

Large surveys conducted in the United States by the Centers for Disease Control and Prevention revealed that around 40% of adults used some form of complementary and alternative medicine in the preceding 12 months for various concerns, including depression (Barnes et al., 2004; 2008). Respondents offered five reasons for their interest in complementary and alternative medicine, the most common of which was the belief it was helpful in combination with standard treatment approaches. The next most common reasons provided were the notion that it was interesting to try (50%), the belief that conventional medical approaches would not be helpful (28%), the exposure to a medical professional who recommended it (26%), and the feeling it was more affordable than conventional medical intervention (13%). The ten complementary and alternative therapies most endorsed by respondents were reported by Barnes et al. (2004; 2008). Three of these ten were selected for examination in this chapter and include natural products, diet-based approaches, and massage.

Dietary Supplements

Some mental health professionals propose that nutritional factors play an important role in the development and maintenance of depressive disorders, and therefore consider them useful treatment targets. Interventions derived from this perspective include the use of nutritional supplements and herbal remedies (e.g., St. John's wort). These interventions have sometimes been recommended as adjuncts to front-line treatments, such as antidepressant medication or psychotherapy, while at other times they have been proposed as monotherapies.

Dietary supplements are defined by federal law as containing these elements: (1) they are taken orally, (2) they are intended to supplement diet, (3) they contain one or more dietary ingredients, and (4) they are labeled as dietary supplements (Food and Drug Administration [FDA], 2005; National Center for Complimentary and Integrative Health, 2020). The volume of scientific evidence for dietary supplements varies considerably.

The National Center for Complimentary and Integrative Health (2020) provides some general conclusions regarding this literature. First, when scientific evidence exists for a supplement, the supplement investigated in studies may differ from those available to consumers for purchase. This makes generalizing from the data available in scientific papers to the consumer market difficult. Second, supplements may interact with medications or may elevate risks during surgery. Consequently, consumers should be sure to disclose any supplements they are taking to all of their healthcare providers. Third, many supplements have not been tested in children, or pregnant or breastfeeding women. Therefore, additional caution should be exercised when considering the use of supplements with these populations. Fourth, what is listed on a dietary label may be inaccurate and may not include every ingredient contained in the product. Fifth, supplements are not as strongly regulated as medication.

The FDA regulates supplements as food rather than as drugs (FDA, 2022). However, this can be misleading because some supplements may have components that interfere with other medications, or they may function as drugs even though they are labeled as supplements. This might lead consumers to underestimate the risks associated with supplements. The FDA does take consumer-protecting action at times, however. For example, they recently announced they sent warning letters to ten companies illegally selling supplements claiming to cure, treat, mitigate, or prevent depression (Food and Drug Administration, 2021). They further stated these supplements were unapproved new drugs and cautioned they could be harmful to consumers because they had not evaluated whether they were effective for their intended use, what the proper dosage might be, whether and how they interact with other drugs, whether they have harmful side effects, or whether they are unsafe in other ways. They also expressed concern that these supplements may be harmful to consumers by interfering with efficacious treatments if they pursued these supplements in lieu of treatments with known efficacy and safety profiles.

Empirical investigation of nutritional factors in mental health conditions, including depressive disorders, has increased over the past two decades (Schefft et al., 2017), with a field dubbed *nutritional psychiatry* (Sarris et al., 2015) organizing around these issues. For example, a systematic review and meta-analysis investigated the efficacy of several supplements as possible ways to augment antidepressant medication (Schefft et al., 2017). These included inositol, vitamin D, folic acid, vitamin B12, *S*-adenosyl-L-methionine (SAMe), omega-3 polyunsaturated fatty acids (n-3 PUFA), and zinc. Efficacy was only found for zinc and n-3 PUFAs for patients without medical or neurological comorbidities. In the case of folic acid, the authors of the review contend that there is sufficient evidence to suggest it is not efficacious. For the remaining substances, the authors conclude the literature was insufficiently mature to support claims of efficacy or to otherwise facilitate drawing conclusions.

Additionally, St. John's wort, or *Hypericum perforatum*, is an herbal remedy used to treat depression. Its scientific support is mixed. In a systematic review, Dhingra and Parle (2012) reported modest effects over placebo in the treatment of mild to moderate depression, stating there was insufficient evidence to draw conclusions about its effects in severe cases. In addition, *Hypericum* may interact with other medications, weakening their effects or increasing their side effects. These interactive effects have been observed with antidepressant medications, oral contraceptives, antiviral agents, and anticoagulants (Clement et al., 2006; Fava et al., 2005).

Ketogenic Diet
The ketogenic diet has been recommended as an adjunctive intervention to medication and psychotherapy in the treatment of depression (Wlodarczyk et al., 2021). The ketogenic diet is characterized by a high fat, moderate protein, and low carbohydrate eating pattern with a primary purpose of producing the metabolic state of ketosis (Masood et al., 2021). This diet is associated with enzymatic changes thought to elevate extracellular GABA levels that positively impact mood (Wlodarczyk et al., 2021). The existing literature examining the impact of the ketogenic diet on depression is limited. It is currently composed of a few rodent studies that demonstrated antidepressant effects (Ari et al., 2016; Scolnick, 2017; Zhang et al., 2015) and a human case report describing a reduction in general depressive symptoms as a result of starvation (von Geijer & Ekelund, 2015). There are no randomized controlled trials that have investigated the effects of this dietary pattern on depression. Thus, there is currently an insufficient empirical basis to conclude the ketogenic diet is efficacious in the treatment of depressive disorders. Additional concerns include association with emergency room

visits for dehydration, electrolyte disturbance, and hypoglycemia (Armeno et al., 2018; Güzel et al., 2016; Wlodarek, 2019).

Massage
Massage therapy has been proposed as an intervention for psychiatric disorders, including depression (Rapaport et al., 2018). The body of evidence is mildly supportive of its utility as an adjunctive intervention for depressive symptoms that are present during acute periods of dysphoria, but there is limited evidence to support its use in the treatment of depressive disorders (Rapaport et al., 2018). In addition, the existing literature suffers from a range of methodological problems compromising what may be confidently gleaned from the published data, including widely varied massage protocols, small and heterogeneous samples, and insufficient use of reliable and valid depression measures.

2.2 Research-Supported Approaches

Several efficacious psychological treatments for depressive disorders are presently available. Division 12 of the American Psychological Association maintains a list of evidence-based interventions. Broadly speaking, the psychological treatments with the strongest research support include cognitive-behavioral therapy (e.g., Butler et al., 2006) and interpersonal psychotherapy (e.g., Cuijpers et al., 2011). Cognitive-behavioral therapy is a skills-based approach that focuses on developing adaptive ways of thinking and behaving. Interpersonal psychotherapy, in contrast, emphasizes the remediation of problematic interpersonal relationships that maintain depression. Additionally, two psychotherapies were specifically designed for depressive disorders that are chronic and refractory, and both have strong empirical support. The first is Radically Open Dialectical Behavior Therapy, which is a transdiagnostic approach that targets skills related to social bonds such as openness, flexible responding, and social signaling (Gilbert et al., 2020; Lynch, 2018). The second is Cognitive Behavioral Analysis System of Psychotherapy. (McCollough, 1999). This approach combines situational analysis (a type of problem-solving), interpersonal discrimination exercises (which examine previous traumatic experiences), and behavioral skills training (such as practicing assertiveness skills). Although beyond the scope of this chapter, some of the other interventions to be considered include antidepressant medications and electroconvulsive therapy for severe depression. See Hupp and Tolin (in press) for more information about research-supported approaches.

2.3 Conclusion

Depressive disorders are common, frequently comorbid with other mental disorders, and impair several domains of functioning. Two primary diagnostic and assessment controversies include whether clinicians can reliably distinguish normative grief reactions from a mood disturbance and whether imaging technology can optimize the identification and treatment of depressive disorders. Several dubious interventions exist, and include apispuncture and various unsupported complementary and alternative medicine approaches. Fortunately, robust psychological treatments are available, including for severe and difficult-to-treat depression. Depressive disorder treatment outcomes are optimized when these treatments are delivered by adequately trained practitioners who deliver them with fidelity. Treatment is further enhanced by avoiding scientifically unsupported assessment and treatment practices.

R. Trent Codd, III, EdS, BCBA, is the VP of Clinical Services for the Carolinas, Refresh Mental Health. He is co-author of the book *Nonlinear Contingency Analysis: Going Beyond Cognition and Behavior in Clinical Practice* (2021).

References

Abd El-Wahab, S. D., & Eita, L. H. (2015). The effectiveness of live bee sting acupuncture on depression. *IOSR Journal of Nursing and Health Science*, *4*, 19–27.

Adinoff, B., & Devous, M. (2010a). Scientifically unfounded claims in diagnosing and treating patients. *American Journal of Psychiatry*, *167*(5), 598–599. https://doi.org/10.1176/appi.ajp.2010.10020157.

Adinoff, B., & Devous Sr,M. D. (2010b). Response to Amen letter. *American Journal of Psychiatry*, *167*(9), 1125–1126. https://doi.org/10.1176/appi .ajp.2010.10050671r.

Allen, J. J., Schnyer, R. N., Chambers, A. S., Hitt, S. K., Moreno, F. A., & Manber, R. (2006). Acupuncture for depression: A randomized controlled trial. *The Journal of Clinical Psychiatry*, *67*(11), 1665–1673.

Amen Clinics. (n.d.a). Brain SPECT. www.amenclinics.com/services/brain-spect/.

Amen Clinics. (n.d.b). Depression. www.amenclinics.com/conditions/depression/

Amen, D. (2008). *Healing the hardware of the soul: How making the brain–soul connection can optimize your life, love, and spiritual growth.* Simon and Schuster.

Amen, D. G., & Easton, M. (2021). A new way forward: How brain SPECT imaging can improve outcomes and transform mental health care into brain health care. *Frontiers in Psychiatry, 12,* 715315.

American Psychiatric Association (APA). (2013). *Diagnostic and statistical manual of mental disorders.* 5th edn. https://doi.org/10.1176/appi.books.9780890425596.

American Psychiatric Association (APA). (2022). *Diagnostic and statistical manual of mental disorders, fifth edition, text revision* (DSM-5-TR). American Psychiatric Association.

Ari, C., Kovács, Z., Juhasz, G., Murdun, C., Goldhagen, C. R., Koutnik, A. P., Poff, A. M., Kesl, S. L., & D'Agostino, D. P. (2017). Exogenous ketone supplements reduce anxiety-related behavior in Sprague-Dawley and Wistar Albino Glaxo/Rijswijk rats. *Frontiers in Molecular Neuroscience, 9,* 137. https://doi.org/10.3389/fnmol.2016.00137.

Armeno, M., Araujo, C., Sotomontesano, B., & Caraballo, R. H. (2018). Update on the adverse effects during therapy with a ketogenic diet in pediatric refractory epilepsy. *Revista de Neurologia, 66*(6), 193–200.

Barkil-Oteo, A. (2013). Collaborative care for depression in primary care: How psychiatry could "troubleshoot" current treatments and practices. *The Yale Journal of Biology and Medicine, 86*(2), 139–146.

Barnes, P. M., Bloom, B., & Nahin, R. L. (2008). Complementary and alternative medicine use among adults and children: United States, 2007. *National Health Statistics Report,* (12), 1–23.

Barnes, P. M., Powell-Griner, E., McFann, K., & Nahin, R. L. (2004). Complementary and alternative medicine use among adults: United States, 2002. *Advance Data from Vital and Health Statistics,* (343), 1–19.

Beck, A. T., Ward, C. H., Mendelson, M., Mock, J., & Erbaugh, J. (1961). An inventory for measuring depression. *Archives of General Psychiatry, 4,* 561–571. https://doi.org/10.1001/archpsyc.1961.01710120031004.

Bernstein, R. (2016). Head case: Why has PBS promoted controversial shrink Dr. Daniel Amen? https://observer.com.

Burton, R. (2008). Brain scam. https://neurocritic.blogspot.com/2008/05/more-brain-scams.html.

Butler, A. C., Chapman, J. E., Forman, E. M., & Beck, A. T. (2006). The empirical status of cognitive-behavioral therapy: A review of meta-analyses. *Clinical Psychology Review, 26*(1), 17–31. https://doi.org/10.1016/j.cpr.2005.07.003.

Clement, K., Covertson, C. R., Johnson, M. J., & Dearing, K. (2006). St. John's wort and the treatment of mild to moderate depression: A systematic review. *Holistic Nursing Practice, 20*(4), 197–203.

Cuijpers, P., Geraedts, A. S., van Oppen, P., Andersson, G., Markowitz, J. C., & van Straten, A. (2011). Interpersonal psychotherapy for depression: A meta-analysis. *American Journal of Psychiatry, 168*(6), 581–592. https://doi .org/10.1176/appi.ajp.2010.10101411.

Dhingra, S., & Parle, M. (2012). Herbal remedies and nutritional supplements in the treatment of depression: A review. *Klinik Psikofarmakoloji Bülteni-Bulletin of Clinical Psychopharmacology, 22*(3), 286–292. https://doi.org/10 .5455/bcp.20120729090446.

Farah, M. J., & Gillihan, S. J. (2012). The puzzle of neuroimaging and psychiatric diagnosis: Technology and nosology in an evolving discipline. *AJOB Neuroscience, 3*(4), 31–41. https://doi.org/10.1080/21507740 .2012.713072.

Fava, M., Alpert, J., Nierenberg, A. A., Mischoulon, D., Otto, M. W., Zajecka, J., Murck, H., & Rosenbaum, J. F. (2005). A double-blind, randomized trial of St John's wort, fluoxetine, and placebo in major depressive disorder. *Journal of Clinical Psychopharmacology, 25*(5), 441–447. https://doi.org/10 .1097/01.jcp.0000178416.60426.29.

Food and Drug Administration (FDA). (2005). Dietary supplement labeling guide: chapter I. General dietary supplement labeling. www.fda.gov.

Food and Drug Administration. (2021, February 19). FDA warns 10 companies for illegally selling dietary supplements claiming to treat depression and other mental health disorders [Press release]. www.fda.gov/news-events /press-announcements/fda-warns-10-companies-illegally-selling-dietary-supplements-claiming-treat-depression-and-other.

Food and Drug Administration (FDA). (2022). Dietary supplements. www .fda.gov/food/dietary-supplements.

Frances, A. (2013). *Essentials of psychiatric diagnosis: Responding to the challenge of DSM-5*. Guilford Publications.

Gilbert, K., Hall, K., & Codd, R. T. (2020). Radically open dialectical behavior therapy: Social signaling, transdiagnostic utility and current evidence. *Psychology Research and Behavior Management, 13*, 19–28. https://doi .org/10.2147/PRBM.S201848.

Güzel, O., Yılmaz, U., Uysal, U., & Arslan, N. (2016). The effect of olive oil-based ketogenic diet on serum lipid levels in epileptic children. *Neurological Sciences, 37*(3), 465–470. https://doi.org/10.1007/s10072-015-2436-2.

Hall, H. (2013). Dr. Amen's love affair with SPECT scans. https://sciencebased medicine.org.

Hupp, S., & Tolin, D. (in press). *Science-based therapy*. Cambridge University Press.

Lynch, T. R. (2018). *Radically open dialectical behavior therapy: Theory and practice for treating disorders of overcontrol*. New Harbinger Publications.

Masood, W., Annamaraju, P., & Uppaluri, K. R. (2021). Ketogenic diet. *StatPearls* [Internet]. www.ncbi.nlm.nih.gov/books/NBK499830/.

McCullough Jr,J. P. (1999). *Treatment for chronic depression: Cognitive behavioral analysis system of psychotherapy (CBASP)*. Guilford Press.

National Center for Complementary and Integrative Health. (2020). Dietary and herbal supplements. www.nccih.nih.gov/health/dietary-and-herbal-supplements.

Novella, S. (2010). Acupuncture for depression. https://sciencebasedmedicine .org.

Rapaport, M. H., Schettler, P. J., Larson, E. R., Carroll, D., Sharenko, M., Nettles, J., & Kinkead, B. (2018). Massage therapy for psychiatric disorders. *Focus, 16*(1), 24–31. https://doi.org/10.1176/appi.focus.20170043.

Sarris, J., Logan, A. C., Akbaraly, T. N., Amminger, G. P., Balanzá-Martínez, V., Freeman, M. P., Hibbeln, J., Matsuoka, Y., Mischoulon, D., Mizoue, T., Nanri, A., Nishi, D., Ramsey, D., Rucklidge, J. J., Sanchez-Villegas, A., Scholey, A., Su, K.-P., & Jacka, F. N. on behalf of the International Society for Nutritional Psychiatry Research. (2015). Nutritional medicine as mainstream in psychiatry. *The Lancet Psychiatry, 2*(3), 271–274. https://doi.org /10.1016/S2215-0366(14)00051-0.

Satel, S. L., & Lilienfeld, S. O. (2013). *Brainwashed: The seductive appeal of mindless neuroscience*. Basic Books.

Schefft, C., Kilarski, L. L., Bschor, T., & Koehler, S. (2017). Efficacy of adding nutritional supplements in unipolar depression: A systematic review and meta-analysis. *European Neuropsychopharmacology, 27*(11), 1090–1109. https://doi.org/10.1016/j.euroneuro.2017.07.004.

Scolnick, B. (2017). Ketogenic diet and anorexia nervosa. *Medical Hypotheses, 109*, 150–152. https://doi.org/10.1016/j.mehy.2017.10.011.

Smith, C. A., Armour, M., Lee, M. S., Wang, L. Q., & Hay, P. J. (2018). Acupuncture for depression. *Cochrane Database of Systematic Reviews*, (3). https://doi.org/10.1002/14651858.CD004046.pub4.

von Geijer, L., & Ekelund, M. (2015). Ketoacidosis associated with low-carbohydrate diet in a non-diabetic lactating woman: A case report. *Journal of Medical Case Reports, 9*(1), 1–3.

Włodarczyk, A., Cubała, W. J., & Stawicki, M. (2021). Ketogenic diet for depression: A potential dietary regimen to maintain euthymia? *Progress in Neuro-Psychopharmacology and Biological Psychiatry, 109*, 1–6. https:// doi.org/10.1016/j.pnpbp.2021.110257.

Włodarek, D. (2019). Role of ketogenic diets in neurodegenerative diseases (Alzheimer's disease and Parkinson's disease). *Nutrients*, *11*(1), 169. https://doi.org/10.3390/nu11010169.

Zhang, Y., Liu, C., Zhao, Y., Zhang, X., Li, B., & Cui, R. (2015). The effects of calorie restriction in depression and potential mechanisms. *Current Neuropharmacology*, *13*(4), 536–542. https://doi.org/10.2174/1570159X1 3666150326003852.

Bipolar Spectrum

Monica Ramirez Basco and Brittany L. Mason

The bipolar spectrum includes the diagnoses of bipolar disorder I, bipolar disorder II, and cyclothymic disorder, as well as mood states somewhere in between these formal diagnoses which do not meet current diagnostic criteria (American Psychiatric Association, 2022). For the purposes of this chapter, we refer to these conditions as bipolar disorder. Bipolar disorder is a psychiatric illness characterized by significant shifts in mood, physical symptoms, cognition, and behavior from the highs of mania to the lows of major depression. The diagnostic labels have changed over time (e.g., manic-depressive illness, bipolar affective disorder) as have the clinical criteria (Mason et al., 2016) in order to incorporate new scientific knowledge. The disorder itself, with its distinctive episodic periods of euphoria and dysphoria, has not changed. However, our awareness of the subtleties and understanding of the variations in its course over time and across individuals has led to greater appreciation for the spectrum of presenting symptoms of this mood disorder (American Psychiatric Association, 2022). This chapter seeks to address common misconceptions about those with bipolar disorder and the benefits for related treatments. In addition, a brief discussion of cognitive-behavioral treatment approaches that are effective for bipolar disorder is included. A major take-home from this chapter is that although bipolar disorder is a serious, lifelong illness, there are effective treatments that can help manage it and provide a good quality of life.

3.1 Pseudoscience and Questionable Ideas

In spite of clinical and scientific breakthroughs in diagnostics, pharmacotherapy, and psychotherapy, bipolar disorder remains difficult to diagnose, especially in its early phases (Evans, 2000), and is often resistant to treatment (Gitlin, 2006). New medications have helped people gain better control over symptoms and psychosocial interventions such as cognitive-behavioral therapy (CBT; Basco & Rush, 2005) have provided tools to help people anticipate and manage symptoms and make full use of interventions to reduce the risk of recurrence. The evidence supporting the use of pharmacological agents like lithium, quetiapine, aripiprazole, and others, both as monotherapies and in combination, is vast (Yatham et al., 2018). However, there still remains a significant gap in the understanding of this mental illness, as well as in the overall efficacy of treatments. Below are a few common misconceptions about bipolar disorder.

3.1.1 Myths That Influence Treatment

3.1.1.1 Myth: Bipolar Symptoms Are Not That Serious

Public awareness of bipolar disorder has increased dramatically (Allister, 2019; Vovou et al., 2021). The upside of this is that with more information, people have come to recognize their mood changes as periods of depression and mania and have sought needed treatment. The downside is that the mood episodes that are part of the illness have been misconstrued as normal day-to-day mood swings that most people experience. Stress affects everyone's moods in one way or another, but only people with severe mood disorders like bipolar disorder will experience major depressive, manic, or hypomanic episodes (National Institute of Mental Health, 2018). These episodes are understood in the context of how difficult they make someone's day-to-day functioning, so even if one person is having a bad day and doesn't cook dinner or do the dishes, they may be able to pick it all back up tomorrow. Frequently, those in an episode will not. Sometimes extremely stressful events will kick off an episode of mania, especially if that stress makes it hard for people to sleep at night as their minds fill with worry. It's also possible for stressful things to occur during periods of depression or mania, and as a result, people may function more poorly at home, work, or in their relationships, which then causes additional problems that lead to high stress. When manic or depressive symptoms have emerged, it doesn't really matter if they came before or after a period of stress; the medical care will be the same to control the symptoms. Adding psychotherapy to the treatment plan can help people plan ahead, recognize the onset of stress, and design strategies to keep it from affecting their lives (Basco, 2015).

3.1.1.2 Myth: Substance Use Is the Primary Cause of Bipolar Disorder

When you hear awful stories in the news about a famous person with bipolar disorder having severe problems or serious consequences from drug and alcohol abuse, it is easy to jump to the conclusion that substances cause the problem or that everyone with the disorder abuses drugs. Studies have shown that about 40% of people with bipolar disorder will have trouble with substance abuse at some time in their lives (Cerullo & Strakowski, 2007), but that doesn't mean they use substances all the time or that substances caused their symptoms. There are several reasons people use substances, one of which is coping with stressors in their lives. During episodes of depression, mania, or mixed states, people can feel extremely irritable and agitated. Sleep loss and racing thoughts can make it hard to concentrate, thus adding to that irritability. For some people, but not the majority, the intensity of those feelings can lead them to act out their anger or hostility toward others (Ballester et al., 2014). This is especially true when faced with extremely stressful circumstances in the face of alcohol and substance abuse (Quigley et al., 2018).

3.1.1.3 Myth: The Patient Should Always Be Blamed for Nonadherence

Cognitive-behavioral therapy for bipolar disorder (Basco, 2000; Basco & Rush, 1996; 2005) was developed to address two notable challenges in its pharmacological treatment: (1) suboptimal effectiveness of commonly used mood stabilizing medications even when taken consistently, and (2) poor adherence to treatment regimens. Both mental health providers and laypersons have proposed pseudoscientific notions to explain these failures. For example, patients are often blamed for their "noncompliance" despite considerable evidence that medications for this illness do not work for everyone and often produce intolerable side effects (Geddes & Miklowitz, 2013), which can lead many to discontinue their use. In addition, between episodes of depression and mania, patients may assume that they only need psychotherapy to manage their residual symptoms. It is not possible to predict the length of asymptomatic times between episodes, but data show that prematurely discontinuing treatment can prompt recurrence of symptoms (Suppes et al., 1991). Some are willing to take this risk for an opportunity to stop treatment until the next episode. Cognitive-behavioral therapy can help people weigh the pros and cons of these decisions before making changes that increase their risk for the next episode.

3.1.1.4 Myth: The Person Wants to Be Impaired

Another common misconception is that people with bipolar disorder have an underlying desire to remain ill, especially if they have experienced euphoric periods of manias that, although transient, bring them creativity and needed energy. While this can occur, people who have experienced euphoric manias are generally aware of the negative consequences such as the way the symptoms can affect their relationships (Bulteau et al., 2018) and do not wish to relive them (Andriakos, 2018). A related misconception, not supported by the scientific literature, is that bipolar disorder is actually a personality disorder not dissimilar to borderline personality disorder (Gunderson et al., 2006). However, numerous scientific studies of bipolar disorder have revealed evidence of underlying neurobiological phenomena (Harrison et al., 2018). Additionally, clinical trials of pharmacological agents have demonstrated effectiveness in reducing symptoms and the risk for recurrence of episodes of both depression and mania (Geddes & Miklowitz, 2013).

3.1.2 Treatment Controversies

In order to sort science from pseudoscience and to describe what is effective for bipolar disorder, one must first define the term "effective." The evidence that determines what treatments and interventions are, and are not, effective are generally taken from randomized controlled clinical trials. Random assignment to a treatment or control group helps to answer the question, "effective compared to what?" Small studies lacking control groups cannot clearly examine what would have happened without the therapy under study, and any determination of how the treatment affected the illness is only weak, if it exists at all. "One-offs" can happen, and therefore, one single research study showing an effect does not mean that if the trial is repeated, the same effects will be found. This is why science requires multiple studies showing similar results before claims of effectiveness can be made. Conversely, one person's experience cannot reasonably be considered as evidence of benefit or harm, without a broad sampling of many people to decide if the noted behavior or treatment response is more common.

Thus, evaluating the effect of a treatment on complex human beings with a complex illness tends to require large numbers of people and large randomized controlled trials. When one trial or multiple trials show a repeatable positive effect beyond the occurrence of chance, it strengthens the case for the treatment. However, biology is complicated and each person's experience of bipolar disorder or their reactions to treatments can differ. It is nearly impossible to test every possibility and thus what large randomized controlled trials can show are broad effects for many, but not necessarily all, participants. Similarly, there may be treatments or interventions that show some benefit to a small handful of people or for a certain group for reasons that scientists cannot yet explain. A treatment's effects on individual people can frequently be overgeneralized. Therefore, unless clinically indicated, the evidence for any treatment should be strongly evaluated before embarking on a regimen. Providers do a service to their patients by listening closely to what they report is helpful even if the effect is unexplained. Several additional controversies related to treatment will be described next.

3.1.2.1 Misconceptions about Treatment

Incomplete responses and treatment failures are not uncommon in bipolar disorder (Baldessarini et al., 2020; Tournier et al., 2019). Treatments that have been shown to be effective in clinical trials do not necessarily work for everyone, symptoms vary greatly from person to person, and even a given individual can present differently across the course of their lives. This is frustrating for people who want clear information and solid answers about best treatments, often leading them to the misconception that nothing can be done about it. This is far from the truth. Contributing to this discouraging view, clinicians may not always appreciate the severity of the disorder when people present with mild symptoms, have good coping strategies that mask symptoms, or have lengthy periods of mental wellness between episodes of depression or mania. When unable to observe their patients on a regular basis, it is easy to assume that symptoms are well-controlled and medications are being taken as prescribed. Misconceptions about the course of the illness and treatment on the parts of both the patient and clinicians can thereby lead to missed opportunities to address needed treatment updates.

3.1.2.2 Adherence to Pharmacological Treatments and Natural Medicines

Bipolar disorder is associated with impaired cognitive functioning, motivation, and perception of treatment in both the depressive and manic phases. Therefore, cognitive and behavioral skills needed to remember to take medications daily may be compromised. Depression can lead to hopelessness about the effectiveness of treatment and low motivation for daily care behaviors, including taking medication. Mania can cause disorganization in thought, disruption in daily routines, and distractibility. If mania produces a euphoric mood, some people will discontinue medications because they simply forget to take them or see no need for treatment. For these reasons, treatment adherence is a significant problem for people with bipolar disorder just as it is with other chronic illnesses (Basco & Rush, 1995; Consoloni et al., 2021; Doane et al., 2021). When medications are discontinued but symptoms remain, it is not uncommon to seek alternative treatments, like supplements or "natural medicines." While these substances do not require a prescription, it is just as important to examine the evidence for their potential efficacy, as many beneficial drugs are modeled on naturally occurring substances such as plant extracts. Complementary and alternative medicine (CAM) is a term used to describe a number of these therapies; however, there is little evidence to support their efficacy. Some "natural therapies" suggested from websites include magnesium, vitamins, fish oil, rhodiola rosea (also known as arctic root or golden root), N-acetylcysteine, and some others as products designed to support mainline treatments, as in the case for choline and inositol. Given the complexity of bipolar disorder, one must question the aspect of the disease for which treatment is sought – reducing acute manic episodes, managing bipolar depression, or preventing relapse. It is possible for a therapy to be effective for one aspect of this illness and perhaps even harmful for another. A good example is the use of anti-depressant medications for bipolar depression that inadvertently induce manic symptoms. There are some CAM agents, including so-called "nutraceuticals" (like branched chain amino acids, L-tryptophan and folic acid), that have been used in conjunction with other antimania agents or N-acetylcysteine for acute bipolar depression (Yatham et al., 2018); however, the evidence supporting them is currently weak.

3.1.2.3 Treatments that Help in One Area but Harm Another

In general, many of these nontraditional and commonly used therapies are ineffective, and in some cases potential side effects or drug interactions increase their harm. Some approaches are effective for treating depression, but not mania, while some can induce rapid cycling (Sharma et al., 2017). Given the amount of time that many people with bipolar disorder experience depressive symptoms, an otherwise effective therapy for depression must not exacerbate other aspects unique to the bipolar disorder.

3.1.2.4 Mislabeled or Misleading Products

There is some evidence of the adjunctive value of dietary supplements in the treatment of mood disorders such as bipolar disorder (Geddes et al., 2016; Stoll et al., 1999). However, one must critically evaluate supplements, as they may not contain the advertised ingredients, possess the ingredients in amounts that differ from the reported levels, or lack scientific evidence for their efficacy (Food and Drug Administration, n.d.). Also, a number of these supplements only show efficacy in the event that a person is deficient in the first place, such as in the case of folate. In some cases, supplements can cause harm if the substance is not simply excreted from the body but instead induces real effects in the system. In summary, supplements are not classified as drugs by the FDA and are thus subject to much lower regulatory standards.

3.2 Research-Supported Approaches

Cognitive-behavioral therapy teaches skills to relieve symptoms, improve treatment adherence, resolve problems, and improve quality of life. This approaches' specific methods aim to correct maladaptive thoughts, improve behavioral coping, and reduce distressing emotions. Cognitive-behavioral therapy was first developed long before randomized controlled trials were performed to test efficacy. Clinical scholars like Aaron T. Beck (1979) and Albert Ellis (1957) treated people with severe depression and noted how significant distortions in thinking worsened patients' emotional symptoms. They experimented with ways to help people reason through these distortions, thus improving mood. Over time, specific treatment strategies were operationalized and documented in manuals (e.g., Beck, 1979) and later tested in randomized controlled trials. Scientific developments such as these often begin with ideas, models, and guesses before they are scientifically tested and verified.

Early studies of adding psychotherapy to medication treatment for bipolar disorder (Benson, 1975; Powell et al., 1977; Shakir et al., 1979) showed promise for reducing the length of depressive and manic episodes and for delaying relapse. Cognitive-behavioral therapy was expanded to include interventions for not only improving adherence, but helping people cope with prodromal (Lam et al., 2000), within-episode (Perry et al., 1999), and residual symptoms of the disorder (Fava et al., 2001). While these therapy protocols initially focused on relieving depressive episodes, the overarching focus of cognitive-behavioral therapy for bipolar disorder is to help people gain better control over the entire course of the illness, reducing the frequency and duration of mood episodes that inevitably recur. The implementation of treatment, therefore, is not limited to a single episode of depression or mania. In fact, studies show that most people utilize cognitive-behavioral therapy for bipolar disorder during the course of ongoing pharmacological treatment of the illness when symptoms are not at their most severe (Chiang et al., 2017). This provides opportunities to educate people and teach skills for monitoring symptoms and intervening when they begin or show signs of worsening.

3.3 Conclusion

Bipolar disorder is a chronic mental illness characterized by recurring periods of depression, mania, and mixed states, often with residual symptoms between episodes. In spite of scientific advances, misconceptions about the disorder and its treatment are still common among people with the illness, their family members, and even clinicians. These include, but are not limited to, incorrect assumptions about the nature of the illness, blaming patients for their symptoms, expecting indefinite, continuous treatment, questioning the effectiveness of psychotherapy, and valuing complementary and alternative medicine as a replacement for pharmacotherapy. Cognitive-behavioral therapy for bipolar disorder has been shown to reduce the risk of relapse, improve manic and depressive symptoms, and improve general psychosocial functioning. Comprehensive treatment including pharmacological and psychotherapeutic intervention helps those struggling with bipolar disorder reduce the risk of recurrence and improve quality of life.

Monica Ramirez Basco, PhD, is a Licensed Clinical Psychologist and Founding Fellow of the Academy of Cognitive Therapy. She is author of the book, *The Bipolar Workbook, Tools for Controlling Your Mood Swings, Second Edition* (2015).

Brittany L. Mason, PhD, is a Scientific Review Officer for the National Institute of Health.

References

Allister, N. (2019). Ups and downs: Social media advocacy of bipolar disorder on world mental health day. *Frontiers in Communication, 4*, 24–32. https://doi.org/10.3389/fcomm.2019.00024.

American Psychiatric Association (2022). *Diagnostic and statistical manual of mental disorders, fifth edition, text revision (DSM-5-TR)*. American Psychiatric Association.

Andriakos, J. (2018). 13 things people with bipolar disorder want you to know. *Mental Health.* www.self.com/story/bipolar-disorder-facts-real-people-stories.

Baldessarini, R.J., Vázquez, G.H. & Tondo, L. (2020). Bipolar depression: A major unsolved challenge. *International Journal of Bipolar Disorders*, *8*(1), 1 https://doi.org/10.1186/s40345-019-0160-1.

Ballester, J., Goldstein, B., Goldstein, T. R., Yu, H., Axelson, D., Monk, K., Hickey, M. B., Diler, R. S., Sakolsky, D. J., Sparks, G., Iyengar, S., Kupfer, D. J., Brent, D. A., &Birmaher, B. (2014). Prospective longitudinal course of aggression among adults with bipolar disorder. *Bipolar Disorders*, *16*(3), 262–269. https://doi.org/10.1111/bdi.12168.

Basco, M. R. (2000). Cognitive-behavior therapy for Bipolar I Disorder. *Journal of Cognitive Psychotherapy*, *14*, 287–304. https://doi.org/10.1891/0889-8391.14.3.287.

Basco, M.R. (2015). *The bipolar workbook, tools for controlling your mood swings* (2nd ed.). Guilford Press.

Basco, M. R., & Rush, A. J. (1995). Compliance with pharmacotherapy in mood disorders. *Psychiatric Annals*, *25*(5), 269–270, 276, 278–279. https://doi.org/10.3928/0048-5713-19950501-03.

Basco, M. R., & Rush, A. J. (1996). *Cognitive-behavioral therapy for bipolar disorder*. Guilford Press.

Basco, M. R., & Rush, A. J. (2005). *Cognitive-behavioral therapy for bipolar disorder* (2nd ed.). Guilford Press.

Beck, A. T. (1979). *Cognitive therapy and emotional disorders*. Penguin Books.

Benson, R. (1975). The forgotten treatment modality in bipolar illness: psychotherapy. *Diseases of the Nervous System*, *36*(11), 634–638. www.ncbi.nlm.nih.gov/pubmed/1183307.

Bulteau, S., Grall-Bronnec, M., Bars, P. Y., Laforgue, E. J., Etcheverrigaray, F., Loirat, J. C., Victorri-Vigneau, C., Vanelle, J.-M., & Sauvaget, A. (2018). Bipolar disorder and adherence: Implications of manic subjective experience on treatment disruption. *Patient Preference and Adherence*, *12*, 1355–1361. https://doi.org/10.2147/ppa.S151838.

Cerullo, M. A., & Strakowski, S. M. (2007). The prevalence and significance of substance use disorders in bipolar type I and II disorder. *Substance Abuse Treatment, Prevention, and Policy*, *2*, 29. https://doi.org/10.1186/1747-597X-2-29.

Chiang, K.-J., Tsai, J.-C., Liu, D., Lin, C.-H., Chiu, H.-L., & Chou, K.-R. (2017). Efficacy of cognitive-behavioral therapy in patients with bipolar disorder: A meta-analysis of randomized controlled trials. *PLoS One*, *12*(5), e0176849. https://doi.org/10.1371/journal.pone.0176849.

Consoloni, J. L., M'Bailara, K., Perchec, C., Aouizerate, B., Aubin, V., Azorin, J. M., Bellivier, F., Correard, N., Courtet, P., Dubertret, C., Etain, B., Gard, S., Haffen, S., Leboyer, M., Llorca, P.-M., Olié, E., Polosan, M., Schwan, R., Samalin, L., ... Group FACE BD. (2021). Trajectories of medication adherence in patients with Bipolar Disorder along 2 years-follow-up. *Journal Affective Disorders*, *282*, 812–819. https://doi.org/10.1016/j.jad.2020.12.192.

Doane, M. J., Ogden, K., Bessonova, L., O'Sullivan, A. K., & Tohen, M. (2021). Real-world patterns of utilization and costs associated with second-generation oral antipsychotic medication for the treatment of bipolar disorder: A literature review. *Neuropsychiatric Disease and Treatment*, *17*, 515–531. https://doi.org/10.2147/NDT.S280051.

Ellis, A. (1957). Rational psychotherapy and individual psychology. *Journal of Individual Psychology*, *13*, 38–44.

Evans, D. L. (2000). Bipolar disorder: Diagnostic challenges and treatment considerations. *Journal of Clinical Psychiatry*, *61*(Suppl 13), 26–31.

Fava, G. A., Bartolucci, G., Rafanelli, C., & Mangelli, L. (2001). Cognitive-behavioral management of patients with bipolar disorder who relapsed while on lithium prophylaxis. *Journal of Clinical Psychiatry*, *62*(7), 556–559. https://doi.org/10.4088/jcp.v62n07a10.

Food and Drug Administration (n.d.). Food and Drug Administration website. www.fda.gov/food/buy-store-serve-safe-food/what-you-need-know-about-dietary-supplements.

Geddes, J. R., Gardiner A., Rendell, J., Voysey, M., Tunbridge, E., Hinds, C., Yu, L.-M., Hainsworth, J., Attenburrow, M.-J., Simon, J., Goodwin, G. M., Harrison, P. J., & CEQUEL Investigators and Collaborators. (2016). Comparative evaluation of quetiapine plus lamotrigine combination versus quetiapine monotherapy (and folic acid versus placebo) in bipolar depression (CEQUEL): A 2 × 2 factorial randomized trial. *Lancet Psychiatry*, *3*(1), 31–39. https://doi.org/10.1016/S2215-0366(15)00450-2.

Geddes, J. R., & Miklowitz, D. J. (2013). Treatment of bipolar disorder. *Lancet*, *381*(9878), 1672–1682. https://doi.org/10.1016/s0140-6736(13)60857-0.

Gitlin, M. (2006). Treatment-resistant bipolar disorder. *Molecular Psychiatry*, *11*(3), 227–240. https://doi.org/10.1038/sj.mp.4001793.

Gunderson, J. G., Weinberg, I., Daversa, M. T., Kueppenbender, K. D., Zanarini, M. C., Shea, M. T., Skodol, A. E., Sanislow, C. A., Yen, S., Morey, L. C., Grilo, C. M., McGlashen, T. H., Stout, R. L., & Dyck, I. (2006). Descriptive and longitudinal observations on the relationship of borderline personality disorder and bipolar disorder. *American Journal of Psychiatry*, *163*(7), 1173–1178. https://doi.org/10.1176/appi.ajp.163.7.1173.

Harrison, P. J., Geddes, J. R., & Tunbridge, E. M. (2018). The emerging neurobiology of bipolar disorder. *Trends in Neurosciences*, *41*(1), 18–30. https://doi.org/10.1016/j.tins.2017.10.006.

Lam, D. H., Bright, J., Jones, S., Hayward, P., Schuck, N., Chisholm, D., & Sham, P. (2000). Cognitive therapy for bipolar illness – A pilot study of relapse prevention. *Cognitive Therapy and Research*, *24*(5), 503–520. https://doi.org/10.1023/A:1005557911051.

Mason, B. L., Brown, E. S., & Croarkin, P. E. (2016). Historical underpinnings of bipolar disorder diagnostic criteria. *Behavioral Sciences (Basel, Switzerland)*, *6*(3), 14. https://doi.org/10.3390/bs6030014.

National Institute of Mental Health. (2018). Bipolar disorder. NIH Publication 19-MH-8088. www.nimh.nih.gov/sites/default/files/documents/health/publications/bipolar-disorder/19-mh-8088.pdf.

Perry, A., Tarrier, N., Morriss, R., McCarthy, E., & Limb, K. (1999). Randomised controlled trial of efficacy of teaching patients with bipolar disorder to identify early symptoms of relapse and obtain treatment. *British Medical Journal*, *318*(7177), 149–153. https://doi.org/10.1136/bmj.318.7177.149.

Powell, B. J., Othmer, E., & Sinkhorn, C. (1977). Pharmacological aftercare for homogeneous groups of patients. *Hospital & Community Psychiatry*, *28*(2), 125–127.

Quigley, B. M., Houston, R. J., Antonius, D., Testa, M., & Leonard, K. E. (2018). Alcohol use moderates the relationship between symptoms of mental illness and aggression. *Psychology of Addictive Behaviors*, *32*(7), 770–778. https://doi.org/10.1037/adb0000390.

Shakir, S. A., Volkmar, F. R., Bacon, S., & Pfefferbaum, A. (1979). Group psychotherapy as an adjunct to lithium maintenance. *American Journal of Psychiatry*, *136*(4A), 455–456. www.ncbi.nlm.nih.gov/pubmed/426116.

Sharma, A., Gerbarg, P., Bottiglieri, T., Massoumi, L., Carpenter, L. L., Lavretsky, H., Muskin, P. R., Brown, R. P., & Mischoulon, D., as Work Group of the American Psychiatric Association Council on Research. (2017). *S*-Adenosylmethionine (SAMe) for neuropsychiatric disorders: A clinician-oriented review of research. *Journal of Clinical Psychiatry*, *78*(6), e656–e667. https://doi.org/10.4088/JCP.16r11113.

Stoll, A.L., Severus, E., Freeman, M.P., Rueter, S., Zboyan H.A., Diamond, E., Cress, K. K., & Marangell, L.B. (1999). Omega 3 fatty acids in bipolar disorder, a preliminary double-blind, placebo-controlled trial. *Archives of General Psychiatry*, *56*(5), 407–412. https://doi.org/10.1001/archpsyc.56.5.407.

Suppes, T., Baldessarini, R. J., Faedda, G. L., & Tohen, M. (1991). Risk of recurrence following discontinuation of lithium treatment in bipolar disorder. *Archives of General Psychiatry*, *48*(12), 1082–1088. https://doi.org/10.1001/archpsyc.1991.01810360046007.

Tournier, M., Neumann, A., Pambrun, E., Weill, A., Chaffiol, J. P., Alla, F., Bégaud, B., Maura, G., & Verdux, H. (2019). Conventional mood stabilizers and/or second-generation antipsychotic drugs in bipolar disorders: A population-based comparison of risk of treatment failure. *Journal of Affective Disorders*, *257*, 412–420. https://doi.org/10.1016/j.jad.2019.07.054.

Yatham, L. N., Kennedy, S. H., Parikh, S. V., Schaffer, A., Bond, D. J., Frey, B. N., Sharma, V., Goldstein, B. I., Rej, S., Beaulieu, S., Alda, M.,

MacQueen, G., Milev, R. V., Ravindran, A., O'Donovan, C., McIntosh, D., Lam, R. W., Vazquez, G., Kapczinski, F., ... Berk, M. (2018). Canadian Network for Mood and Anxiety Treatments (CANMAT) and International Society for Bipolar Disorders (ISBD) 2018 guidelines for the management of patients with bipolar disorder. *Bipolar Disorders, 20* (2), 97–170. https://doi.org/10.1111/bdi.12609.

Vovou, F., Hull, L. & Hull, L. (2021). Mental health literacy of ADHD, autism, schizophrenia, and bipolar disorder: A cross-cultural investigation. *Journal of Mental Health, 30*(4), 470–480. https://doi.org/10.1080/09638237 .2020.1713999.

4

Anxiety

Dean McKay

Anxiety disorders are, collectively, among the most common psychiatric conditions, and are widely considered stress-induced. This class of disorders accounts for significant medical and mental health burden as well as reduced occupational and social functioning (Baxter et al., 2014). The recent COVID-19 pandemic illustrates how influential stress is in evoking anxiety conditions. In a large-scale census-controlled epidemiology study, it was found that 8.2% of the population reported at least one anxiety disorder in 2019, and the rate was almost three times higher the following year due to the COVID-19 pandemic (Twenge & Joiner, 2020). To further highlight the stress-inducing nature of anxiety disorders, worldwide analyses of prevalence rates during the COVID-19 pandemic showed a high rate of these disorders, with a rate of approximately 27.6% (Santomauro et al., 2021).

The *Diagnostic and Statistical Manual of Mental Disorders* (DSM, 5th edition, text revision, DSM-5-TR; American Psychiatric Association, 2022) lists the following conditions in the broad category of anxiety disorders: specific phobia, social anxiety disorder, panic disorder, agoraphobia, generalized anxiety disorder, as well as two which are most commonly diagnosed in childhood, namely separation anxiety disorder and selective mutism. There is also substance/medication-induced anxiety disorder, and anxiety disorder due to another medical condition.

Although less well investigated, research has also shown that anxiety disorders have a substantial adverse effect on subjective wellbeing, particularly for panic disorder, generalized anxiety disorder, and social anxiety disorder (Cramer et al., 2005). While wellbeing may impel individuals to seek treatment, it has also been found that deficits in mental health literacy interferes with individuals seeking any treatment, and more specifically, interferes with finding effective treatment (Johnson & Coles, 2013). As a result, individuals with anxiety disorders are at particularly high risk of receiving pseudoscientific interventions.

Anxiety disorders share the common feature of excessive threat response. These excessive threat reactions can be based on exaggerated threat from the external environment (i.e., social anxiety, specific phobia). Exaggerated threat reactions can also stem from interoceptive experiences such as worries (in generalized anxiety disorder) or unexpected changes in physiological reactions (in panic disorder). Thus, mechanisms for the etiology for anxiety disorders can be determined based on structured and testable hypotheses regarding how these excessive anxiety reactions might occur, what would maintain them, and how to intervene to alleviate them.

4.1 Pseudoscience and Questionable Ideas

Theoretical and clinical management of anxiety has been a central focus in mental health treatment for centuries. The range of conceptualizations for anxiety expression has been highly varied and generally not ground in falsifiable theories. To be fair, many questionable notions of anxiety conditions were in the pre-scientific method era, and include: reproductive organs being misaligned, most especially with the idea of the "wandering uterus" in women (discussed in Santoro, 2019); terrors from ancient gods (such as Pan, in ancient Greece); and that there was insufficient holiness that necessitated a "shock" treatment involving being pushed unexpectedly into holy water (Schullian & Lewis, 1981).

More recently, there has been a proliferation of dubious remedies that purport to alleviate anxiety and stress. As with the variety of ancient remedies, these also lack any scientific basis, but do not have the justification of appearing before the development of the scientific method. This chapter is not an exhaustive review of the pseudoscientific and questionable approaches for anxiety relief, but only a sampling of prominent ones. Given the ubiquity of anxiety problems, it is likely that dubious treatments will continue to proliferate, particularly given the current state of science education in professional therapy training.

4.1.1 Core Issues and Controversies

Anxiety disorders cause incredible pain. These conditions are associated with significant suicide ideation and attempts (Sareen et al., 2005). There is substantial disability associated with anxiety disorders (Hendricks et al., 2014), and poor subjective quality of life (Mendelowicz & Stein, 2000; Olatunji et al., 2007). It therefore comes as little surprise that people with anxiety disorders are often desperate for relief, and thus are susceptible to the efficacy claims that often accompany pseudoscientific treatments. Often, these treatments, touted as providing extremely rapid relief, typically failed to maintain any benefit or produced no change (Rosen et al., 1998). Further, at the present time, the most efficacious treatments for anxiety disorders involve exposure therapy with or without cognitive therapy. The descriptions of these treatments can sometimes emphasize facets related to anxiety evocation as part of the curative process. As a result, clinicians and people with anxiety disorders can be hesitant, out of concern that the intervention may worsen symptoms (Deacon et al., 2013).

Clinicians' holding erroneous concerns about the risk of exposure therapy is not the only issue that may contribute to the proliferation of pseudoscientific methods in the treatment of anxiety. Another significant challenge is the basic scientific knowledge among clinicians. Indeed, the minimum competency exam, the Examination for Professional Practice in Psychology (EPPP), has not been carefully validated (Sharpless & Barber, 2009). The original EPPP covered the full gamut of psychology, and not solely content areas relevant to clinical practice. In lieu of validation research, the exam has been updated to include a focus on competency-based assessment (discussed in Callahan et al., 2020). McFall (2006) lamented that scientific training in clinical psychology was insufficient, and laid out the foundations for more rigorous scientific education through a different training model, the clinical scientist, to address the limitations in how the scientist-practitioner model had been implemented. In furtherance of ensuring a workforce trained in the scientific grounding of cognitive-behavioral methods, a taskforce was formed that developed specific guidelines for doctoral education (Klepac et al., 2012). The success of these efforts in improving the scientific literacy of the clinician workforce has not yet been appraised. Of course, this is all restricted to the scientific knowledge of doctoral level psychologists, and does not address the science competency of a wide range of other mental health practitioners, ones who have less rigorous training programs, or are degrees less historically tied to scientific bases of mental health.

Where this leaves us is with a set of disorders that affect a very large proportion of the general population, across all ages, and with significant disability and poor subjective wellbeing. And while there's efficacious treatment, it is technically demanding to properly administer. Thus, clinicians who have not received training in scientifically informed therapy are far more likely to turn to dubious interventions or ones with fantastical claims even if their mechanisms are questionable or benefits no greater than due to non-specific effects.

4.1.2 Dubious Approaches

While there is a preponderance of questionable assessment and treatment approaches for anxiety disorders, there are several that are highly visible. Most of those listed here are heavily promoted through continuing education offerings and marketing campaigns, and advertised by practitioners as modalities offered. These approaches are typically based on mechanisms of action that have not been empirically tested, are not based on sound theoretical bases, and have not been subjected to rigorous investigations. The absence of these features has not stopped their most ardent supporters from making fantastic claims of validity or efficacy. These are all hallmarks of pseudoscientific methods (discussed in Lohr et al., 2012).

Further, it is worth noting that the psychological literature is surprisingly limited in evaluation of adverse treatment effects. It is only recently that this has begun to receive attention (Dimidjian & Hollon, 2010; Lilienfeld, 2007), but still at a more conceptual rather than data-driven level. Nevertheless, there are several treatments for anxiety disorders for which harms are reasonably known, and these will also be identified below.

4.1.2.1 Genetic Profiles to Determine Rates of Neurotransmitter Metabolism

In recent years, there have been several assessment approaches developed for anxiety disorders that lack a sound scientific basis. Fortunately, the most widely used psychology-based assessment instruments are based on existing models of psychopathology. However, one prominent assessment method that has emerged recently purports to evaluate one's genetic profile to determine rates of neurotransmitter metabolism, in order to offer greater precision in dosing medication. Reports have indicated that these medical assessment batteries are not based on any sound available evidence showing genetic determination of neurotransmitter metabolism, and that numerous other factors (diet, exercise, age, to name a few) are better determinants of metabolic function (Cohen & Zubenko, 2019). The American Psychiatric Association even concluded that these tests should not be ordered, and were potentially hazardous to patient care given the risk of improper dosing based on unsupported medical evidence (Zeier et al., 2018). Even when considering genome-wide association studies, there remains limited evidence for any single gene or set of genes in predicting anxiety disorders (Otowa et al., 2016), never mind such specificity as for neurotransmitter metabolism.

4.1.2.2 Neurofeedback

Among psychological interventions, neurofeedback has been promoted as a potential intervention for anxiety. This treatment is based on the assumption that specific brain waves are associated with anxiety expression, and through direct biofeedback-modeled interventions, alteration of these brain waves lead to anxiety reduction. At the present time there is no consensus regarding which brain waves to target, or what level of change might be necessary, to alleviate anxiety symptoms (Papo, 2018). Neurofeedback does have the benefit of being a science-oriented treatment, even if it lacks the underlying scientific bases. That is, at the present time, neurofeedback for anxiety disorders can be rightly considered a dubious method. To be fair, and like many pseudoscientific approaches, neurofeedback has been associated with benefits for clients. For example, one meta-analysis of 26 studies showed that neurofeedback was associated with a one standard deviation reduction in anxiety symptoms (Russo et al., 2022). However, it has been noted that the benefits of neurofeedback are likely best attributed to non-specific effects, rather than a particular mechanism of the intervention (Tolin et al., 2020).

4.1.2.3 Energy Therapies/Emotional Freedom Techniques

There are several interventions that are collectively referred to as energy therapies or emotional freedom techniques. Most of these treatments were originally developed to address trauma reactions, but have been widely used for anxiety disorders. The purported mechanism of psychopathology stems from imbalances in electrical fields surrounding the body, and in particular emanate from specific physical points (sometimes called Meridian Points). The purported mechanism of treatment is through "tapping," or application of pressure, on these specific points during therapy, usually in conjunction with other therapies such as exposure (Church & Brooks, 2010). There are other variants of these treatments. For example, Thought Field Therapy suggests that the key pressure points need to be tapped in specific sequences (Irgens et al., 2012). One other that has been used extensively among practitioners is Tapas Acupressure Therapy, which focuses the mechanisms of action on pressure points solely on the face (Mollon, 2007).

As noted before, these interventions are lacking in sound theoretical formulations, specifically the lack of any conceptual rationale for acupressure points being associated with anxiety expression. There is also no known valid method for assessing purported electrical fields around the body. This has not stopped the proponents of these methods from developing research protocols to test the efficacy of these interventions. As these therapies now formally advocate linking these methods with exposure therapies, the independent value of these treatments remains in question.

4.1.2.4 Brainspotting

Developed originally for trauma, brainspotting emphasizes the importance of the direction of eye gaze, and the promoters of this approach have even developed a slogan to engage clinicians and clients – "Where you look affects how you feel" (Brainspotting Trainings, LLC, 2017). The developers of brainspotting suggest that the mechanism of anxious expression comes from connections between learned events and "spots" in the visual field that have projections to emotional processing sections of the midbrain (Corrigan & Grand, 2013; Corrigan et al., 2015). The authors suggest several specific brain areas that they implicate in this regard, in a specific sequence. In developing this chapter, no supporting basic neuroscience research could be found that supported the association between the purported brain areas and anxiety (or trauma).

With no specific underlying pathophysiology to support the above claims, the mechanism of treatment is on questionable ground. Specifically, the clinician instructs the client to develop imagery of the anxiety-evoking situation. Following this, the clinician instructs the client to slowly track the finger (or pointer or other object), and when the clinician observes a disruption in eye gaze, this is hypothesized to correspond to a "spot" associated with the neural path to the associated brain areas. While workshops and certification programs are available, as of this writing there appear to be only uncontrolled case illustrations claiming the treatment is beneficial.

4.1.2.5 Accelerated Resolution Therapy

As with brainspotting, Accelerated Resolution Therapy relies on eye movements as part of the core methods of intervention. While developed initially for posttraumatic stress disorder, it has also been promoted for treatment of phobias, generalized anxiety, and other psychiatric conditions. The promotional literature on Accelerated Resolution Therapy highlights that treatment is rapid, with symptom resolution in three to five sessions; the treatment does not require between-session homework; and the treatment has a more formal structure with a specific number of eye movements. These features provide an important selling point for the therapy that emphasizes less required decision making, which alleviates the cognitive burden associated with providing conceptually driven therapy (described on a related website). Examination of the available literature shows limited controlled research. The most recent review was published in 2017, with anecdotal and case reports only since then. In the 2017 review article (Waits et al., 2017), the authors noted that while there was limited available research, plenty of clinicians reported in personal communications that it was highly efficacious. The purported mechanism of action, focusing primarily on emotional reactivity and the distressing image, is largely in line with available research on etiological factors in anxiety disorders (i.e., Foa & Kozak, 1986). However, the protocol specifically indicates that providers may develop imagery related to metaphors, and somatic reactions, which are not grounded in any available theory or evidence for anxiety disorders.

4.1.2.6 Thought Stopping

As treatments go, thought stopping seems the most intuitively obvious, and yet lacks any substantive mechanism to support its application in the alleviation of anxiety symptoms. The mechanism of action derives from operant models of punishment, where the application of an aversive stimulus would weaken the experience of unwanted thoughts (such as unrealistic fears). The model of thought stopping comes from covert conditioning (Cautela & Wisocki, 1977), and even recently has been defended as a plausible intervention for a wide array of problems (Bakker, 2009). However, it has been determined to be harmful due to experimental research demonstrating the deliberate efforts to suppress unwanted thoughts typically results in "rebound" effects, whereby the thoughts are worsened (Abramowitz et al., 2001). Accordingly, thought stopping should be considered a harmful treatment for anxiety disorders.

4.1.2.7 Autonomous Sensory Meridian Response

A recently developed approach involves using the autonomous sensory meridian response (ASMR) to produce relaxation and induce sleep. Advocates of the ASMR approach rely on a library of videos depicting individuals, usually whispering or speaking in quiet somnolent tones, and engaged in some form of repetitive action (such as popping bubble paper) or engaged in gustatory actions (such as eating soft foods). The seemingly reasonable assumption is that promoting relaxation in anxious individuals is palliative. Further, experimental research shows that ASMR videos can result in changes in heart rate, blood pressure, and skin conductance (Poerio et al., 2018). The faulty assumption, one now long known, is that relaxation alone is not an adequate treatment for anxiety disorders, and is often used as a control condition in treatment trials (i.e., Norton, 2012). Further, for some anxiety conditions, such as generalized anxiety disorder, relaxation often paradoxically worsens anxiety and can be used to serve as an exposure procedure (Heide & Borkovec, 1984; Kim & Newman, 2019; see the Research-Supported Approaches section below). What makes the use of ASMR as a treatment potentially harmful is that it demands the user call up videos that are intended to specifically induce the relaxation response; provides no method for users to develop skills in activating relaxation independently; and in some individuals may elicit aversive reactions to specific sounds (i.e., misophonia; Rabasco & McKay, 2021).

4.1.2.8 Animal-Assisted Therapy

Incorporating animals into treatment has become a popular method for alleviating anxiety disorders. The most frequently cited animal-assisted treatments are canine and equine therapies (Young & Horton, 2019). The treatment is predicated on a mechanism of human bonding with the animal, and that through repeated interactions, the bonding impact has lasting palliative effects on anxiety (Shen et al., 2018). The enthusiasm for this form of treatment comes from correlative findings that interactions with animals result in lowered blood pressure, heart rate, and other biological markers of anxiety. However, as Shen et al. (2018) show, the popularity of animal-assisted therapy may be more a result of subjective enjoyment of interacting with animals, and not due to a unique quality of bonding from the treatment. In reviewing the available research for a specific form of animal-assisted therapy, namely equine-related treatment, Anestis et al. (2014) found no benefit for any psychiatric condition.

4.1.2.9 Essential Oils

A range of essential oils have been described as anxiety relievers. Commercially marketed expressly to promote calmness, these remedies are typically blends of oils, such as peppermint, spearmint, ginger, cardamom, fennel, rose, chamomile, valerian root, lavender, jasmine, basil, and many more (far too many to list here). Users of essential oils are typically encouraged to use drops of the fluid in a diffuser, and promoters of this approach indicate its benefits accrue from being inhaled. Aside from many essential oils being toxic to pets (who lack the necessary enzymes to metabolize many of the oils), there is no mechanism whereby the phenols from essential oils promote anxiety relief. While research does show that essential oils may have the potential to relieve acute anxiety there are many problems in the existing research, such as a lack of comparison control oils and limited information on dosage (Gong et al., 2020). Additionally, the research typically examines anxiety in general rather than specific anxiety disorders. Further, the mechanisms are highly speculative. The purported mechanism centers on the oils triggering an olfactory response that in turn stimulates serotonin and dopamine release. This mechanism of action is, at this point, so speculative that there is no hypothesized specific brain area for neurotransmitter action, nor is there specificity of essential oil that might promote anxiety relief. Much of the available research is in rodent models of psychopathology, which remain inconclusive (Zhang & Yao, 2019). As with many other pseudoscientific methods of treatment, this has not prevented the marketing of these compounds to the public. Further, there are numerous oils that are purported to alleviate anxiety, but no single one has been recommended as superior to any other, despite widely varied chemical properties.

4.2.1.10 Crystals

Numerous crystals have been promoted for anxiety reduction and overall wellness. For example, the precious gem amethyst has been suggested to promote calmness (Grant, 2011). Other gems have also been described as anxiety-alleviating, and are marketed in some forms (i.e., bracelets, necklaces) specifically for this purpose. At the present time, there are no coherent models of anxiety disorders, or anxiety and stress generally, that describe mechanisms whereby crystals of any type would provide relief. Most proponents of crystals draw on Sanskrit and anecdotal results to support their use (Todd, 2021). The majority of the available research suggests any psychological benefit results from placebo effects, rather than any unique properties of the crystals. Defenders of the use of crystals point to the necessity of using them in specific places, such as "the vortex" in Sedona, Arizona, where energy from the earth aggregates in these locations to interact with crystals to promote healing. The vortexes (according to material from websites offering vacation wellness packages; note that "vortices" is rarely used in this context) are also promoted as healing locations even without the crystals.

4.2 Research-Supported Approaches

Anxiety disorders have been the subject of intense research scrutiny for the past 50 years. As a result, there are several well established mechanisms of anxiety onset and maintenance, as well as mechanisms of treatment effect. Given the extensity of this line of research, the current discussion will focus on three of the most prominent approaches.

Behavioral inhibition has been proposed as an individual-difference variable that puts children at risk for developing anxiety disorders. One facet of behavioral inhibition is that individuals with high levels of this attribute are more sensitive to punishment, and react with anxiety and apprehension in future situations where there is a risk of aversive consequences (Gray & McNaughton, 1982). Since the time the behavioral inhibition system was hypothesized, extensive research has demonstrated that the system predicts anxiety symptoms and disorders, whereby the conditioning of fear and anxiety is facilitated (Sandstom et al., 2020). Prior to the hypothesized behavioral inhibition model of anxiety disorders, conditioning theory provided the basis for the application of exposure therapy, which has grown to be the dominant evidence-based method of treatment (Garner et al., 2021). Targeting the memory structures associated with fear learning has been considered the central mechanism of efficacy (Foa & Kozak, 1986). More recently, the methods of exposure have changed to suggest a wide range of methods of altering the memory structure, so that the corrective information can accrue through multiple methods. This is referred to as the inhibitory learning model (for a detailed discussion, see Craske et al., 2014).

The central mechanism of action in the *cognitive model* for anxiety disorders is a persistent misinterpretation of situations as dangerous (Beck et al., 1985). Refinements in this model have followed, and one of the most robust cognitive indicators of anxiety disorders is intolerance of uncertainty (Carleton, 2014). Individuals with anxiety disorders often find the general range of uncertainty the general population accepts is lower, and thus the perceived risk of danger is elevated. Treatment targeting this construct, and associated cognitions (i.e., overestimation of threat), form the basis of cognitive therapy for anxiety disorders. It should be noted that most practitioners no longer draw firm distinctions in the application of cognitive and behavioral (i.e., exposure) therapy, and favor the more blended approach of cognitive-behavioral therapy. This is due to the role of exposure in activating specific cognitions (via behavioral experiments) and the expected change in cognition that comes from direct exposure therapy.

Given that anxiety disorders are based, in part, on perceived risks, one way it may be mitigated is through social connections, and this is done in the *interpersonal models* of therapy. As interpersonal function declines, perceived vulnerability to danger worsens. Evolutionary models support a role for social connectedness as a feature of improving survival, and thus as the perception of interpersonal rejection becomes more sensitive, anxiety reactions increase (Leary, 2022). Although interpersonal therapies were not developed directly from these evolutionary models, long-standing evolved mechanisms serve as useful and evidence-based frameworks for the mechanisms of anxiety disorders. Interpersonal psychotherapy (IPT), originally developed for depression (Klerman et al., 1984), has since been modified for anxiety disorders. The central mechanisms of change revolve principally around improved social support and lower general interpersonal stress (Lipsitz & Markowitz, 2013). Over the past 20 years, IPT has been formally incorporated in anxiety disorder treatment, most notably for generalized anxiety disorder (Newman et al., 2011) and social anxiety disorder (Lipsitz et al., 2008).

4.3 Conclusion

Anxiety disorders are a broad class of diagnoses, and are experienced by a large proportion of the population. As such, the demand for treatment for these disorders is extremely high. Further, pursuit of treatment represents a high individual economic burden (Konnopka & König, 2020). This economic burden is exacerbated by the wide marketing of pseudoscientific and questionable interventions. Specifically, Dimidjian and Hollon (2010) cited resource loss as a significant harm of treatment, even if the intervention results in no change in symptoms.

Complicating the therapeutic landscape is the comparably low proportion of practitioners who practice evidence-based methods for anxiety disorders. Recent surveys are in short supply, but as of 2009, over two-thirds of anxiety disorder sufferers did not receive evidence-based treatment (Shafran et al., 2009). In a survey of 51 practitioners in Wyoming who reported regularly treating anxiety disorders, it was found that exposure was rarely practiced despite the wide recognition of its efficacy (Hippol & Deacon, 2013). It is unclear whether the level of evidence-based treatment delivery has improved in the past ten years, but given the widespread availability of the pseudoscientific methods described in this chapter, it is reasonable to predict that large proportions of sufferers continue to receive inappropriate care.

Addressing this problem requires targeting at least three major areas. First, the public needs to be better informed about scientific methods of treatment, as well as interventions that are dubious or improbable in producing change. Recent surveys show that demand for anxiety disorder treatment has risen (American Psychological Association, 2021), and thus the opportunity exists to ensure the public is informed regarding appropriate care.

Second, practitioners would benefit from a stronger educational program regarding efficacious treatments. Large proportions of providers are from a wide range of mental health fields. Many of these fields educate clinicians in methods of intervention without corresponding education in appraising false and unrealistic claims around efficacy. These practitioners, often in an effort to stand out in a competitive marketplace, are susceptible to clever marketing promotions for treatments that claim incredible benefits but that fail to deliver in practice.

Third, across every level of mental health subfield, evidence-based methods need to be more widely disseminated. Considering the widespread levels of anxiety disorders in the general population, it is safe to state that the majority of practitioners will encounter this class of diagnoses in the course of their career. Generalists will need to be well equipped with the means to assess and provide treatment, or at least recommend practitioners who deliver appropriate care, to their clients.

Dean McKay, PhD, ABPP, is a Professor of Psychology at Fordham University. He is co-editor of the book *Training and Supervision in Specialized Cognitive Behavior Therapy: Methods, Settings, and Populations* (2022).

References

Abramowitz, J. S., Tolin, D. F., & Street, G. P. (2001). Paradoxical effects of thought suppression: A meta-analysis of controlled studies. *Clinical Psychology Review, 21*, 683–703.

American Psychiatric Association. (2022). *Diagnostic and statistical manual of mental disorders (5th ed., text revision)*. Author.

American Psychological Association. (2021). *Demand for mental health treatment continues to increase, say psychologists*. Author. www.apa.org/news/press/releases/2021/10/mental-health-treatment-demand.

Anestis, M. D., Anestis, J. C., Zawilinski, L. L., Hopkins, T. A., & Lilienfeld, S. O. (2014). Equine-related treatments for mental disorders lack empirical support: A systematic review of empirical investigations. *Journal of Clinical Psychology, 70,* 1115–1132.

Bakker, G. M. (2009). In defence of thought stopping. *Clinical Psychologist, 13,* 59–68.

Baxter, A. J., Vos, T., Scott, K. M., Ferrari, A. J., & Whiteford, H. A. (2014). The global burden of anxiety disorders in 2010. *Psychological Medicine, 44,* 2363–2374.

Beck, A. T., Emery, G., & Greenberg, R. L. (1985). *Anxiety disorders and phobias: A cognitive perspective.* Basic Books.

Brainspotting Trainings, LLC. (2017). https://brainspotting.com/.

Callahan, J. L., Bell, D. J., Davila, J., Johnson, S. L., Strauman, T. J., & Yee, C. M. (2020). The enhanced examination for professional practice in psychology: A viable approach? *American Psychologist, 75*(1), 52–65.

Carleton, R. N. (2014). The intolerance of uncertainty construct in anxiety disorders: Theoretical and practical perspectives. *Expert Review of Neurotherapeutics, 12,* 937–947.

Cautela, J. R., & Wisocki, P. A. (1977). The thought stopping procedure: Description, applications, and learning theory interpretations. *Psychological Record, 27,* 255–264.

Church, D., & Brooks, A. J. (2010). Application of emotional freedom techniques. *Integrative Medicine, 9,* 46–48.

Cohen, B. M., & Zubenko, G. S. (2019). Gene testing to guide antidepressant treatment: Has its time arrived? Harvard Health Blog. www.health.harvard.edu/blog/gene-testing-to-guide-antidepressant-treatment-has-its-time-arrived-2019100917964.

Corrigan, F., & Grand, D. (2013). Brainspotting: Recruiting the midbrain for accessing and healing sensorimotor memories of traumatic activation. *Medical Hypotheses, 80,* 759–766.

Corrigan, F. M., Grand, D., & Raju, R. (2015). Brainspotting: Sustained attention, spinothalamic tracts, thalamocortical processing, and the healing of adaptive orientation truncated by traumatic experience. *Medical Hypotheses, 84,* 384–394.

Cramer, V., Torgersen, S., & Kringlen, E. (2005). Quality of life and anxiety disorders: A population study. *Journal of Nervous and Mental Disease, 193,* 196–202.

Craske, M. G., Treanor, M., Conway, C. C., Zbozinek, T., & Vervliet, B. (2014). Maximizing exposure therapy: An inhibitory learning approach. *Behaviour Research & Therapy, 58,* 10–23.

Deacon, B. J., Farrell, N. R., Kemp, J. J., Dixon, L. J., Sy, J. T., Zhang, A. R., & McGrath, P. B. (2013). Assessing therapist reservations about exposure therapy for anxiety disorders: The Therapist Beliefs about Exposure Scale. *Journal of Anxiety Disorders, 27,* 772–780.

Dimidjian, S., & Hollon, S. D. (2010). How would we know if psychotherapy were harmful? *American Psychologist, 65,* 21–33.

Foa, E. B., & Kozak, M.J. (1986). Emotional processing of fear: Exposure to corrective information. *Psychological Bulletin, 99,* 20–35.

Garner, L., Steinberg, E., & McKay, D. (2021). Exposure therapy. In A. Wenzel (Ed.), *Handbook of cognitive behavioral therapy* (pp. 275–312). American Psychological Association Press.

Gong, M., Dong, H., Tang, Y., Huang, W., & Lu, F. (2020). Effects of aromatherapy on anxiety: A meta-analysis of randomized controlled trials. *Journal of Affective Disorders, 274,* 1028–1040.

Grant, G. (2011). Measuring stress reduction using the infrared negative ions amethyst biomat. *Prime-Journal, 1,* 50–56.

Gray, J. A., & McNaughton, N. (1982). *The neuropsychology of anxiety: An inquiry into the septo-hippocampal system.* Oxford University Press.

Heide, F. J., & Borkovec, T. D. (1984). Relaxation-induced anxiety: Mechanisms and theoretical implications. *Behaviour Research and Therapy, 22,* 1–12.

Hendricks, S. M., Spijker, J., Licht, C. M. M., Beekman, A. T. F., Hardeveld, F., de Graaf, R., Batelaan, N.M., & Penninx, B. W. J. H. (2014). Disability in anxiety disorders. *Journal of Affective Disorders, 166,* 227–233.

Hippol, L. J., & Deacon, B. J. (2013). Dissemination of evidence-based practices for anxiety disorders in Wyoming: A survey of practicing psychotherapists. *Behavior Modification, 37,* 170–188.

Irgens, A., Dammen, T., Nysaeter, T. E., & Hoffart, A. (2012). Thought field therapy (TFT) as a treatment for anxiety symptoms: A randomized controlled trial. *Explore, 8,* 331–338.

Johnson, E. M., & Coles, M. E. (2013). Failure and delay in treatment-seeking across anxiety disorders. *Community Mental Health Journal, 49*(6), 668–674.

Kim, H., & Newman, M. G. (2019). The paradox of relaxation training: Relaxation induced anxiety and mediation effects of negative contrast sensitivity in generalized anxiety disorder and major depressive disorder. *Journal Affective Disorders, 259,* 271–278.

Klepac, R. K., Ronan, G. F., Andrasik, F., Arnold, K. D., Belar, C. D., Berry, S. L., Christoff, K. A., Craighead, L. W., Dougher, M. J., Dowd, E. T., Herbert, J. D., McFarr, J. D., Rizu, S. L., & Strauman, T. J. (2012). Guidelines for cognitive behavioral training within doctoral psychology programs in the United States: Report of the Inter-Organizational Task Force of Cognitive Behavioral Psychology Doctoral Education. *Behavior Therapy, 43,* 687–697.

Klerman, G. L., Weissman, M. M., Rounsaville, B. J., & Chevron, E. S. (1984). *Interpersonal psychotherapy of depression.* Basic Books.

Konnopka, A. & König, H. (2020). Economic burden of anxiety disorders: A systematic review and meta-analysis. *PharmacoEconomics, 38*, 25–37.

Leary, M. R. (2022). Emotional responses to interpersonal rejection. *Dialogues in Clinical Neuroscience, 17*, 435–441.

Lilienfeld, S. O. (2007). Psychological treatments that cause harm. *Perspectives on Psychological Science, 2*, 53–70.

Lipsitz, J. D., Gur, M., Vermes, D., Petkova, E., Cheng, J., Miller, N., Laino, J., Liebowitz, M. R., & Fyer, A. J. (2008). A randomized trial of interpersonal therapy versus supportive therapy for social anxiety disorder. *Depression and Anxiety, 25*, 542–553.

Lipsitz, J. D., & Markowitz, J. C. (2013). Mechanisms of change in interpersonal therapy (IPT). *Clinical Psychology Review, 33*, 1134–1147.

Lohr, J. M., Lilienfeld, S. O., & Rosen, G. M. (2012). Anxiety and its treatment: Promoting science-based practice. *Journal of Anxiety Disorders, 26*, 719–727.

McFall, R. M. (2006). Doctoral training in clinical psychology. *Annual Review of Clinical Psychology, 2*, 21–49.

Mendlowicz, M. V., & Stein, M. B. (2000). Quality of life in individuals with anxiety disorders. *American Journal of Psychiatry, 157*, 669–682.

Mollon, P. (2007). Thought field therapy and its derivatives: Rapid relief of mental health problems through tapping on the body. *Primary Care and Community Psychiatry, 12*, 123–127.

Newman, M. G., Castonguay, L. G., Borkovec, T. D., Fisher, A. J., Boswell, J. F., Szkodny, L. E., & Nordberg, S. S. (2011). A randomized controlled trial of cognitive behavior therapy for generalized anxiety disorder with integrated techniques from emotion-focused and interpersonal therapies. *Journal of Consulting and Clinical Psychology, 79*, 171–181.

Norton, P. J. (2012). A randomized controlled trial of transdiagnostic cognitive-behavioral treatments for anxiety disorder by comparison to relaxation training. *Behavior Therapy, 43*, 506–517.

Olatunji, B. O., Cisler, J. M., & Tolin, D. F. (2007). Quality of life in the anxiety disorders: A meta-analytic review. *Clinical Psychology Review, 27*, 572–581.

Otowa, T., Hek, K., Lee, M., Byrne, E. M., Mirza, S. S., Bigdeli, T., Aggen, S. H., Adkins, D., Wolen, A., Fanous, A., Keller, M. C., Castelao, E., Kutalik, Z., der Auwera, S. V., Homuth, G., Nauck, M., Teumer, A., Milaneschi, Y., … Hettema, J. M. (2016). Meta-analysis of genome-wide association studies of anxiety disorders. *Molecular Psychiatry, 21*, 1391–1399.

Papo, D. (2018). Neurofeedback: Principles, appraisal, and outstanding issues. *European Journal of Neuroscience, 49*, 1454–1469.

Poerio, G. L., Blakey, E., Hostler, T. J., & Veltri, T. (2018). More than a feeling: Autonomous sensory meridian response (ASMR) is characterized by reliable changes in affect and physiology. *PLoS One, 13*, e0196645.

Rabasco, A., & McKay, D. (2021). Exposure therapy for misophonia: Concepts and procedures. *Journal of Cognitive Psychotherapy*, *35*, 156–166.

Rosen, G. M., Lohr, J. M., McNally, R. J., & Herbert, J. D. (1998). Power therapies, miraculous claims, the cures that fail. *Behavioural and Cognitive Psychotherapy*, *26*, 99–101.

Russo, G. M., Balkin, R. S., & Lenz, A. S. (2022). A meta-analysis of neurofeedback for treating anxiety-spectrum disorders. *Journal of Counseling and Development*, *100*, 236–251.

Sandstrom, A., Uher, R., & Pavlova, B. (2020). Prospective association between childhood behavioral inhibition and anxiety: A meta-analysis. *Research on Child and Adolescent Psychopathology*, *48*, 57–66.

Santomauro, D. F., Herrera, A. M. M., Shadid, J., Zheng, P., Ashbaugh, C., Pigott, D. M., Abbafati, C., Adolphe, A., Amlaug, J. O., Aravkin, A. Y., Bang-Jensen, B. L., Bertolacci, G. J., Bloom, S. S., Castellano, R., Castro, E., Chakrabarti, S., Chattopadhyay, J., Cogen, R. M., Collins, J. K., ... Ferrari, A. J. (2021). Global prevalence and burden of depressive and anxiety disorders in 204 countries and territories in 2020 due to the COVID-19 pandemic. *The Lancet*, *398*, 1700–1712.

Santoro, N. F. (2019). A role for the wandering uterus? *Endocrinology*, *160*, 55–56.

Sareen, J., Cox, B. J., & Afifi, T. O. (2005). Anxiety disorders and risk for suicidal ideation and attempts: A population-based longitudinal study of adults. *Archives of General Psychiatry*, *62*, 1249–1257.

Schullian, D. M., & Lewis, T. H. (1981). Richard Carew on the treatment of a 'Franticke Person' in medieval Cornwall. *Journal of the History of Medicine and Allied Sciences*, *36*, 64–66.

Shafran, R., Clark, D. M., Fairburn, C. G., Arntz, A., Barlow, D. H., Ehlers, A., Freeston, M., Garety, P. A., Hollon, S. D., Ost, L. G., Salkovskis, P. M., Williams, J. M. G., & Wilson, G. T. (2009). Mind the gap: Improving the dissemination of CBT. *Behaviour Research and Therapy*, *47*, 902–909.

Sharpless, B. A., & Barber, J. P. (2009). The Examination for Professional Practice in Psychology (EPPP) in the era of evidence-based practice. *Professional Psychology: Research and Practice*, *40*, 333–340.

Shen, R. Z. Z., Xiong, P., Chou, U. I., & Hall, B. J. (2018). "We need them as much as they need us": A systematic review of the qualitative evidence for possible mechanisms of effectiveness of animal-assisted intervention. *Complementary Therapies in Medicine*, *41*, 203–207.

Todd, L. (2021). Do crystals work for anxiety and depression? *Medical News Today*. www.medicalnewstoday.com/articles/crystals-for-anxiety-and-depression.

Tolin, D. F., Davies, C. D., Moskow, D. M., & Hofmann, S. G. (2020). Biofeedback and neurofeedback for anxiety disorders: A quantitative and qualitative systematic review. In Y. K. Kim (Ed.), *Anxiety disorders; Rethinking and understanding recent discoveries* (pp. 265–289). Springer Nature-Singapore.

Twenge, J. M., & Joiner, T. E. (2020). U.S. Census Bureau-assessed prevalence of anxiety and depressive symptoms in 2019 and during the 2020 COVID-19 pandemic. *Depression & Anxiety, 37*, 954–956.

Waits, W., Marumoto, M., & Weaver, J. (2017). Accelerated Resolution Therapy (ART): A review and research to date. *Current Psychiatry Reports, 19*, 18.

Young, C., & Horton, J. (2019). Canine and equine therapy for mental health: A review of clinical effectiveness. *Canadian Agency for Drugs and Technologies in Health, 26*, 31553551.

Zeier, Z., Carpenter, L. L., Kalin, N. H., Rodriguez, C. I., McDonald, W. M., Widge, A. S., & Nemeroff, C. B. (2018). Clinical implementation of pharmacogenetic decision support tools for antidepressant drug prescribing. *American Journal of Psychiatry, 175*, 873–886.

Zhang, N., & Yao, L. (2019). Anxiolytic effect of essential oils and their constituents: A review. *Agriculture and Food Chemistry, 67*, 13790–13808.

5

Obsessions and Compulsions

Dean McKay

Obsessive-compulsive disorder (OCD) is a complex and heterogeneous condition. Hallmark symptoms include unwanted, persistent, and intrusive thoughts and images of harm or other undesirable ideas, called obsessions. Ritualized behaviors, called compulsions, may also be present that are designed to alleviate the obsessions. In the fifth edition of the Diagnostic and Statistical Manual (DSM-5; American Psychiatric Association, 2013), a new category of diagnoses, the Obsessive-Compulsive Related Disorders (OCRDs), was introduced. This category of disorders has been hypothesized to share a common feature, namely a breakdown in behavioral inhibition that may manifest in persistent thoughts and repetitive behaviors. The disorders in the OCRDs include: body dysmorphic disorder, hoarding disorder, trichotillomania, and excoriation disorder. Given the wide variation in symptom presentations of OCD, as well as the diversity of symptom profiles for the other disorders in the OCRDs, interested readers are referred to Abramowitz, McKay, and Storch (2017) and Storch, Abramowitz, and McKay (2017) for detailed information on the full scope of these conditions.

Each of the conditions in the OCRDs is marked by significant disability (i.e., Markarian et al., 2010; Stein et al., 2019). Individuals with OCRDs experience intense anxiety, and the drive to complete ritualistic behavior consumes large portions of their days. As a result, individuals with OCRDs are often eager to seek help. There are current evidence-based treatments for each of the OCRDs (discussed in Abramowitz et al., 2017, and Storch et al., 2017). However, there is also a limited number of providers who are knowledgeable and qualified to deliver these interventions (discussed in Lattie & Stamatis, 2022). There are currently programs available to train mental health professionals in scientifically informed therapy (such as the Behavior Therapy Training Institute from the International Obsessive-Compulsive Disorder Foundation [IOCDF]), although these programs cannot match the level of need in the public. Considering that OCD alone affects approximately 2% of the population, there are large numbers of people who cannot access appropriate care.

When conditions of high need without commensurate appropriate care exists, practitioners of questionable and pseudoscientific methods typically rush in to fill the void. As this chapter will document, the challenge in OCD related to evidence-based care is actually more serious than just lack of sufficient numbers of qualified scientifically trained professionals. There are also several interventions that have been promoted as scientifically based but whose foundations are built on dubious theoretical concepts and methodologies that have little justification.

5.1 Pseudoscience and Questionable Ideas

Before delving into the range of pseudoscientific notions that have infected treatment approaches for the OCRDs, it is worth starting on a positive note. Namely, any Google search of effective treatment for OCD, and its derivations, consistently results in large numbers of pages suggesting exposure with response prevention in particular, and cognitive-behavior therapy in general. This is consistently the dominant evidence-based treatment for this class of disorders, so people who might be searching for information about the best treatments will most likely be led to the right methods. As noted earlier, the IOCDF runs behavior therapy training programs, and in general has been an effective voice in getting the message out regarding the best treatments (Szymanski, 2012).

Sadly, the positive feature of wide dissemination of information about evidence-based treatment has not been matched by the availability of knowledgeable and suitably trained practitioners. Further, longstanding clinical lore suggests the majority of psychopathology stems from unresolved traumatic reactions. This is based in large measure on the lingering dominance of psychodynamic concepts that emphasize unresolved unconscious conflicts, ones that may result in the kinds of conflictual behavior seen in OCD, where the inner unwanted images and urges run in opposition to declarative cognitions regarding their social acceptability (discussed in Moritz et al., 2012). While indeed there are cases where traumatic events may spark onset of OCD symptoms (reviewed in McKay & Leone, under review), there is little evidence that OCD is primarily the result of trauma. As discussed in the Trauma chapter of this book, the trauma subfield of mental health specialties is suffused with pseudoscientific methods. These approaches have also found their way into the treatment histories of many people with OCD.

In addition to the problematic mental health legacy that all psycho-pathology emerges from trauma, OCD and associated disorders have been long associated with Obsessive-Compulsive Personality Disorder (OCPD). Again, while there are certainly overlapping features, and even diagnostic confusion in prior iterations of the DSM (see, for example, Wu et al., 2006), it is not accurate to assume that a diagnosis of OCD is determinative for a diagnosis of OCPD. Given this persistent diagnostic assumption among clinicians, many people with OCD receive treatments more suited for general personality disorders, such as emotion regulation strategies. These may be helpful in general emotional functioning, but do not address the acute behavioral and anxiety-related pathology that is the hallmark of these disorders.

While some psychological models give rise to pseudoscientific interven-tions, the dominance of the medical models in OCD has also resulted in highly questionable approaches. Worse, these questionable methods have garnered large funding for investigations that, unsurprisingly, had low payoff. The former director of the National Institute of Mental Health (NIMH), Dr. Tom Insel, was a particularly aggressive proponent of bio-medical models of mental illness from 2002 until 2015. Research on fund-ing trends showed that during Dr. Insel's time as director, the allocation of funding toward biomedical research in mental illness far outpaced that for psychosocial approaches (Teachman et al., 2019). In the context of OCD, the NIMH had online resources to aid the public. During Dr. Insel's time as NIMH head, these online "fact sheets" typically emphasized medical interventions and de-emphasized evidence-based psychological treat-ments. The OCD fact sheet had listed numerous interventions, including some questionable ones such as exploratory pharmacological compounds, and then listed general psychotherapy when at the time clearly established evidence-based treatment was known and available. This state of affairs only changed following submission of a detailed letter publicizing this erroneous information (Taylor et al., 2010). Following Dr. Insel's time as NIMH director, he acknowledged that the biomedical emphasis has not resulted in significant progress. Specifically, in an interview with *Wired* magazine in 2017, shortly after he concluded his time at NIMH, he said the following: "I spent 13 years at NIMH really pushing on the neuroscience and genetics of mental disorders, and when I look back on that I realize that while I think I succeeded at getting lots of really cool papers published by cool scientists at fairly large costs – I think $20 billion – I don't think we moved the needle in reducing suicide, reducing hospitalizations, improv-ing recovery for the tens of millions of people who have mental illness" (Rogers, 2017, *Wired Magazine*).

One potential explanation for the limited progress can be due to the highly speculative nature of the medical research in OCD. Again, with respect to medical models in general, Kendler (2008) lamented that psychiatric interventions were overly reliant on monomethod approaches, and that there was no sound guiding conceptual framework. Kendler further lamented the methods of psychiatric models of illness by drawing attention to the medical model tendency to overlook the full gamut of contributory factors for diagnoses, and called for models to account for the full range of causal influences, from genes up through environment and culture (Kendler, 2013). Sadly, the field has not heeded Kendler's call to action, and as a result, this chapter devotes significant space to medically questionable and pseudoscientific methods that have been applied to OCD.

5.1.1 Core Issues and Controversies

While OCD and OCRDs are increasingly recognized by mental health providers, there remain persistent challenges in assessment and diagnosis. A significant problem underpinning this comes from a general lack of knowledge of the full gamut of symptoms of the disorder. For example, in a vignette study where 208 physicians were presented with common OCD symptoms, over half misdiagnosed the presentation (Glazier et al., 2015). In a further review, it was shown that practitioners across the full spectrum of healthcare professionals have a high rate of misdiagnosing the disorder (Stahnke, 2021).

5.1.1.1 Urges and Intentionality

A core feature of many obsessions that individuals with OCD report are unwanted urges, such as the thought that the individual might harm a loved one, or may act on the urge to harm themselves. This is a complicated matter to properly assess, and demands practitioners possess nuanced clinical judgment where they can discern an intrusive thought that many in the population may routinely experience from one marked by a genuine intention to cause harm. In this regard, practitioners who encounter these obsessions must be able to assess for cognitive features of OCD. For example, someone suffering from bona fide harm obsessions is likely to also report concerns over the extent their thoughts represent a risk factor for them to act on the urge, even if accidentally. This is sometimes referred to as overimportance of thoughts (Calamari et al., 2006). Practitioners who hew to classic notions of psychopathology as described earlier might be unfamiliar with these cognitive dimensions, and instead assume a higher risk of dangerousness than is suitable. This erroneous conceptualization would also likely signal to the individual with OCD that their belief is reasonable, despite the reality that the OCD diagnosis is not a risk factor that is predictive of threat to others.

5.1.1.2 Assumptions of Pseudoscientific Medical Interventions

The prevailing assumption among medical interventions for OCD centers on dysfunction in putative neural circuitry that regulates repetitive actions (i.e., Welter et al., 2011). The available research has emphasized that circuitry dysfunction is in an interconnected system of neural structures, the cortico-striatal–thalamo-cortical (CSTC) in OCD (reviewed in Ting & Feng, 2011). Dysfunction in this circuit has led to an assumption that the system is underactivated, and thus stimulation would promote improved functioning. Interestingly, there is evidence that stimulation of this area may actually *promote* compulsive behavior (Ahmari et al., 2013). More refined recent reviews suggest that underactivation is associated with behavioral control, while overactivation is associated with emotion-based tasks (Rasgon et al., 2017). As a result, models of OCRDs collectively have emphasized a breakdown in behavioral inhibition, and have generally assumed that emotional functioning improves with better behavioral control. This assumption overlooks the consistent finding that evidence-based psychological interventions demonstrate high efficacy, and focus specifically on emotional reactions to feared and avoided situations. These neural models are also based on *ex post facto* reasoning, rather than on models of behavior and emotion that would be later subjected to hypothesis testing.

5.1.1.3 Assumptions of Pseudoscientific Psychological Interventions

There are several pseudoscientific treatments for OCD. Most of these emphasize the aforementioned assumed underlying traumatic beginnings of OCD and related conditions. There are also pseudoscientific models of OCD that focus on assumed breakdowns in energy fields, or lowered stimulation in neural areas connected to olfactory systems. These interventions do not have any empirical foundation in basic psychopathology research, nor do they have any comprehensive testable models that would allow for hypothesis testing.

5.1.2 Dubious Approaches

The OCRDs represent a complex and varied set of psychological conditions. Treatment demands highly specialized training and a nuanced understanding of the varied ways symptoms may be present. Just over 50 years ago, OCD was considered an untreatable condition (Kringlen, 1965). Since that time, extensive careful research has shown that exposure with response prevention, a highly specialized form of cognitive therapy, is effective in alleviating symptoms. OCRDs that are marked by primarily repetitive behaviors without associated feared consequences (such as trichotillomania) have been shown to respond well to habit reversal, an intervention that focuses on developing competing responses for the repetitive behavior. Despite the availability of these well-established evidence-based methods, there are several treatments that should be considered dubious.

5.1.2.1 Energy Therapies

There are a collection of treatments that purport to adjust hypothetical energy fields around an individual, on the assumption that these fields regulate emotional reactions and behavior. These energy therapies include therapeutic intervention of tapping specific points on the body, with or without imagery associated with the presenting symptoms. Problematic in all of these interventions is that there are no testable models of psychopathology that would connect putative energy fields and intrusive thoughts or repetitive behaviors. In the case of OCD, the application of energy therapies also includes exposure-based components, which already have substantial empirical support. As a result, reviews of the research suggest a benefit from the energy therapy protocols, but these do not isolate the unique contribution of the energy therapy intervention, nor does the extant research compare treatments with or without the unique energy therapy features (i.e., Clond, 2016). This issue of combining an ineffective component (e.g., tapping) to an effective component (e.g., exposure) and then touting the effectiveness of the combined approach has been characterized as a *purple hat therapy* (see the Trauma chapter for a more detailed discussion).

5.1.2.2 Neurofeedback

Brain waves observed through electroencephalography (EEG) have been associated with a wide range of psychopathology. In the case of OCRDs, the key wave is referred to as error-related negativity (ERN), which is a heightened response that occurs following perceived errors. This response in EEG assessment is consistent with neurobiological models whereby individuals with OCD (and anxiety disorders) are more sensitive to aversive experiences (Gray & McNaughton, 1982). Reviews of the research suggest that ERN waves are consistently observed in individuals with OCD (Riesel, 2019).

One might therefore assume, considering the available testing hypothesis and robust ERN indicators, that a direct bio-feedback approach using EEG would target ERN. Unfortunately, this is not the case. Instead, neurofeedback focuses on training individuals to control beta-waves, which are associated with a wide range of attention and cognitive activity (reviewed in Newson & Thiagarajan, 2019). While available as a treatment for over two decades, as of this writing there are no comprehensive models for neurofeedback and OCD, nor controlled research on this intervention, nor even adequate uncontrolled case research to conduct a systematic review (Weber et al., 2020).

5.1.2.3 Thought Stopping

In the early 1970s, behavioral theory was ascendant in clinical psychology. As such, both reinforcement-based methods and interventions derived from aversive control were evaluated. On the aversive conditioning side, thought stopping was an acceptable and compelling method for addressing problems such as obsessions. The basic method for intervention was to progress from mild aversive physical sensations (i.e., snapping a rubber band on the wrist when the thought occurred) to less overt aversive responses (such as internally stating to oneself "stop!"; Cautela & Wisocki, 1977). It seems simplistic, and intuitive. However, in light of contemporary knowledge of OCD, it is also harmful (McKay et al., 2021).

Since the time that thought stopping was developed, research on the natural etiology of obsessions revealed that many people with OCD spontaneously attempt to employ similar approaches. Further, research into deliberate suppression of thoughts reveals that as effort to block thoughts increases, their availability also increases. This suppression effect has been observed in OCD, in particular where mood is adversely affected for failures to exert control over thoughts (Purdon et al., 2005). Worse, a core dysfunctional belief associated with OCD is need for control over thoughts (Kim et al., 2016; Taylor et al., 2005).

5.1.2.4 Psychodynamic Therapy

Doubting is a central problem in OCRDs (Lazarov et al., 2015). That is, an individual with OCD is often uncertain of their actions, so they seek reassurance that their actions work to alleviate their feared outcomes. Interestingly, the first detailed OCD case described in psychotherapy was the "rat man" by Freud (1909/1997). In this case description, Freud highlighted the centrality of doubting as part of the pathological features of rat man's intrusive thoughts. Despite this early conceptualization that focused on doubting, psychodynamic methods of intervention rest on intrapsychic exploration of potential unconscious conflicts. As such, the treatment leads frequently to *possible* explanations for the resultant behavior, but little in the way of definitive answers. This in turn fosters doubt, rather than ameliorates it. As there are presently no conceptual or testable models of psychodynamic treatments for OCD, this approach to treatment should be considered harmful.

5.1.2.5 Ketamine

Originally used as a tranquilizer for large animals, ketamine has recently emerged as a potential medical therapeutic for a wide range of psychiatric conditions (Krystal et al., 2019). As a therapeutic approach, most of the research activity has focused on its application for depression (see Krystal et al., 2019). The central mechanism of action involves the glutamergic system. The rush to apply a new medical therapeutic to other psychiatric conditions has led to the application of ketamine for OCD. This rush, however, is without consideration for the lack of any comprehensive models that involve glutamate in OCD. Indeed, it is only recently that basic medical research has begun to examine the glutamergic system in OCD, so far based largely on speculation based on the embeddedness of glutamate tracts within the CSTC (i.e., Vlček et al., 2018). As of this review, the available research shows that ketamine has no lasting benefit on OCD symptoms.

5.1.2.6 Magnetic Stimulation

For close to two decades, medical research on OCRDs has suggested that stimulation of the brain areas associated with the neural circuitry of these disorders would have a palliative effect. Much of this research has been based on electrical stimulation, with or without accompanying cognitive-behavior therapy. A recent meta-analysis of data on electrical stimulation of brain areas associated with any psychiatric conditions shows minimal effect (Homan et al., 2021). Included in this review were studies relying on transcranial magnetic stimulation (TMS).

The inclusion of TMS as a dubious approach to avoid derives from at least two factors. One is the assumption that magnetic action on neural systems has any demonstrable effect. It has long been established that the iron level in blood is not impacted by magnets (Pauling & Coryell, 1936). Similarly, neuronal tissue has not been found to react to magnets (Dubiel et al., 1999). So, there is little reason to expect magnetic stimulation to impact neural circuitry. Second, as noted earlier, the existing research on neural circuits in OCD remains speculative and unconnected to a meaningful model of the disorder. Without this foundation, there is no compelling reason to expect stimulation, electrical or magnetic, to have any meaningful effect on symptoms.

5.1.2.7 New Age Wellness Remedies

New age wellness remedies have centered on essential oils to promote calmness and crystals for purported energy properties. These methods connect well with structured pseudoscientific methods described earlier under the heading of energy therapies. The list of potential palliative oils is too lengthy to list here, but the collective set of compounds remains speculative in their impact on neurotransmitter systems associated with OCD. Indeed, in a review of the effectiveness of any essential oil in alleviating OCD symptoms, the authors note that the benefits remained unclear, and no direct link between any oil and any potential neurotransmitter system was yet known (Ayati et al., 2020).

Essential oils at least have the property of existing as a vapor that enters the bloodstream, and thus have a chance of impacting the neural system. Another New Age wellness remedy – crystals, such as amethyst, quartz, and others – have also been promoted as potential remedies for OCD. These are primarily marketed to the public without any supporting scientific findings, no matter how questionable. A search on the literature for this chapter showed that crystals in OCD primarily exist as a scientific area of inquiry as it relates to minerals in the bloodstream. However, a search online for crystal remedies for OCD reveals a vast marketplace promoting a large array of stones purported to aid in OCD.

5.1.2.8 Relaxation Training

From 1980 up until the DSM-5 that was published in 2013, OCD was classified as an anxiety disorder. As a result, psychological models emphasized reducing sympathetic arousal as a means of treating these disorders. However, research has shown that relaxation training is an ineffective method for treating OCD (i.e., Lindsay et al., 1997), and at this point is often relied on in research trials as a credible control condition.

5.1.2.9 Generic Cognitive Therapy

The basic underlying approach to cognitive therapy involves identifying dysfunctional beliefs and then formulating challenges to these beliefs based on evidence that the client gathers in collaboration with the therapist (see, for example, Beck, 1976). Cognitive therapy is a helpful approach for many disorders; however, in the OCRDs, the person already has a frank acknowledgment that the underlying beliefs are irrational. As a result, generic cognitive therapy is an exercise in accumulating evidence to counter beliefs the person already fully recognizes as irrational. Additionally, most contemporary models of OCD emphasize the role of doubting, where the person is uncertain of their actions and then seeks reassurance that their behaviors were sufficient to alleviate the feared outcomes. Thus, generic cognitive therapy may also be construed as an elaborate reassurance-supporting intervention that fails to provide any lasting benefit for people with OCD (see McKay et al., 2021).

5.2 Research-Supported Approaches

Shortly after Kringlen (1965) observed that all available treatments to that point were ineffective in treating OCD, Meyer (1966) reported on the application of *exposure with response prevention* (ERP) to treat the condition. Since then, ERP has been subjected to hundreds of trials to address the full range of symptom presentations of OCD, and extended to several related conditions such as body dysmorphic disorder (see Abramowitz et al., 2017).

As a therapeutic intervention, ERP appears simplistic: Identify the situations that might provoke rituals, gradually present these situations to the client, followed by blocking rituals. As the distress naturally dissipates, the client and therapist may proceed with more challenging avoided situations. While seemingly simple, the execution of this treatment is highly technical. Clients often automatically engage in avoidance strategies during exposure that interferes with habituation. There are also factors related to clinician willingness to engage in exposure, given that the procedure has the potential to result in intense emotional reactions. There is also the challenge of clinicians moving too quickly through situations without sufficient attention to habituation to prior steps in the process. All of these are potential risks for harm associated with ERP (discussed in McKay et al., 2021). Nonetheless, ERP is a highly efficacious method of treatment, one associated with large effect sizes and durable gains for the majority adults (McKay et al., 2015) and children (Franklin et al., 2015) with OCD.

Although ERP is a well-established and efficacious treatment for OCD, recent additional theoretical conceptualizations of exposure itself indicates that there may be additional modifications in how this treatment is delivered. Specifically, the recent inhibitory learning model of exposure (Craske et al., 2014) has set in motion a great deal of excitement in the anxiety disorder treatment community, as this approach does not require elicitation of anxiety in order to produce change. The author of this chapter has referred to inhibitory learning as a "clinician's model" because the various approaches to implementing exposure are likely how full-time practitioners of the approach implicitly developed treatment programs (Frank & McKay, 2019). Therefore, interested readers may want to remain current on trends in ERP to watch for advances in implementation of the approach based on formal adoption of the inhibitory learning model.

The collection of OCRDs includes conditions that were previously classified as impulse control disorders, such as trichotillomania, or new disorders that are likewise marked by impulsivity, namely excoriation disorder. In the case of these conditions, the behavior is considered a habit or automatic process. As a result, treatment focuses on heightening awareness of the circumstances and physical sensations that prompt the behavior, followed by competing muscle tensing (such as making a fist, pushing toes into soles of shoes). Collectively, this is referred to as habit reversal, and it is a well-studied and highly efficacious method for treating these conditions (Bate et al., 2011).

The cognitive model of OCD emerged in the late 1980s and is based on several central constructs associated with the disorder (Taylor et al., 2005). These include inflated responsibility, overimportance and control of thoughts, overestimation of threat, perfectionism, and intolerance of uncertainty. These core cognitive dimensions of the disorder are the focus of cognitive therapy, and are part of evidence-based treatment, with well-developed clinician-oriented protocols (i.e., Wilhelm & Steketee, 2006). Most practitioners integrate this tailored form of cognitive therapy with ERP to develop comprehensive psychological intervention (McKay et al., 2015).

5.3 Conclusion

The OCRDs are a major category of psychiatric conditions. These disorders are marked by significant impairment in functioning as well as lowered subjective wellbeing. While there are several well-established evidence-based methods of intervention, the availability of qualified practitioners is inadequate relative to the demand for care. Filling this void are a wide range of questionable, unscientific, and untested remedies. Included in this list of questionable remedies are several medically based interventions that have the appearance of being based on science, but on closer inspection lack a conceptual foundation that would support their use.

Efforts to train a qualified and scientifically informed workforce of mental health practitioners are underway, although progress is slow. This is largely due to the highly complex nature of the OCRDs, and the technical demands of evidence-based treatment for these disorders. An important step in this process, however, is educating the existing mental health workforce of the questionable methods on the market and their lack of efficacy, while concurrently ensuring that junior level professionals are armed with the knowledge and skills to provide proper treatment.

Dean McKay, PhD, ABPP, is a Professor of Psychology at Fordham University. He is co-editor of the book *Complexities in Obsessive Compulsive and Related Disorders: Advances in Conceptualization and Treatment* (2021).

References

Abramowitz, J. S., McKay, D., & Storch, E. A. (Eds.) (2017). *Wiley handbook of obsessive compulsive disorders: Vol. 1: Obsessive-compulsive disorder across the lifespan.* Wiley.

Ahmari, S. E., Spellman, T., Douglass, N. L., Kheirbek, M. A., Simpson, H. B., Diesseroth, K., Gordon, J.A., & Hen, R. (2013). Repeated cortico-striatal stimulation generates persistent OCD-like behavior. *Science, 340,* 1234–1239.

American Psychiatric Association. (2013). *Diagnostic and statistical manual of mental disorders* (5th ed.). Author.

Ayati, Z., Sarris, J., Chang, D., Emami, S. A., & Rahimi, R. (2020). Herbal medicines and phytochemicals for obsessive-compulsive disorder. *Phytotherapy Research, 34,* 1889–1901.

Bate, K. S., Malouff, J. M., Thorseteinsson, E. T., & Bhullar, N. (2011). The efficacy of habit reversal therapy for tics, habit disorders, and stuttering: A meta-analytic review. *Clinical Psychology Review, 31,* 865–871.

Beck, A. T. (1976). *Cognitive therapy and the emotional disorders.* Plume.

Calamari, J. E., Cohen, R. J., Rector, N. A., Szacun-Shimizu, K., Riemann, B. C., & Norberg, M. M. (2006). Dysfunctional belief-based obsessive-compulsive disorder subgroups. *Behaviour Research and Therapy, 44,* 1347–1360.

Cautela, J. R., & Wisocki, P. A. (1977). The thought stopping procedure: Description, applications, and learning theory interpretations. *Psychological Record, 27,* 255–264.

Clond, M. (2016). Emotional freedom techniques for anxiety: A systematic review with meta-analysis. *Journal of Nervous and Mental Disease, 204,* 388–395.

Craske, M. G., Treanor, M., Conway, C. C., Zbozinek, T., & Vervliet, B. (2014). Maximizing exposure therapy: An inhibitory learning approach. *Behaviour Research & Therapy, 58,* 10–23.

Dubiel, S. M., Zablotna-Rypien, B., Mackey, J. B., & Williams, J. M. (1999). Magnetic properties of human liver and brain ferritin. *European Biophysics Journal, 28,* 263–267.

Frank, B., & McKay, D. (2019). The suitability of an inhibitory learning approach in exposure when habituation fails: A clinical application to misophonia. *Cognitive and Behavioral Practice, 26,* 130–142.

Franklin, M. S., Dingfelder, H. E., Freeman, J. B., Ivarsson, T., Heyman, I., Sookman, D., McKay, D., Storch, E.A., & March, J. (2015). Cognitive behavioral therapy for pediatric Obsessive-Compulsive Disorder: Empirical review and clinical recommendations. *Psychiatry Research, 227,* 78–92.

Freud, S. (1909/1997). Theoretical (from "Notes upon a case of obsessional neurosis"). In D. J. Stein & M. H. Stone (Eds.), *Essential papers on obsessive-compulsive disorder* (pp. 45–64). New York University Press.

Glazier, K., Swing, M., & McGinn, L. K. (2015). Half of obsessive-compulsive disorder cases misdiagnosed: Vignette-based survey of primary care physicians. *Journal of Clinical Psychiatry, 76,* 761–767.

Gray, J. A., & McNaughton, N. (1982). *The neuropsychology of anxiety: An inquiry into the septo-hippocampal system.* Oxford University Press.

Homan, S., Muscat, W., Joanlanne, A., Marousis, N., Cecere, G., Hofmann, L., Ji, E., Neumeier, M., Vetter, S., Seifritz, E., Dierks, T., & Homan, P.

(2012). Treatment effect variability in brain stimulation across psychiatric disorders: A meta-analysis of variance. *Neuroscience and Biobehavioral Reviews, 124,* 54–62.

Kendler, K. S. (2008). Explanatory models for psychiatric illness. *American Journal of Psychiatry, 165,* 695–702.

Kendler, K. S. (2013). Decision making in the pathway from genes for psychiatric and substance use disorders. *Molecular Psychiatry, 18,* 640–645.

Kim, S. K., McKay, D., Taylor, S., Tolin, D., Olatunji, B., Timpano, K., & Abramowitz, J. (2016). The structure of obsessive compulsive symptoms and beliefs: A correspondence and biplot analysis. *Journal of Anxiety Disorders, 38,* 79–87.

Kringlen, E. (1965). Obsessional neurotics: A long-term follow-up. *British Journal of Psychiatry, 111,* 709–722.

Krystal, J. H., Abdallah, C. G., Sanacora, G., Charney, D. S., & Duman, R. S. (2019). Ketamine: A paradigm shift for depression research and treatment. *Neuron, 101,* 774–778.

Lattie, E. G., & Stamatis, C. A. (2022). Focusing on accessibility of evidence-based treatments for obsessive-compulsive disorder. *JAMA Open Network, 5,* e221978.

Lazarov, A., Cohen, T., Liberman, N., & Dar, R. (2015). Can doubt attenuate access to internal states? Implications for obsessive-compulsive disorder. *Journal of Behavior Therapy and Experimental Psychiatry, 49* (Part B), 150–156.

Lindsay, M., Crino, R., & Andrews, G. (1997). Controlled trial of exposure and response prevention in obsessive-compulsive disorder. *British Journal of Psychiatry, 171,* 135–139.

Markarian, Y., Larson, M. J., Aldea, M. A., Baldwin, S. A., Good, D., Berkeljon, A., Murphy, T. K., Storch, E. A., & McKay, D. (2010). Multiple pathways to functional impairment in obsessive-compulsive disorder. *Clinical Psychology Review, 30,* 78–88.

McKay, D., Abramowitz, J. S., & Storch, E. A. (2021). Mechanisms of harmful treatments for obsessive-compulsive disorder. *Clinical Psychology: Science & Practice, 28,* 52–59.

McKay, D., & Leone, L. (under review). *Trauma and obsessive-compulsive disorder: Cognitive-behavioral complications and considerations for treatment.*

McKay, D., Sookman, D., Neziroglu, F., Wilhelm, S., Stein, D., Kyrios, M., Mathews, K., & Veale, D. (2015). Efficacy of cognitive-behavior therapy for obsessive-compulsive disorder. *Psychiatry Research, 227,* 104–113.

Meyer, V. (1966). Modification of expectations in cases with obsessional rituals. *Behavior Research and Therapy, 4,* 273–280.

Moritz, S., Kempke, S., Luyten, P., Randjbar, S., & Jelinek, L. (2012). Was Freud partly right on obsessive-compulsive disorder (OCD)? Investigation of latent aggression in OCD. *Psychiatry Research, 187*, 2–15.

Newson, J. J., & Thiagarajan, T. C. (2019). EEG frequency bands in psychiatric disorders; A review of resting state studies. *Frontiers in Human Neuroscience, 12*, 521.

Pauling, L., & Coryell, C. D. (1936). The magnetic properties and structure of hemoglobin, oxyhemoglobin, and carbonoxyhemoglobin. *Proceedings of the National Academy of Sciences, 22*, 210–216.

Purdon, C., Rowa, K., & Antony, M. M. (2005). Thought suppression and its effects on thought frequency, appraisal and mood state in individuals with obsessive-compulsive disorder. *Behaviour Research and Therapy, 43*, 93–108.

Rasgon, A., Lee, W. H., Leibu, E., Laird, A., Glahn, D., Goodman, W., & Frangou, S. (2017). Neural correlates of affective and non-affective cognition in obsessive compulsive disorder: A meta-analysis of functional imaging studies. *European Psychiatry, 46*, 25–32.

Riesel, A. (2019). The erring brain: Error-related negativity as an endophenotype for OCD – A review and meta-analysis. *Psychophysiology, 56*, e13348.

Rogers, A. (2017). Star neuroscientist Tom Insel leaves the Google-Spawned Verily for … a startup? Wired Magazine. www.wired.com/2017/05/star-neuroscientist-tom-insel-leaves-google-spawned-verily-startup/?mbid=social_twitter_onsiteshare.

Stahnke, B. (2021). A systematic review of misdiagnosis in those with obsessive-compulsive disorder. *Journal of Affective Disorder Reports, 6*, 100231.

Stein, D. J., Costa, D. L., Lochner, C., Miguel, E. C., Reddy, Y. J. C., Shavitt, R. G., van den Heuvel, O. A., & Simpson, H. B. (2019). Obsessive-compulsive disorder. *Nature Review Disease Primers, 5*, 52.

Storch, E. A., Abramowitz, J. S., & McKay, D. (Eds.) (2017). *Wiley handbook of obsessive compulsive disorders: Vol. 2: Obsessive-compulsive related disorders*. Wiley.

Szymanski, J. (2012). Using direct-to-consumer marketing strategies with obsessive-compulsive disorder in the nonprofit sector. *Behavior Therapy, 41*, 251–256.

Taylor, S., McKay, D., & Abramowitz, J. S. (2005). Hierarchical structure of dysfunctional beliefs in obsessive-compulsive disorder. *Cognitive Behaviour Therapy, 34*, 216–228.

Taylor, S., McKay, D., & Abramowitz, J. S. (2010). More on the brain disease model of mental disorders. *The Behavior Therapist, 33*, 16–17.

Teachman, B. A., McKay, D., Barch, D. M., Prinstein, M. J., Hollon, S. D., & Chambless, D. L. (2019). How psychosocial research can help the National

Institute of Mental Health achieve its grand challenge to reduce the burden of mental illnesses and psychological disorders. *American Psychologist, 74,* 415–431.

Ting, J., & Feng, G. (2011). Neurobiology of obsessive-compulsive disorder: Insights in neural circuitry dysfunction through mouse genetics. *Current Opinion in Neurobiology, 21,* 842–848.

Vlček, P., Polák, J., Brunovsky, M., & Horáček, J. (2018). Role of glutamergic system in obsessive-compulsive disorder with possible therapeutic implications. *Pharmacopsychiatry, 51,* 229–242.

Weber, L. A., Ethofer, T., & Ehlis, A. C. (2020). Predictors of neurofeedback training outcome: A systematic review. *NeuroImage: Clinical, 27,* 102301.

Welter, M. L., Burbaud, P., Fernandez-Vidal, S., Bardinet, E., Coste, J., Piallat, B., Besnard, S., Sauleau, P., Devaux, B., Pidoux, B., Chaynes, P., Tézenas du Montcel, S., Bastian, A., Langbour, N., Teillant, A., Haynes, W., Yelnik, J., Karachi, C., & Mallet, L. (2011). Basal ganglia dysfunction in OCD: Subthalamic neuronal activity correlates with symptoms severity and predicts high-frequency stimulation efficacy. *Translational Psychiatry, 1,* e5.

Wilhelm, S., & Steketee, G. S. (2006). *Cognitive therapy for obsessive compulsive disorder: A guide for professionals.* New Harbinger.

Wu, K. D., Clark, L. A., & Watson, D. (2006). Relations between obsessive-compulsive disorder and personality: Beyond Axis I–Axis II comorbidity. *Journal of Anxiety Disorders, 20,* 695–717.

6

Trauma

Gerald M. Rosen, Henry Otgaar, and Harald Merckelbach

Posttraumatic stress disorder (PTSD) appeared as a new diagnosis in the third edition of the American Psychiatric Association's *Diagnostic and Statistical Manual* (DSM; American Psychiatric Association (APA), 1980). Essentially, the diagnosis was carved out of the field of stress studies, which previously held to the notion that all stressors created risk for a wide range of negative health consequences (Holmes & Rahe, 1967; Seyle, 1946). In contrast to this conceptualization of stress-related disorders, the framers of PTSD advanced the assumption of a specific etiology: namely, that a distinct subset of traumatic stressors created risk for the development of a distinct clinical syndrome. This linkage between a class of events (Criterion A in the DSM-III) and a defined disorder (symptom Criteria B through D) provided a rationale to separate PTSD from general stress studies and create the new field of traumatology.

Robert Spitzer, a Columbia University psychiatrist, served as chair of the DSM-III when PTSD was introduced to its nosology (Decker, 2013). Decades later, Spitzer and colleagues (2007) revisited the diagnosis and observed, "no other DSM diagnosis, with the exception of Dissociative Identity Disorder (a related disorder), has generated so much controversy in the field as to the boundaries of the disorder, diagnostic criteria, central assumptions, clinical utility, and prevalence in various populations" (p. 233). In this chapter, we consider the issues and controversies that have plagued the PTSD diagnosis since its inception, examine questionable and implausible trauma-related therapies, and highlight problematic real-world applications of the PTSD construct.

6.1 Pseudoscience and Questionable Ideas

6.1.1 Core Issues and Controversies

Without questioning the very real distress and psychiatric impairments experienced by those faced with life-threatening or other emotionally traumatic events, we can ask whether PTSD as a construct within the domain of stress reactions best carves nature at its joints (see Gangestad & Snyder, 1985; MacCorquodale & Meehl, 1948; Morey, 1991). A related question is whether the diagnosis of PTSD possesses substantial incremental validity (Sechrest, 1963) above and beyond extant and possibly better validated diagnoses (e.g., depression, anxiety disorders). To address these issues, we consider a variety of external validating criteria that have been evoked to support the diagnostic construct: (1) the idea that a specific etiology underlies PTSD, (2) the belief that PTSD constitutes a taxon, and (3) the hope that a specific biomarker might distinguish PTSD from other diagnoses.

6.1.1.1 Challenges to the Assumption of a Specific Etiology

Following the rules of the DSM, PTSD cannot be diagnosed in the absence of a traumatic event (Breslau & Davis, 1987). Yet, numerous publications have demonstrated that the full range of PTSD symptoms can manifest after non-Criterion A events such as divorce (Dreman, 1991), money problems (Scott & Stradling, 1994), and even bed bug attacks (Goddard & de Shazo, 2012). It also has been demonstrated that factors extraneous to trauma contribute more variance to clinical outcomes than the event itself (Bowman & Yehuda, 2004; Brewin et al, 2000; Ozer et al., 2003). Cross-cultural variability in PTSD lifetime prevalence rates (e.g., 4.4% for trauma-exposed individuals in Iraq, 9.6% for Australians, and 14.5% for individuals from Northern Ireland) further demonstrates the need to consider variables beyond Criterion A events (Koenen et al., 2017). In short, it seems that Criterion A events are neither necessary nor sufficient to cause PTSD symptoms (O'Donnell et al., 2010; Rosen & Lilienfeld, 2008). In the face of these findings and so many more, it is reasonable that clinicians and researchers ask this question: How is it possible that violent rape, horrific accidents, divorce, and exposure to bed bugs can be lumped together in a single class of stressors? Our view on this is in total agreement with Shephard's (2004) observation that any unit of classification that simultaneously encompasses such diverse events, "must, by any reasonable lay standard, be a nonsense, a patent absurdity" (p. 37).

6.1.1.2 Does PTSD Represent a Distinct Syndrome?

With controversy surrounding the assumption of a specific etiology, the question of diagnostic validity turns to the clinical syndrome itself and whether PTSD symptom criteria are distinguishable from other, already extant disorders. Here too, there have been multiple challenges to the PTSD construct. First, there is the issue of high comorbidity rates

(Institute of Medicine, 2006; Young, 2004) and disorders being defined by the same symptom criteria (Spitzer et al, 2007). Compare, for example, PTSD's symptom criteria D5 in the DSM-5-TR ("Markedly diminished interest or participation in significant activities," APA, 2022, p. 302) with symptom A2 for major depressive disorder ("Markedly diminished interest or pleasure in all, or almost all, activities most of the day, nearly every day," p. 183). Next, studies have demonstrated that patients with clinical disorders such as major depression (Bodkin et al., 2007) and social phobia (Erwin et al., 2006) endorse the symptoms of PTSD without reporting Criterion A events. Challenges to PTSD also arise from the 636,120 symptom combinations by which one may receive the diagnosis (Galatzer-Levy & Bryant, 2013), and changing criteria over various editions of the DSM that give the appearance of an ever-expanding laundry list of stress-related reactions, without specificity to any single diagnostic construct (Herbert & Forman, 2010). To make matters more complicated, studies suggest that PTSD and depression arise from similar predictive variables and a shared vulnerability (Breslau et al., 2000; O'Donnell et al., 2004). Such findings are consistent with conceptualizing PTSD as the upper end of a stress–response continuum rather than a taxon or discrete clinical syndrome (Broman-Fulks et al., 2007; Forbes et al., 2005; Ruscio et al., 2002). These findings also align with recent conceptual models in which mental disorders are viewed as complex networks of interacting symptoms, rather than latent entities that cause symptoms to emerge (e.g., Armour et al., 2017; Fried et al., 2017; McNally et al., 2015).

Finally, there have been numerous attempts to identify an underlying mechanism or distinct marker that might validate PTSD. These efforts include research on low cortisol levels, small hippocampal volumes, other alterations in brain structures, neurocircuitry, physiologic reactivity, inflammatory markers, and most recently, the possibility of genetic markers. In almost every instance, if not all, these efforts have been hampered by inconsistent findings, lack of specificity, and/or conceptual issues that challenge the very logic of the proposed mechanism (Rosen & Lilienfeld, 2008; Uttal, 2001). To this day, an assessment offered by the Institute of Medicine (2006) holds true: "No biomarkers are clinically useful or specific in diagnosing PTSD, assessing the risk of developing it, or charting its progression" (p. 46). Considering the failed efforts to establish PTSD as a distinct disorder we find ourselves in agreement with North et al. (2009), who stated: "It is still not established whether or not there are specific types of traumatic events and levels of exposure to them that are associated with a syndrome that is cohesive in clinical characteristics, biological correlates, familial patterns, and longitudinal diagnostic stability" (p. 34).

6.1.1.3 *Expansion of the Trauma Narrative*

Despite failed attempts to validate PTSD as a distinct clinical syndrome with a specific etiology, the reach of traumatology has extended to an increasing array of events and stress-related symptoms (Haslam, 2016). Even expected reactions to stressful events are now referred to as PTSD symptoms, as occurred after the 9/11 attack in the United States (e.g., Silver et al., 2002). Yet, labeling situation-based emotional reactions as "symptoms" is akin to suggesting that coughing in a smoky tavern is a symptom of lung cancer (Rosen et al., 2008; Wakefield & Horwitz, 2010). In a further extension of the PTSD narrative, the DSM-5 (APA, 2013) introduced two new diagnostic categories: Other Specified Trauma- and Stressor-Related Disorder, and Unspecified Trauma- and Stressor-Related Disorder. When one applies criteria for these disorders, most any clinically significant distress after most any upsetting event can be diagnosed as a mental disorder. The irony of this situation should not go unnoticed: what once was a singular diagnosis carved out of general stress studies has now been placed within an expanding narrative that subsumes the entire field from which it came.

6.1.2 Ineffective and/or Potentially Harmful Treatments

PTSD has been viewed as a social construction created in the political aftermath of the Vietnam War for the purpose of bringing relief to war veterans and survivors of other life-threatening trauma (Scott, 1990; Shephard, 2001; Summerfield, 2001). Within this context the impetus to help victims was particularly strong and new therapies were promoted with the best of intentions. Perhaps these positive sentiments also conspired with the talents of charismatic and ambitious clinicians who prematurely marketed their methods. Cuijpers et al. (2010) considered factors that might have motivated academicians in this climate: "Researchers of psychological treatments do have personal interests in publication of (larger) effects, as these are more likely to lead to tenure and lucrative workshop fees" (p. 177).

Several of the new treatments were informed by existing interventions for anxiety disorders, such as exposure-based methods. Other treatments were derived from newly formed assumptions and novel methods. Among these new methods were Emotional Freedom Techniques,

Thought Field Therapy, Tapas Acupuncture Technique, Whole-Life Healing, Traumatic Incident Reduction, Eye Movement Desensitization and Reprocessing, Critical Incident Stress Debriefing, Recovered Memory Therapy, Visual/Kinesthetic Dissociation, and Sensory Motor Psychotherapy. For the purposes of the present chapter, we will consider a few examples of therapies that are harmful or based on scientifically implausible theories.

6.1.2.1 Harmful Therapies Based on Faulty Assumptions

On multiple occasions, mental health practitioners have learned that good intentions are not enough because unsubstantiated mental health techniques can be harmful (Lilienfeld et al., 2015). Here, we review two examples of this truism.

Crisis Incident Stress Debriefing (and Management)
Critical Incident Stress Debriefing (CISD) was introduced in the 1980s as a preventive intervention for emergency personnel who witnessed trauma (Mitchell, 1983). Its methods were based on the assumption that providing emotional assistance in the immediate aftermath of trauma could substantially reduce risk for later psychiatric disorder. Contrary to early enthusiasm and positive claims, research began to indicate that group debriefings not only failed to prevent future disorder (e.g., Marchand et al., 2006), but might for some individuals interfere with processes of natural recovery (e.g., Carlier et al., 2000; Kenardy et al., 1996). The direction of these negative effects was affirmed in meta-analyses (e.g., van Emmerik et al., 2002) and comprehensive reviews of the literature (McNally et al., 2003; Rose et al., 2005). In the face of negative findings, proponents of CISD changed the name of their methods to Critical Incident Stress Management (CISM) and proposed that a debriefing was just one component of a multi-method comprehensive intervention strategy (Everly & Mitchell, 1999; Mitchell & Everly, 1998). However, changing methods in this manner creates a moving target that is unfalsifiable and therefore outside the realm of science.

Nowadays, the typical recommendation to clinicians, professional agencies, and emergency personnel is to avoid compulsory group debriefings (e.g., Gist & Devilly, 2010; McNally et al., 2003). Nevertheless, CISM remains heavily promoted through proprietary training workshops and journals that continue to tout its success (e.g., Swab, 2020). This resistance to disconfirming evidence further moves CISM into the realm of pseudoscience.

Recovered Memory Techniques

Assumptions regarding trauma memories (how they are stored, pro-
cessed and retrieved), form the basis for what Young (2004) called the
"inner logic" of PTSD. Resting on the questionable view that such
memories can fragment, and through dissociation or repression are
banned from consciousness, there arose various recovery memory techniques intended to facilitate awareness and post-traumatic healing. What
followed was a debate among trauma experts so contentious that it came
to be known as the "memory wars" (Crews, 1995). On one side of this
debate were scholars who cited evidence in support of repressed memories (e.g., Brown et al., 1999; Kopelman, 2002; Pope & Brown, 1996). On
the other side were those who contended that trauma was remembered
all too well, apart from normal processes of forgetting and memory decay
(McNally, 2003; 2022). The fires around these issues were fueled by
widely publicized cases in which therapists' suggestions of buried memories led to patients recalling past trauma, filing criminal charges against
their alleged abusers, and pursuing civil lawsuits (Loftus & Ketcham,
1994). But then some patients recanted their recovered memories and,
supported by research that induced memories of never-experienced
events (e.g., Scoboria et al., 2017), successfully sued therapists for malpractice (Lief, 1999; Ost et al., 2002).

Over time a type of consensus emerged in which it was acknowledged
that the existence of repressed memories could be questioned but not
disproved (Ost, 2003) and suggestive recovery techniques were to be
used with caution, if not avoided entirely (Lynn et al., 2015). Within this
framework, some observers optimistically posited that the memory wars
had been settled (e.g., Barden, 2016; McHugh, 2003; Paris, 2012).
Unfortunately, just as with the stubborn resilience demonstrated by
CISD/M proponents, debates over repressed and recovered memories
are far from over. Recent studies demonstrate that many therapists and
members of the public continue to believe in the existence of unconscious
repressed memories; therapists continue to discuss the topic with clients;
and patients continue to recover memories while in therapy (Dodier
et al., 2019; Houben et al., 2020; Otgaar et al., 2019; 2021; Patihis et al.,
2019; 2020). One treatment approach discussed later in this chapter, Eye
Movement Desensitization and Reprocessing (EMDR), demonstrates
a continuing and dangerous mix of findings wherein the majority of
EMDR practitioners endorse the concept of repressed memories
(Houben et al., 2019), while research demonstrates the possibility that
a task such as eye movements facilitates the production of false memories
(e.g., Houben et al., 2018; 2020; Kenchel et al., 2020; but see also van

Schie & Leer, 2019). Further contributing to ongoing concerns, the DSM-5 introduced the phrase "dissociative amnesia," a synonym for repressed memory as problematic as the original and a cause of much debate (Brand et al., 2018; McNally, 2007; Merckelbach & Patihis, 2018; Patihis et al., 2019). In the face of this history and continuing controversy, clinicians should stay informed of practice guidelines (American Medical Association Council on Scientific Affairs, 2008; American Psychological Association, 1998), avoid inappropriately suggestive techniques, and proceed with caution when exploring a patient's trauma history.

6.1.2.2 Implausible Therapies Based on Quirky Methods

Several novel methods promoted for the treatment of PTSD became known as the "Power Therapies." These techniques often advanced implausible theories accompanied by miraculous claims of cure (Devilly, 2005; Rosen et al., 1998). Here we consider the most well-publicized of the power therapies: interventions that employ tapping on energy acupoints (Thought Field Therapy, Emotional Freedom Techniques) or rely on some form of bilateral stimulation (Eye Movement Desensitization and Reprocessing).

Energy Tapping Therapies
Roger Callahan popularized Thought Field Therapy (TFT) in his book *The Five Minute Phobia Cure* (Callahan, 1985). Callahan's methods employed various algorithms based on ancient Chinese acupoints to balance the body's energy and promote nature's healing. Specific tapping sequences (algorithms) were tailored to treat specific disorders, even though the theoretical and empirical basis for these prescribed methods remained uncertain. In the only controlled study comparing specific individualized treatment sequences as recommended by Callahan to random sequences, no significant differences were found (Pignotti, 2005). This null effect goes to the central assumption that prescribed patterns are required to obtain successful treatment outcomes. Relatedly, one of Callahan's students developed a variant of TFT called Emotional Freedom Techniques (EFT) that did not rely on disorder-specific procedures (Craig & Fowlie, 1995). Instead, EFT employs the same set of acupoints for any and all disorders. Therefore, any reports of rapid and powerful treatment effects associated with EFT, if accepted, would provide further evidence that specific algorithms are unnecessary. This state of affairs leaves open the more basic question of whether tapping itself is an active or inert component in energy-based methods.

It is beyond the scope of any single chapter to resolve debates regarding the status of energy tapping therapies. One leading proponent of these methods has claimed that EFT has been validated in over 100 clinical trials (Church et al., 2020). Skeptics, on the other hand, have questioned the tapping therapies for being based on implausible theories, advancing extraordinary claims, relying on weak tests or case reports, failing to rule out placebo effects, and disregarding negative findings (e.g., Gaudiano & Herbert, 2000; Lohr et al., 2008; Pignotti & Thyer, 2009). This ongoing back-and-forth between proponents and skeptics on the status of tapping therapies was demonstrated in an exchange of papers published in the *Journal of Nervous and Mental Disease*. Church and colleagues (2018) claimed that a meta-analysis supported tapping as an active ingredient in EFT. Spielmans and colleagues (2020) found that the reported analysis was flawed, used incorrect statistics, and provided no such support for tapping. Church and colleagues (2020) then published a corrigendum in which they abandoned their original *a priori* hypothesis and reported that a new post-hoc analysis using different time point measures found even larger effects in support of tapping. In response, Spielmans and Rosen (2022) observed that the new meta-analysis by Church and colleagues violated basic precepts of science and failed to remedy multiple method flaws. In effect, the proponents of tapping therapies had taken on the imprimatur of science without accepting its necessary rigors. Despite this reality, there is every reason to believe that energy practitioners will continue tapping with their clients: that is, until professional and licensing authorities provide science-based practice guidelines that are clear and enforceable.

Eye Movement Desensitization and Reprocessing (a Purple Hat Therapy)

EMDR was developed by Francine Shapiro in the late 1980s (Shapiro, 1989a; 1989b). While most everyone agrees that EMDR can be beneficial in the treatment of PTSD, the question remains as to what the method's active components are (e.g., eye movements, bilateral stimulation, exposure, imagery, cognitive framing, allegiance effects). Debates over this central question (e.g., Herbert et al., 2000) have challenged the very foundations for using empirically supported treatments as a guide to sound clinical practice.

As originally crafted (Chambless & Hollon, 1998; Chambless & Ollendick, 2001), treatment methods were labeled as "possibly efficacious" if found to be more effective than no treatment in a single randomized controlled trial, and "efficacious" if support was obtained in a second trial conducted by an independent research team. It is within this framework that EMDR became a recognized intervention in the treatment of PTSD. Yet, as observed by McNally (1999): "what is effective in EMDR is not new and what is new is not effective" (p. 619). Rosen and Davison (2003) considered how this situation left considerable room for mischief:

Experience with EMDR demonstrates that current decision rules for determining ESTs are inadequate. Furthermore, the current system makes psychology vulnerable to any treatment innovator or savvy charlatan who puts a novel method through a single randomized controlled trial with a no-treatment comparison. Hypothetically, a doctor could ask clients with driving phobias to wear a large purple hat while applying relaxation and cognitive coping skills to *in vivo* practice. The practitioner places a band of magnets in the purple hats, claiming that particular algorithms for positioning the magnets are determined by age, sex, and personality structure of the client. When properly placed, so the practitioner claims, the magnets reorient energy fields, accelerate information processing, improve interhemispheric coherence, and eliminate phobic avoidance. The inventor might call his method "purple hat therapy" (PHT) or "*e*lectro Magnetic Desensitization and Remobilization" (eMDR), conduct a single RCT against no treatment, and apply for listing as an EST. (p. 305)

Lilienfeld and colleagues have considered the limitations of ESTs and recommended that treatments be evaluated within a science-based framework that takes into account a method's theoretical plausibility (Lilienfeld, 2011; Lilienfeld et al., 2018; Lohr et al., 2012; Rosen et al., 2020; Washburn et al., 2019). Within this framework, EMDR or any other novel method would not receive any sort of recognition until it was demonstrated that *what was new was effective*. Recognizing this issue, researchers have tried to identify what if anything about eye movements contributes to treatment outcome. For example, it has been suggested that eye movements elicit an orienting response (Barrowcliff et al., 2004; Lee & Cuijpers, 2013; Schubert et al., 2010) or impact the limited capacity of working memory (deVoogd & Phelps, 2020). These newer models have persuaded some (see Carey, 2019 regarding McNally's views), but others are less sanguine (Cuijpers et al., 2020). Further, before accepting the role of eye movements, it would seem necessary to explain studies that have reported equal treatment effects for finger tapping and/or eyes-fixed conditions (Renfrey & Spates, 1994).

On balance, everything about EMDR brings us back to a central and science-based question: namely, how can clinicians best structure known therapeutic processes to maximize treatment outcome (Lohr et al., 2012)? Within this framework, we might ask if some individuals most benefit from direct confrontation with real-life exposures while others experience greater gains using imagery with a competing task that reduces the intensity of exposure. Notice that we can ask this type of question, and so many others, without ever mentioning EMDR or its insulated use of specialized terms and implausible constructs (Shapiro, 1995). In this science-based world grounded in plausible theory, we can repeatedly recite this mantra about the power therapies: *While EFT involves finger tapping and EMDR involves finger wagging, a clearheaded clinician does well to do neither.* We also can keep in mind two sayings popularized, although not originated, by Carl Sagan (1996). First, extraordinary claims require extraordinary evidence. Second, while it may be a virtue to keep an open mind, don't let it be so open that your brains fall out.

6.1.3 Real-World Challenges to Traumatology

6.1.3.1 PTSD in the Courtroom

Because the etiology of PTSD is tied to specific events, the diagnosis has been particularly attractive in cases that involve personal injury claims or disability payments (Lees-Haley, 1986; Slovenko, 1994; Trimble, 1985). Two additional considerations complicate the assessment of these types of cases. First, PTSD symptoms are well-publicized, subjective, and easily feigned (Eldrige, 1991; Sparr & Atkinson, 1986). Second, it is widely recognized that clinicians are poorly equipped to serve as lie detectors when tasked with identifying falsified presentations of psychiatric disorder (Ekman & O'Sullivan, 1991; Raifman, 1983). As if this wasn't sufficiently troubling, unusually high rates of PTSD have been reported among groups of litigants, thereby raising the concern that feigned symptom reporting has impacted the PTSD database (Frueh et al., 2005; Rosen, 2006).

In the midst of these issues, forensic experts are informed by best practice guidelines (e.g., Wettstein, 2010), ethical standards (American Academy of Psychiatry and the Law, 2005; American Psychology–Law Society, 2013), and the use of tests and protocols used to detect feigned

PTSD (Matto et al., 2019). Clinicians, on the other hand, act as advocates for their patients and can find themselves in alien territory if they are called upon to testify at trial. When a situation arises with a client involved in litigation, clinicians are encouraged to consider limitations that result from their reliance on a patient's self-reporting (Greenberg & Shuman, 1997; Strasburger et al., 1997). Even with the use of broader assessment methods (Taylor et al., 2007), mental health professionals may be unable to recognize feigned presentations of PTSD (Hickling et al., 2002; Rosen, 1995).

6.1.3.2 Vanity Credentials

Specialty certifications in the treatment of PTSD are offered by several organizations including the American Academy of Experts in Traumatic Stress (AAETS, 2021), the Association of Traumatic Stress Specialists (2021), the International Association of Trauma Professionals (2021), and the Trauma Institute International (2021). Looking at just one of these organizations, the AAETS offers Certification in Bereavement Trauma, Certification in Domestic Violence, Certification in Disability Trauma, Certification in Rape Trauma, and ten others. Each of these certifications carries an acronym that can be placed after one's name, creating the possibility of representing oneself as Dr. John Doe, PhD, CBT, CDV, CDT, CRT. To qualify for any of AAETS's credentials it is only necessary to fill out a form and check various items for which you can be awarded points. For example, having a doctoral level education will earn you 60 points. If you are licensed, add another 40. With a total of 200 points and payment of $250, without having to pass a test or submit a work product, and absent a felony record or other professional liability issue, you will have fulfilled the credentialing criteria.

We do not question the appropriateness of professionals who represent their competencies by obtaining a degree, meeting requirements for state licensure, or listing recognized qualifications through the American Board of Professional Psychology (Hill & Packard, 2013; Nezu et al., 2009). At the same time, concerns are raised when dubious specialty certifications mislead the public with false impressions of authority and expertise (Rosen et al., 2020). The problem of dubious and bogus credentials has been discussed for decades (e.g., Dawes, 1994; Koocher, 1979; Woody, 1997), but now is particularly pressing when one considers the ever-expanding trauma industry (Dineen, 1996).

6.2 Research-Supported Approaches

McNally (2006) observed: "Advocacy for victims must rest on the best science possible" (p. 924). It is in this spirit that we provide the following guidance. With regard to immediate assistance offered to trauma survivors, mental health professionals are discouraged from conducting critical incident stress debriefings or imposing their own views on how recovery "should" take place. Instead, an alternative model known as Psychological First Aid now guides the efforts of mental health professionals. The core elements of this approach include support for an individual's immediate needs (e.g., safety, comfort, food, housing, other practical assistance), encouragement to maintain connections with available social supports (e.g., friends, family, spiritual resources), provision of simple practical tips on coping, information on community resources, and emergency referrals using a stepped care approach (Gist & Devilly, 2010; Watson et al., 2011). The astute observer will notice that these recommendations largely fall outside the purview of psychology or psychiatry and likely can be addressed without the involvement of mental health professionals.

After the immediate aftermath of trauma when individuals present for treatment, we urge clinicians to be judicious in their use of this diagnosis. As cautioned by Sparr (1990): "PTSD should be diagnosed if the facts fit, but only if they fit. To do otherwise dilutes and trivializes the diagnosis" (p. 259). If a patient reports phobic avoidance after a traumatic event absent other symptom complaints then the diagnosis should be specific phobia, not PTSD. If a patient reports low mood and sleep difficulties after trauma but fails to endorse nightmares, flashbacks, or exaggerated startle, a diagnosis of adjustment disorder may be indicated, not PTSD. In the context of these considerations, Bryant (2010) cautioned: "It is important to consider the full range of symptom criteria that constitute a PTSD diagnosis, and not reflexively apply the diagnosis whenever posttraumatic anxiety presents" (pp. 212–213).

When it comes to planning treatment for patients diagnosed with PTSD, we encourage clinicians to consider the benefits of leaving behind the DSM. In its place, clinicians are encouraged to conceptualize a client's presenting problems in terms of networks of interacting symptoms (Armour et al., 2017; Fried et al., 2017; McNally et al., 2015). Rather than conceptualizing post-traumatic distress as a diagnostic taxon (i.e., a category in nature; Meehl & Golden, 1982), a more fruitful and scientifically supportable position gives consideration to a broad range of possible reactions to adverse events.

A corollary to avoiding the DSM's listing of post-trauma disorders is the recommendation that clinicians abandon any allegiance to treatment-based acronyms, particularly those founded on implausible theories (e.g., Lilienfeld, 2011). Instead, clinicians are encouraged to plan treatment interventions around science-based and empirically supported principles of behavior change (Castonguay & Beutler, 2006; Lilienfeld et al., 2018; Lohr et al., 2012; Rosen & Davison, 2003). For example, if a patient presents with anxiety reactions and phobic avoidance, principles of exposure-based methods can be employed irrespective of the diagnosis submitted to insurance. Cognitive restructuring, imagery rescripting, relaxation, mindfulness, response prevention, and behavioral activation also transcend diagnoses and procedural acronyms. Each of these intervention efforts, some of which do not require expertise in psychology, can be provided without mention of the DSM or debates over the construct validity of PTSD.

6.3 Conclusion

In this chapter, we have considered numerous and perhaps insurmountable issues that challenge whether PTSD carves nature at its joints and advances our understanding of human reactions to adversity. Despite these challenges, the field of traumatology has expanded a western-centric narrative that blurs distinctions between normal reactions and symptoms of disorder (Summerfield, 1999; Wakefield & Horwitz, 2010; Watters, 2010). This narrative also focuses on a distinct diagnostic construct rather than a complex network of reactions that more likely reflects post-traumatic psychiatric distress. Feeding on this narrative is a growing industry of trauma counselors who are encouraged to bolster their standing with vanity credentials while practicing proprietary treatments based on implausible theory. It is not an encouraging picture. As observed by the English historian Ben Shephard (2004):

> If "trauma" could now be broken up into its constituent parts, it would return to its social contexts and be de-medicalized. But for that to happen, psychiatry would have to surrender ground, and history teaches us that such acts of professional self-denial are indeed rare. Besides, it is now too late. Trauma has been vectored into the wider society by the law and the media. (pp. 57–58)

While we are not blinded by optimism, we remain hopeful that Shephard's less than sanguine appraisal was premature. Should it turn out that a post-traumatic disorder exists in nature, one that disrupts normal functioning after extreme adversity, we expect a better under-standing of its features and boundaries to emerge over time. We have confidence in the self-correcting methods of scientific inquiry. In the meantime, clinicians are encouraged to pair conceptually sound case formulations with empirically supported and theoretically plausible prin-ciples of change.

Gerald M. Rosen, PhD, is a Clinical Professor Emeritus of Psychology at the University of Washington. He is co-editor of the book *Clinician's Guide to Posttraumatic Stress Disorder* (2010).

Henry Otgaar, PhD, is a Professor of Psychology at Maastricht University in the Netherlands. He is co-editor of the book *Finding the Truth in the Courtroom: Dealing with Deception, Lies, and Memories* (2017).

Harald Merckelbach, PhD, is a Professor of Psychology at Maastricht University in the Netherlands. He is author of the book *Good Stories Are Rarely True* (written in Dutch; 2020).

References

American Academy of Experts in Traumatic Stress (AAETS) (2021). www.aaets.org.

American Academy of Psychiatry and the Law (2005). Ethics guidelines for the practice of forensic psychiatry. www.aapl.org/ethics.htm.

American Medical Association Council on Scientific Affairs (2008). Report on memories of childhood abuse: American Medical Association Council on Scientific Affairs. *International Journal of Clinical and Experimental Hypnosis*, *43*, 114–117.

American Psychiatric Association (APA) (1980). *Diagnostic and statistical man-ual of mental disorder* (3rd ed.). Author.

American Psychiatric Association (APA) (1994). *Diagnostic and statistical man-ual of mental disorders* (4th ed.). Author.

American Psychiatric Association (APA) (2013). *Diagnostic and statistical man-ual of mental disorder* (5th ed.). Author.

American Psychiatric Association (APA) (2022). *Diagnostic and statistical man-ual of mental disorder* (5th ed., text revision). Author.

American Psychological Association (1998). Final conclusions of the American Psychological Association working group on investigation of memories of child abuse. *Psychology, Public Policy, and Law*, *4*, 933–940.

American Psychology–Law Society: Division 41 of the American Psychological Association (2013). Specialty guidelines for forensic psychology. *American Psychologist*, *68*, 7–19.

Armour, C., Fried, E. I., & Olff, M. (2017). PTSD symptomics: Network analyses in the field of psychotraumatology. *European Journal of Psychotraumatology, 8* (suppl 3), 1398003. https://doi.org/10.1080/20008198.2017.1398003.

Association of Traumatic Stress Specialists (2021). www.aaets.org.

Barden, R. C. (2016). Memory and reliability: Developments and controversial issues. In P. Radcliffe, A. Heaton-Armstrong, G. Gudjonsson, & D. Wolchover (Eds.), *Witness testimony in sex cases* (pp. 343–359). Oxford University Press.

Barrowcliff, A. L., Gray, N. S., Freeman, T. C .A., & MacCullock, M. J. (2004). Eye movements reduce the vividness, emotional valence and electrodermal arousal associated with negative autobiographical memories. *Journal of Forensic Psychiatry and Psychology, 15,* 325–345.

Bodkin, J. A., Pope, H. G., Detke, M. J., & Hudson, J. I. (2007). Is PTSD caused by traumatic stress? *Journal of Anxiety Disorders, 21,* 176–182.

Bowman, M. L., & Yehuda, R. (2004). Risk factors and the adversity-stress model. In G. M. Rosen (Ed.), *Posttraumatic stress disorder: Issues and controversies* (pp. 39–61). John Wiley & Sons.

Brand, B. L., Dalenberg, C. J., Frewen, P. A., Loewenstein, R. J., Schielke, H. J., Brams, J. S., & Spiegel, D. (2018). Trauma-related dissociation is no fantasy: Addressing the errors of omission and commission in Merckelbach and Patihis (2018). *Psychological Injury and Law, 11,* 377–393.

Breslau, N., & Davis, G. C. (1987). Posttraumatic stress disorder: The stressor criterion. *The Journal of Nervous and Mental Disease, 175,* 255–264.

Breslau, N., Davis, G. C., Peterson, E. L., & Schultz, L. R. (2000). A second look at comorbidity in victims of trauma: The posttraumatic stress disorder-major depression connection. *Biological Psychiatry, 48,* 902–909.

Brewin, C. R., Andrews, B., & Valentine, J. D. (2000). Meta-analysis of risk factors for posttraumatic stress disorder in trauma-exposed adults. *Journal of Consulting and Clinical Psychology, 68,* 748–766.

Broman-Fulks, J. J., Ruggiero, K. J., Green, B. A., Kilpatrick, D. G., Danielson, C. K., Resnick, H. S., & Saunders, B. E. (2007). Taxometric investigation of PTSD: Data from two nationally representative samples. *Behavior Therapy, 37,* 364–380.

Brown, D., Scheflin, A. W., & Whitfield, C. L. (1999). Recovered memories: The current weight of the evidence in science and in the courts. *Journal of Psychiatry and Law, 27,* 5–156.

Bryant, R. A. (2010). Treating the full range of posttraumatic reactions. In G. M. Rosen & B. C. Frueh (Eds.), *Clinician's guide to posttraumatic stress disorder* (pp. 205–234). Wiley.

Callahan, R. J. (1985). *Five minute phobia cure: Dr. Callahan's treatment for fears, phobias and self-sabotage.* Enterprise Publishing, Inc.

Carey, B. (2019, July 11). Francine Shapiro, Developer of Eye Movement Therapy, dies at 71. *New York Times*. www.nytimes.com/2019/07/11/science/francine-shapiro-dead.html.

Carlier, I. V. E., Voerman, A. E., & Gersons, B. P. R. (2000). The influence of occupational debriefing on post-traumatic stress symptomatology in traumatized police officers. *British Journal of Medical Psychology*, *73*, 87–98.

Castonguay, L. G., & Beutler, L. E. (Eds.) (2006). *Principles of therapeutic change that work*. Oxford University Press.

Chambless, D. L., &Hollon, S. D. (1998). Defining empirically supported therapies. *Journal of Consulting and Clinical Psychology*, *66*, 7–18.

Chambless, D. L., & Ollendick, T. H. (2001). Empirically supported psychological interventions: Controversies and evidence. *Annual Review of Psychology*, *52*, 685–716.

Church, D., Stapleton, P., Kip, K., & Gallo, F. (2020). Corrigendum to: Is tapping on acupuncture points an active ingredient in Emotional Freedom Techniques: A systematic review and meta-analysis of comparative studies. *Journal of Nervous and Mental Disease*, *208*, 632–635.

Church, D., Stapleton, P., Yang, A., & Gallo, F. (2018). Is tapping on acupuncture points an active ingredient in Emotional Freedom Techniques? A systematic review and meta-analysis of comparative studies. *Journal of Nervous and Mental Disease*, *206*, 783–793.

Craig, G., & Fowlie, A. (1995). *Emotional freedom techniques: The manual*. Authors.

Crews, F. (1995). *The memory wars: Freud's legacy in dispute*. New York Review of Books.

Cuijpers, P., Smit, F., Bohlmeijer, E., Hollon, S. D., & Andersson, G. (2010). Efficacy of cognitive–behavioural therapy and other psychological treatments for adult depression: Meta-analytic study of publication bias. *British Journal of Psychiatry*, *196*, 173–178.

Cuijpers, P., van Veen, S. C., Sijbrandij, M., Yoder, W., & Cristea, I. A. (2020). Eye movement desensitization and reprocessing for mental health problems: A systematic review and meta-analysis. *Cognitive Behaviour Therapy*, *49*, 165–180.

Dawes, R. M. (1994). *House of cards: Psychology and psychotherapy built on myth*. The Free Press.

Decker, H. S. (2013). *The making of DSM-III: A diagnostic manual's conquest of American psychiatry*. Oxford University Press.

Devilly, G. J. (2005). Power therapies and possible threats to the science of psychology and psychiatry. *Australian and New Zealand Journal of Psychiatry*, *39*, 437–445.

deVoogd, L. D., & Phelps, E. A. (2020). A cognitively demanding working-memory intervention enhances extinction. *Scientific Reports*, *10*, 7020. https://doi.org/10.1038/s41598-020-63811-0.

Dineen, T. (1996). *Manufacturing victims: What the psychology industry is doing to people*. Robert Davies Publishing.

Dodier, O., Patihis, L., & Payoux, M. (2019). Reports of recovered memories of childhood abuse in therapy in France. *Memory, 27*, 1283–1298.

Dreman, S. (1991). Coping with the trauma of divorce. *Journal of Traumatic Stress, 4*, 113–121.

Ekman, P., & O'Sullivan, M. (1991). Who can catch a liar? *American Psychologist, 46*, 913–920.

Eldridge, G. (1991). Contextual issues in the assessment of posttraumatic stress disorder. *Journal of Traumatic Stress, 4*, 7–23.

Erwin, B. A., Heimberg, R. G., Marx, B. P., & Franklin, M. E. (2006). Traumatic and socially stressful life events among persons with social anxiety disorder. *Journal of Anxiety Disorders, 20*, 896–914.

Everly, Jr., G. S., & Mitchell, J. T. (1999). *Critical Incident Stress Management (CISM): A new era and standard of care in crisis intervention*. 2nd ed. Chevron.

Forbes, D., Haslam, N., Williams, B. J., & Creamer, M. (2005). Testing the latent structure of posttraumatic stress disorder: A taxometric study of combat veterans. *Journal of Traumatic Stress, 18*, 647–656.

Fried, E. I., van Borkulo, C. D., Cramer, A. O. J., Boschloo, L., Schoevers, R. A., & Borsboom, D. (2017). Mental disorders as networks of problems: A review of recent insights. *Social Psychiatry and Psychiatric Epidemiology, 52*, 1–10.

Frueh, B. C., Elhai, J.D., Grubaugh, A. L., Monnier, J., Kashdan, T. B., Sauvageot, J. A., Hamner, M. B., Burkett, B. G., & Arana, G. (2005). Documented combat exposure of U.S. veterans seeking treatment for combat-related post-traumatic stress disorder. *British Journal of Psychiatry, 186*, 467–472.

Galatzer-Levy, I. R., & Bryant, R. A. (2013). 636,120 ways to have posttraumatic stress disorder. *Perspectives in Psychological Science, 8*, 651–62.

Gangestad, S., & Snyder, M. (1985). "To carve nature at its joints": On the existence of discrete classes of personality. *Psychological Review, 92*, 317–349.

Gaudiano, B. A., & Herbert, J. D. (2000). Can we really tap our problems away? A critical analysis of Thought Field Therapy. *Skeptical Inquirer, 24*, 29–33.

Gist, R., & Devilly, G. J. (2010). Early intervention in the aftermath of trauma. In G. R. Rosen & B. C. Frueh (Eds.), *Clinician's guide to posttraumatic stress disorder* (pp. 153–176). Wiley.

Goddard, J., & de Shazo, R. (2012). Psychological effects of bed bug attacks (*Cimex lectularius* L.). *American Journal of Medicine, 125*, 101–103.

Greenberg, S. A., & Shuman, D. W. (1997). Irreconcilable conflict between therapist and forensic roles. *Professional Psychology: Research and Practice, 28*, 50–57.

Haslam, N. (2016). Concept creep: Psychology's expanding concepts of harm and pathology. *Psychological Inquiry*, *27*, 1–17.

Herbert, J. D., & Forman, E. M. (2010). Cross-cultural perspectives on posttraumatic stress. In G. M. Rosen & B. C. Frueh (Eds.), *Clinician's guide to posttraumatic stress disorder* (pp. 235–261). John Wiley & Sons.

Herbert, J. D., Lilienfeld, S. O., Lohr, J. M., Montgomery, R. W., O'Donahue, W. T., Rosen, G. M., & Tolin, D. F. (2000). Science and pseudoscience in the development of Eye Movement Desensitization and Reprocessing: Implications for clinical psychology. *Clinical Psychology Review*, *20*, 945–971.

Hickling, E. J., Blanchard, E. B., Mundy, E., & Galovski, T. E. (2002). Detection of malingered MVA related posttraumatic stress disorder: An investigation of the ability to detect professional actors by experienced clinicians, psychological tests, and psychophysiological assessment. *Journal of Forensic Psychology Practice*, *2*, 33–54.

Hill, R. D., & Packard, T. (2013). Specialty certification in professional psychology. In M. J. Prinstein (Ed.), *The portable mentor: Expert guide to a successful career in psychology*. 2nd ed. (pp. 235–243). Springer Science.

Holmes, T. H., & Rahe, R. H. (1967). The Social Readjustment Rating Scale. *Journal of Psychosomatic Research*, *11*, 213–218.

Houben, S. T. L., Otaar, H., Roelofs, J., & Merckelbach, H. (2018). Lateral eye movements increase false memory rates. *Clinical Psychological Science*, *6*, 610–616.

Houben, S. T. L., Otgaar, H., Roelofs, J, Smeets, T., & Merckelbach, H. (2020). Increases of correct memories and spontaneous false memories due to eye movements when memories are retrieved after a time delay. *Behaviour Research and Therapy*, *125*, 103546. https://doi.org/10.1016/j.brat.2019.103546.

Houben, S. T. L., Otgaar, H., Roelofs, J, Wessel, I., Patihis, L., & Merckelbach, H. (2019). Eye movement desensitization and reprocessing (EMDR) practitioner's beliefs about memory. *Psychology of Consciousness: Theory, Research and Practice*, *8*, 258–273. https://doi.org/10.1037/cns0000211.

Institute of Medicine (2006). *Posttraumatic stress disorder: Diagnosis and assessment*. The National Academies Press.

International Association of Trauma Professionals (2021). https://iitap.com/#.

Kenardy, J. A., Webster, R. A., Lewin, T. J., Carr, V. J., Hazell, P. L., & Carter, G. L. (1996). Stress debriefing and patterns of recovery following a natural disaster. *Journal of Traumatic Stress*, *9*, 37–49.

Kenchel, J. M., Domagalski, K., Butler, B. J., & Loftus, E. F. (2020). The messy landscape of eye movements and false memories. *Memory*, *30*(6), 678–685. http://dx.doi.org.offcampus.lib.washington.edu/10.1080/09658211.2020.1862234.

Koenen, K. C., Ratanatharathorn, A., Ng, L., McLaughlin, K. A., Bromet, E. J., Stein, D. J., Karam, E. G., Meron Ruscio, A., Benjet, C., Scott, K., Atwoli, L., Petukhova, M., Lim, C. C. W., Aguilar-Gaxiola, S., Al-Hamzawi, A., Alonson, J., Bunting, B., Ciutan, M., de Girolamo, G., ... Kessler, R. C. (2017). Posttraumatic stress disorder in the world mental health surveys. *Psychological Medicine*, *47*, 2260–2274.

Koocher, G. F. (1979). Credentialing in psychology: Close encounters with competence? *American Psychologist*, *34*, 696–702.

Kopelman, M. D. (2002). Disorders of memory. *Brain*, *125*, 2152–2190.

Lee, C. W., & Cuijpers, P. (2013). A meta-analysis of the contribution of eye movements in processing emotional memories. *Journal of Behavior Therapy and Experimental Psychiatry*, *44*, 231–239.

Lees-Haley, P. R. (1986). Pseudo post-traumatic stress disorder. *Trial Diplomacy*, Winter: 17–20.

Lief, H. I. (1999). Patients versus therapists: Legal actions over recovered memory therapy. *Psychiatric Times*, *16*(11).

Lilienfeld, S. O. (2011). Distinguishing scientific from pseudoscientific psychotherapies: Evaluating the role of theoretical plausibility, with a little help from Reverend Bayes. *Clinical Psychology Science and Practice*, *18*, 105–112.

Lilienfeld, S. O., Lynn, S. J., & Bowden, S. C. (2018). Why evidence-based practice isn't enough: A call for science-based practice. *Behavior Therapist*, *41*, 42–47.

Lilienfeld, S. O., Lynn, S. J., & Lohr, J. M. (2015). Science and pseudoscience in clinical psychology: Initial thoughts, reflections, and considerations. In S. O. Lilienfeld, S. J. Lynn, & J. M. Lohr (Eds.), *Science and pseudoscience in clinical psychology* (2nd ed., pp. 1–16). The Guilford Press.

Loftus, E., & Ketcham, K. (1994). *The myth of repressed memory: False memories and allegations of sexual abuse*. St. Martin's Griffin.

Lohr, J. M., Lilienfeld, S. O., & Rosen, G. M. (2012). Anxiety and its treatment: Promoting science-based practice. *Journal of Anxiety Disorders*, *26*, 719–727.

Lohr, J. M., Olatunji, B. O., & Devilly, G. J. (2008). Threats to evidence-based treatment of trauma: Professional issues an implications. *International Review of Victimology*, *15*, 125–149.

Lynn, S. J., Krackow, E., Loftus, E. F., Locke, T. G., & Lilienfeld, S. O. (2015). Constructing the past: Problematic memory recovery techniques in psychotherapy. In S. O. Lilienfeld, S. J. Lynn, & J. M. Lohr (Eds.), *Science and pseudoscience in clinical psychology* (2nd ed., pp. 210–244). The Guilford Press.

MacCorquodale, K., & Meehl, P. E. (1948). On a distinction between hypothetical constructs and intervening variables. *Psychological Review*, *55*, 95–107.

Marchand, A., Guay, S., Boyer, R., Iucci, S., Martin, A., & St-Hilaire, M. H. (2006). A randomized controlled trial of an adapted form of individual critical incident stress debriefing for victims of an armed robbery. *Brief Treatment and Crisis Intervention*, 6, 122–129.

Matto, M., McNiel, D. E., & Binder, R. L. (2019). A systematic approach to the detection of false PTSD. *Journal of the American Academy of Psychiatry and the Law*, 47, 1–10.

McHugh, P. R. (2003). The end of a delusion: The psychiatric memory wars are over. *Weekly Standard*, 36, 31–34.

McNally, R. J. (1999). On eye movements and animal magnetism: A reply to Greenwald's defense of EMDR. *Journal of Anxiety Disorders*, 13, 617–620.

McNally, R. J. (2003). *Remembering trauma*. The Belknap Press of Harvard University Press.

McNally, R. J. (2006). Psychiatric casualties of war. *Science*, 313, 923–924.

McNally, R. J. (2007). Dispelling confusion about traumatic dissociative amnesia. *Mayo Clinic Proceedings*, 82, 1083–1087.

McNally, R. J. (2022). Are memories of sexual trauma fragmented? *Memory*, 30, 26–30. https://doi.org/10.1080/09658211.2020.1871023.

McNally, R. J., Bryant, R. A., & Ehlers, A. (2003). Does early psychological intervention promote recovery from posttraumatic stress? *Psychological Science in the Public Interest*, 4, 45–79.

McNally, R. J., Robinaugh, D. J., Wu, G. W. Y., Wang, L., Deserno, M. K., & Borsboom, D. (2015). Mental disorders as causal systems: A network approach to posttraumatic stress disorder. *Clinical Psychological Science*, 3, 836–849.

Meehl, P. E., & Golden, R. (1982). Taxometric methods. In P. Kendall & J. Butcher (Eds.), *Handbook of research methods in clinical psychology* (pp. 127–181). Wiley.

Merckelbach, H., & Patihis, L. (2018). Why "Trauma-related dissociation" is a misnomer in courts: A critical analysis of Brand et al. (2017a, b). *Psychological Injury and Law*, 11, 370–376.

Mitchell, J. T. (1983). When disaster strikes … The critical incident stress debriefing team. *Journal of Emergency Medical Services*, 8, 36–39.

Mitchell, J. T., & Everly Jr., G. S. (1998). Critical incident stress management: A new era in crisis intervention. *Traumatic Stress Points*, 12, 6–11.

Morey, L. C. (1991). Classification of mental disorder as a collection of hypothetical constructs. *Journal of Abnormal Psychology*, 100, 289–293.

Nezu, C. M., Finch, A. J. & Simon, N. P. (Eds.) (2009). *Becoming board certified by the American Board of Professional Psychology*. Oxford University Press.

North, C. S., Suris, A. M., Davis, M., & Smith, R. P. (2009). Toward validation of the diagnosis of posttraumatic stress disorder. *American Journal of Psychiatry*, *166*, 34–41.

O'Donnell, M. L., Creamer, M., & Cooper, J. (2010). Criterion A: Controversies and clinical implications. In G. M. Rosen & B. C. Frueh (Eds.), *Clinician's guide to posttraumatic stress disorder* (pp. 51–75). John Wiley & Sons.

O'Donnell, M. L., Creamer, M., & Pattison, P. (2004). Posttraumatic stress disorder and depression following trauma: Understanding comorbidity. *American Journal of Psychiatry*, *161*, 1390–1396.

Ost, J. (2003). Seeking the middle ground in the 'memory wars.' *British Journal of Psychology*, *94*, 125–139.

Ost, J., Costall, A., & Bull, R. (2002). A perfect symmetry? A study of retractors' experiences of making and then repudiating claims of early sexual abuse. *Psychology: Crime and Law*, *8*, 155–181.

Otgaar, H., Howe, M. L., Dodier, O., Lilienfeld, S., Loftus, E., Lynn, S. J., Merckelbach, H., & Patihis, L. (2021). Belief in unconscious repressed memory persists. *Perspectives on Psychological Science*, *16*, 454–460.

Otgaar, H., Howe, M. L., Patihis, L., Merckelbach, H., Lynn, S. J., Lilienfeld, S. O., & Loftus, E. F. (2019). The return of the repressed: The persistent and problematic claims of long-forgotten trauma. *Perspectives on Psychological Science*, *14*, 1072–1095.

Ozer, E. J., Best, S. R., Lipsey, T. L., & Weiss, D. S. (2003). Predictors of posttraumatic stress disorder and symptoms in adults: A meta-analysis. *Psychological Bulletin*, *129*, 52–73.

Paris, J. (2012). The rise and fall of dissociative identity disorder. *Journal of Nervous and Mental Disease*, *200*, 1076–1079.

Patihis, L, Otgaar, H., & Merckelbach, H. (2019). Expert witnesses, dissociative amnesia, and extraordinary remembering: Response to Brand et al. *Psychological Injury and Law*, *12*, 281–285.

Patihis, L., Wood, R. S., Pendergrast, M. H., & Herrera, M. E. (2022). Reports of recovered memories in therapy in undergraduate students. *Psychological Reports*, *125*, 129–147. https://doi.org/101177/0033294120971756.

Pignotti, M. (2005). Thought Field Therapy Voice Technology vs. random meridian point sequences: A single-blind controlled experiment. *The Scientific Review of Mental Health Practice*, *4*, 72–81.

Pignotti, M., & Thyer, B. (2009). Some comments on "Energy psychology: A review of the evidence": Premature conclusions based on incomplete evidence? *Psychotherapy: Theory, Research, and Practice*, *46*, 257–261.

Pope, K. S., & Brown, L. S. (1996). *Recovered memories of abuse: Assessment, therapy, forensics*. American Psychological Association.

Raifman, L. (1983). Problems of diagnosis and legal causation in courtroom use of posttraumatic stress disorder. *Behavioral Sciences and the Law, 1,* 115–130.

Renfrey, G., & Spates, C.R. (1994). Eye movement desensitization: A partial dismantling study. *Journal of Behavior Therapy and Experimental Psychiatry, 25,* 231–239.

Rose, S., Bisson, B., & Wessely, S. (2005). A systematic review of brief psychological interventions ("debriefing") for the treatment of immediate trauma related symptoms and the prevention of Post-traumatic Stress Disorder. *The Cochrane Collaboration* (database online). Updated issue 3. Wiley.

Rosen, G. M. (1995). The *Aleutian Enterprise* sinking and Posttraumatic Stress Disorder: Misdiagnosis in clinical and forensic settings. *Professional Psychology: Research and Practice, 26,* 82–87.

Rosen, G. M. (2006). DSM's cautionary guideline to rule out malingering can protect the PTSD data base. *Journal of Anxiety Disorders, 20,* 530–535.

Rosen, G. M., & Davison, G. C. (2003). Psychology should list empirically supported principles of change (ESPs) and not credential trademarked therapies or other treatment packages. *Behavior Modification, 27,* 300–312.

Rosen, G. M., & Lilienfeld, S. O. (2008). Posttraumatic stress disorder: An empirical analysis of core assumptions. *Clinical Psychology Review, 28,* 836–868.

Rosen, G. M., Lohr, J. M., McNally, R., & Herbert, J. (1998). Power therapies, miraculous claims, and the cures that fail. *Behavioural and Cognitive Psychotherapy, 26,* 97–99.

Rosen, G. M., Spitzer, R. L., & McHugh, P. R. (2008). Problems with the PTSD diagnosis and its future in DSM-V. *British Journal of Psychiatry, 192,* 3–4.

Rosen, G. M., Washburn, J. J., & Lilienfeld, S. O. (2020). Specialty certifications for mental health practitioners: A cautionary case study. *Professional Psychology: Research and Practice, 51,* 545–549.

Ruscio, A. M., Ruscio, J., & Keane, T. M. (2002). The latent structure of posttraumatic stress disorder: A taxometric investigation of reactions to extreme stress. *Journal of Abnormal Psychology, 111,* 290–301.

Sagan, C. (1996). *The demon-haunted world: Science as a candle in the dark.* Ballantine Books.

Schubert, S. J., Lee, C. W., & Drummond, P. D. (2010). The efficacy and psychophysiological correlates of dual-attention tasks in eye movement desensitization and reprocessing (EMDR). *Journal of Anxiety Disorders, 25,* 1–11.

Scoboria, A., Wade, K. A., Lindsay, D. S., Azad, T., Strange, D., Ost, J., & Hyman, I. E. (2017). A mega-analysis of memory reports from eight peer-reviewed false memory implantation studies. *Memory, 25,* 146–163.

Scott, M. J., & Stradling, S. G. (1994). Post-traumatic stress disorder without the trauma. *British Journal of Clinical Psychology*, *33*, 71–74.

Scott, W. (1990). PTSD in DSM-III: A case in the politics of diagnosis and disease. *Social Problems*, *37*, 294–310.

Sechrest, L. (1963). Incremental validity: A recommendation. *Educational and PsychologicalMeasurement*, *23*, 153–158.

Seyle, H. (1946). The general adaptation syndrome and the diseases of adaptation. *Journal of Clinical Endocrinology*, *6*, 117–230.

Shapiro, F. (1989a). Efficacy of the Eye Movement Desensitization procedure in treatment of traumatic memories. *Journal of Traumatic Stress*, *2*, 199–223.

Shapiro, F. (1989b). Eye Movement Desensitization: A new treatment for post-traumatic stress disorder. *Journal of Behavior Therapy and Experimental Psychiatry*, *20*, 211–217.

Shapiro, F. (1995). *Eye Movement Desensitization and Reprocessing: Basic principles, protocols, and procedures*. Guilford.

Shephard, B. (2001). *A war of nerves: Soldiers and psychiatrists in the twentieth century*. Harvard University Press.

Shephard, B. (2004). Risk factors and PTSD: A historian's perspective. In G. M. Rosen (Ed.), *Posttraumatic stress disorder: Issues and controversies* (pp. 39–61). John Wiley & Sons.

Silver, R. C., Holman, E. A., McIntosh, D. N., Poulin, M., & Gil-Rivas,V. (2002). Nationwide longitudinal study of psychological responses to September 11. *JAMA*, *288*, 1235–1244.

Slovenko, R. (1994). Legal aspects of post-traumatic stress disorder. *The Psychiatric Clinics of North America*, *17*(2), 439–446.

Sparr, L. F. (1990), Legal aspects of posttraumatic stress disorder: uses and abuses. In M. E. Wolf & A. D. Mosnain (Eds.), *Posttraumatic stress disorder: Etiology, phenomenology, and treatment* (pp. 239–264). American Psychiatric Press.

Sparr, L. F. & Atkinson, R. M. (1986). Post-traumatic stress disorder as an insanity defense: Medico-legal quicksand. *American Journal of Psychiatry*, *143*, 608–613.

Spielmans, G. I., & Rosen, G. M. (2022). Church's (2020) corrigendum compounds errors and fails to support the specificity of acupoint tapping. *Journal of Nervous and Mental Disease*, *210*, 139–142.

Spielmans, G. I., Rosen, G. M., & Spence-Sing, T. (2020). Tapping away at a misleading meta-analysis: No evidence for specificity of acupoint tapping. *Journal of Nervous and Mental Disease*, *206*, 628–631.

Spitzer, R. L., First, M. B., & Wakefield, J. C. (2007). Saving PTSD from itself in DSM-V. *Journal of Anxiety Disorders*, *21*, 233–241.

Strasburger, L. H., Gutheil, T. G., & Brodsky, A. (1997). On wearing two hats: Role conflict in serving as both psychotherapist and expert witness. *American Journal of Psychiatry*, *154*, 448–456.

Summerfield, D. (1999). A critique of seven assumptions behind psychological trauma programmes in war-affected areas. *Social Science and Medicine*, *48*, 1449–1462.

Summerfield, D. (2001). The invention of post-traumatic stress disorder and the social usefulness of a psychiatric category. *British Medical Journal*, *322*, 95–98.

Swab, J. (2020). Critical incident stress management: Perspectives on its history, frequency of use, efficacy, and success. *Crisis, Stress, and Human Resilience: An International Journal*, *1*, 215–226.

Taylor, S., Frueh, B. C., & Asmundson, G. J. G. (2007). Detection and management of malingering in people presenting for treatment of posttraumatic stress disorder: Methods, obstacles, and recommendations. *Journal of Anxiety Disorders*, *21*, 22–41.

Trauma Institute International (2021). https://traumainstituteinternational.com /certifications/.

Trimble, M. (1985). Post-traumatic stress disorder: history of a concept. In C. Figley (Ed.), *Trauma and its wake* (pp. 5–14). Brunner/Mazel.

Uttal, W. R. (2001). *The new phrenology: The limits of localizing cognitive processes in the brain*. The MIT Press.

van Emmerik, A. A. P., Kamphuis, J. H., Hulsbosch, A. M., & Emmelkamp, P. M. G. (2002). Single session debriefing after psychological trauma: A meta-analysis. *The Lancet*, *360*, 776–771.

van Schie, K., & Leer, A. (2019). Lateral eye movements do not increase false-memory rates: A failed direct-replication study. *Clinical Psychological Science*, *7*, 1159–1167. https://doi.org/10.1177/2167702619859335.

Wakefield, J. C., & Horwitz, A. V. (2010). Normal reactions to adversity or symptoms of disorder? In G. M. Rosen & B. C. Frueh (Eds.), *Clinician's guide to posttraumatic stress disorder* (pp. 33–49). John Wiley & Sons.

Washburn, J. J., Lilienfeld, S. O., Rosen, G. M., Gaudiano, B. A., Davidson, G. C., Hollon, S. D., Otto, M. W., Penberthy, J. K., Sher, K. J., Teachman, B. A., Peris, T., & Weinand, J. (2019). Reaffirming the scientific foundations of psychological practice: Recommendations of the Emory meeting on continuing education. *Professional Psychology: Research and Practice*, *50*, 77–86.

Watson, P. J., Brymer, M. J., & Bonanno, G. A. (2011). Post disaster psychological intervention since 9/11. *American Psychologist*, *66*, 484–494.

Watters, E. (2010). *The globalization of the American psyche: Crazy like us*. Free Press.

Wettstein, R. M. (2010) The forensic psychiatric examination and report. In R. I. Simon & L. H. Gold (Eds.), *Textbook of forensic psychiatry*. 2nd ed. American Psychiatric Publishing.

Woody, R. H. (1997). Dubious and bogus credential in mental health practice. *Ethics and Behavior, 7*, 337–345.

Young, A. (2004). When traumatic memory was a problem: On the historical antecedents of PTSD. In G. M. Rosen (Ed.), *Posttraumatic stress disorder: Issues and controversies* (pp. 127–146). John Wiley & Sons.

7

Dissociation

Steven Jay Lynn, Fiona Sleight, Craig P. Polizzi, Damla Aksen,
Lawrence Patihis, Henry Otgaar, and Olivier Dodier

Dissociative disorders have intrigued, confounded, and provoked debate for more than a century (Janet, 1889/1973). In recent decades, dissociative disorders have entered the mainstream of psychological science, been the target of psychotherapeutic interventions, and captured the imagination of the general public in a litany of highly dramatized television, film, and internet portrayals. From the early academy award-winning films, *Three Faces of Eve* (1957) and *Sybil* (1976), to more recent films such as *Split* (2016), media accounts of dissociation have become widely enmeshed in cultural narratives that are as compelling as they are often misleading.

In this chapter, we present competing explanations regarding dissociative experiences alongside interventions for dissociative disorders that lack scientific support, potentially risk harm, and may create the very symptoms they seek to alleviate. We pay special attention to dissociative identity disorder (DID), previously known by many names including hysterical neurosis, dissociative type, double consciousness, and multiple personality disorder. Dissociative disorders have received scant attention in randomized clinical trials. Nevertheless, before we close, we will note promising interventions that integrate empirically supported change mechanisms. Evidence-based treatments for dissociation are an especially high priority, as these disorders exact a high personal and societal cost (Polizzi et al., 2022) and have not received the attention that they deserve.

Dissociative disorders are described in the extant psychological nomenclature as "disruption of and/or discontinuity in the normal integration of consciousness, memory, identity, emotion, perception, body representation, motor control, and behavior" (DSM-5-TR; American Psychological Association, 2022, p. 329). DID is defined as the existence of (a) "two or more distinct personality states, which may be described in some cultures as an experience of possession" (p. 330), in conjunction with (b) "recurrent gaps in the recall of everyday events, important personal information, and/or traumatic events that are inconsistent with ordinary forgetting" (p. 330). Dissociative amnesia is characterized by "an inability to recall important autobiographical information, usually of a traumatic or stressful nature, that is inconsistent with ordinary forgetting" (p. 337). Finally, depersonalization/derealization disorder is characterized by clinically significant persistent or recurring experiences of "being an outside observer with respect to one's thoughts, feelings, sensations, body or actions" (depersonalization, p. 343) or "experiences of unreality or detachment with respect to surroundings" (derealization, p. 343).

7.1 Pseudoscience and Questionable Ideas

7.1.1 Controversies and Conflicts

Dissociative experiences often represent stark, disturbing, and puzzling departures from everyday consciousness, which accounts, in part, for why they are among the most, if not *the* most, controversial disorders in the field of psychology. Controversy is heavily centered on two intertwined areas of dispute: (a) the origin of dissociative symptoms, as rooted in a traumatic past (e.g., Dalenberg et al., 2012; 2014; Gleaves, 1996) versus sociocognitive influences (e.g., Lilienfeld et al., 1999; Lynn et al., 2022; Spanos, 1994), and (b) the treatment of dissociative symptoms, which will be the focus of our discussion. These conflicts are embedded in broader forays in the so-called memory wars in the late 1980s and 1990s regarding the authenticity of memories that cleaved the psychological community into two rival camps (see Otgaar et al., 2019; Patihis et al., 2014). In fact, the reliability of purportedly dissociated or repressed memories and attempts to exhume them in psychotherapy were close to the epicenter of the debate.

7.1.1.1 Dissociation and Repressed Memories

In one camp were proponents of the idea that repression and dissociation originate as a defensive response to traumatic events to mitigate their emotional repercussions and banish them from awareness (e.g., Dalenberg et al., 2012; 2014; Gleaves, 1996; see Loftus, 1993). Based on this premise, it follows that psychotherapies should uncover or at least process the dissociated memories and experiences before full integration of dissociated or repressed elements of the personality can be achieved.

These notions are widely represented in the popular media as sampled in the following statements that tout different treatments. According to the Traumatic Incident Reduction (TIR) Association's (2015) website, "When something happens that is . . . painful, one has the option of either confronting it fully and feeling the pain, or trying in some way to block one's awareness of it . . . in the second case, the action of experiencing that incident is blocked . . . in the great majority of cases, TIR correctly applied results in the complete and permanent elimination of PTSD symptomatology."

Similarly, the Janov Primal Center (2021) website, which espouses primal therapy (colloquially termed primal scream therapy) states, "We have found a way into those early emotional archives and have learned to have access to those memories, to dredge them up from the unconscious, allowing us to re-experience them in the present, integrate them and no longer be driven by the unconscious . . . The number one killer in the world today is not cancer or heart disease, it is repression."

Otgaar and colleagues (2019) have argued that the term *dissociative amnesia* now substitutes for *repressed memory* "whereby traumas are rendered inaccessible." The authors contend that "after the 1990s, when the term 'repressed memory' was widely critiqued, proponents began to favor dissociative amnesia instead" (p. 1079). In keeping with Otgaar and colleagues (2019), we will treat the terms dissociative amnesia and repressed memories as largely interchangeable with the recognition that the term dissociative amnesia is often specifically associated with treatments for dissociative conditions, particularly those that involve memory retrieval. A sizable percentage of contemporary clinical psychologists still believe that repressed or dissociated memories occur in the face of trauma and translate these beliefs into the practice of memory recovery (see Houben et al., 2021; Otgaar et al., 2019; Patihis & Pendergrast, 2019).

7.1.1.2 The Memory Wars

The memory wars were marked by strong concerns and outright skepticism regarding (a) dramatic increases in reports of repressed/dissociated memories of child sexual abuse, and (b) concerns about the iatrogenic (i.e., therapy-induced) effects of suggestive techniques in psychotherapy that potentially create rather than uncover purportedly distinct indwelling personalities (called alters) among patients. Scholars aligned with the sociocognitive perspective, as noted above, ascribed the genesis of DID mostly to sociocognitive influences like suggestive methods in psychotherapy, media and sociocultural narratives, suggestibility, fantasy-proneness, cognitive failures. Proponents of this view voiced particular concern about the potentially harmful effects of excavating traumatic memories, which they argued were typically well-remembered rather than forgotten (McNally, 2005).

The following three highly publicized legal cases in the midst of the memory wars illustrate concerns about the harmful effects of iatrogenic psychotherapeutic methods related to DID. The first such cases date to the mid-1980s, when Ms. Nadean Cool, a nurse's aide in Wisconsin, entered psychotherapy suffering from common problems including mild depression, family conflict, and symptoms of bulimia (see Lynn et al., 2003). After five years of treatment with psychiatrist Dr. Kenneth Olson, she recovered supposedly "repressed memories of having been in a satanic cult, of eating babies, of being raped, of having sex with animals and of being forced to witness the murder of her eight-year-old friend" (Loftus, 1997a, p. 70). It was not only memories that emerged; more than 130 "personalities" were retrieved as well. Her therapist reportedly subjected her to guided imagery and repeated hypnosis to recover memories of alleged abuse, 15-hour therapy marathon sessions, and even an exorcism. During and after these sessions, Nadean came to believe she housed a parade of personalities that included demons, angels, children, and a duck. Nadean sued Dr. Olsen for malpractice and the case was settled out-of-court for $2.4 million in a trial in which one of this chapter's authors (S.J.L.) testified as an expert.

When Sheri J. Storm read a newspaper article that recounted the eerily familiar Nadean Cool story, she realized that she and Ms. Cool shared not only the same therapist and diagnosis, but also similar horrifying memories (see Lambert & Lilienfeld, 2007). Like Ms. Cool, her initial problems were unremarkable – mild anxiety and insomnia. After recovered memory therapy, Ms. Storm was burdened with images of abuse, bestiality, and satanic ritual abuse involving murder and consumption of human babies, and she believed that she harbored more than 200 personalities. Despite appeals to the Wisconsin Supreme Court, Ms. Storm was never able to succeed in her complaint against Dr. Olson, because it was ruled that her complaint was made after the statute of limitations expired.

More recently, one headline proclaimed, "Therapist Brainwashed Woman Into Believing She was in Satanic Cult, Attorney Says" (Caron, 2011, ABC News). In this case, the woman is Lisa Nasseff, who was treated for 15 months in 2007 for anorexia at the Castlewood Treatment Center in St. Paul, Minnesota. She settled a lawsuit with her former therapist, Mark Schwartz, for allegedly hypnotizing her to falsely believe she possessed 20 multiple personalities, participated in a satanic cult involving her parents, and even engaged in rituals in which a child was sacrificed for members of the cult to eat. According to media reports (Caron, 2011, ABC News), other patients treated at the center settled a lawsuit with Dr. Schwartz claiming similar treatment.

The cases share three notable elements. First, the patients did not embark on therapy with a diagnosis of multiple personality disorder, as it was called at the time, consistent with findings that only about a fifth of DID patients exhibit clear-cut alters before treatment (Kluft, 1991). Such observations provided fodder for the argument that the cases we discussed were the by-product of psychotherapy. Second, the cases involved highly implausible so-called "recovered memories" that were not retrieved until years after the events supposedly occurred. Although therapists have implemented recovered memory therapies in treating diverse conditions, such interventions are particularly relevant in DID, as dissociative amnesia is often a prominent aspect of the diagnosis. Finally, the individuals were subjected to suggestive memory recovery methods like hypnosis, journaling, and calling out different alter personalities by name. Today, it is widely acknowledged that suggestive procedures can instantiate false memories. Estimates of the percentage of the time that such interventions instate false memories range from around 15% to 50%, depending on how a false memory is defined (see Otgaar et al., 2019; Scoboria et al., 2017). Moreover, few would disagree that reports of satanic ritual abuse are the product of imagination and represent false memories, as the FBI has investigated such reports and found no evidence for activities that match the incredible claims (Lanning, 1991).

7.1.2 Diagnostic Issues

Questions about the treatment of dissociative disorders begin with diagnosis. The prevalence of the diagnosis of dissociative conditions varies widely (see Lynn et al., 2019). The reasons for this variability include different base rates of disorders across different settings (e.g., inpatient/ outpatient) and populations (e.g., college students versus individuals with posttraumatic stress disorder (PTSD), substance users), therapist or assessor biases related to the diagnosis, and ambiguity surrounding what defines a "personality state" in DID and what is "non-ordinary forgetting" in dissociative amnesia. The question that divides rival camps is not limited to whether certain individuals meet the criteria for dissociative disorders, but rather what is the genesis of dissociative conditions?

Still, many reports of dissociative amnesia are not credible, can be accounted for by brain injury or neurological conditions, and contradict evidence that memories for highly aversive events are typically disturb-ing and intrusive, rather than dissociated or repressed (see Bernsten & Rubin, 2014). In a review of 128 case studies of purported dissociative amnesia, Mangiulli et al. (2022) contended that empirical support for the diagnosis was often weak, and most case studies failed to rule out alter-native explanations, such as malingering, ordinary forgetting, or brain injury. Of course, if individuals are unlikely to forget or dissociate mem-ories in the face of traumatic stressors in the first place, then a rationale for extensive attempts to recover such memories is dubious. Indeed, such memory recovery attempts risk the construction of false memories.

Different "personality states," which can be observed by others or reported by the individual, figure into the diagnosis in the most recent diagnostic scheme (DSM-5-TR, APA, 2022, p. 320). Unfortunately, what exactly constitutes a behavioral manifestation of a different "personality state" is neither specified nor well-validated. In the guidelines for the treatment of DID advanced by the International Society for the Study of Trauma and Dissociation (ISSTD, 2011), signs of dissociation and "switching" of identities can refer to any number of commonly occurring behaviors including changes in posture, dress, fixed gaze, eyes fluttering, and fluctuations in the style of speech (p. 124). These vague signs are subject to potential treatment biases, false positives, and misdiagnoses. Well-validated structured interviews, trait, and state measures of disso-ciation are available to assist in diagnosis and preferred to poorly speci-fied indicators, such as those described by the ISSTD (Lynn et al., 2019). Nevertheless, whether the features of DID are the product of socio-cognitive influences versus a response to trauma remains debatable.

7.1.3 A Sampling of Memory Recovery Techniques

Contemporary memory recovery interventions often lack empirical sup-port and are considered pseudoscientific, as their evidence base is mostly or exclusively anecdotal. Additionally, they rely on scientifically unsup-ported beliefs that memory is stored permanently and accessible via the use of special techniques vital to positive therapy outcomes. Memory recovery interventions encompass a gamut of empirically unsupported or untested interventions including neurolinguistic programming, sensorimo-tor psychotherapy, somatic experiencing therapy, hypnosis specifically for memory retrieval, guided imagery, alien abduction therapy, energy manip-ulation approaches (e.g., thought field therapy), experiential integration, reenactment protocol, and internal family systems therapy (Lynn et al., 2019; Thyer & Pignotti, 2015).

The mistaken idea of the permanence of memory and the need to recover walled-off memories to heal from trauma is vividly captured in the notion of *body memories*, as described in a manual for sexual abuse survivors (Mack, 2019): "Your body, believe it or not, remembers everything. Sounds, smells, touches, tastes. But the memory is not held in your mind, locked somewhere in the recesses of your brain. Instead, it's held in your body, all the way down at the cellular level" (para. 1). In van der Kolk's (1994) words, "The body keeps the score" (p. 53). The implication is that if somatic experiences are not recovered and "dealt with," complete recovery from a traumatic event such as sexual abuse is difficult or impossible. According to the ISSTD treatment guidelines, "attention to the movement and sensation of the body can teach the therapist about past traumas" (2011, p. 162).

The internet is a conspicuous source of misinformation regarding memory recovery and DID, as the following examples illustrate. The technique called brainspotting seeks to determine the supposed location of unavailable experiences and symptoms of trauma at the "unconscious body brain" and release them. A brainspot is defined as the "the eye position which is related to the energetic/emotional activation of a traumatic/emotionally charged issue within the brain, most likely in the amygdala, the hippocampus, or the orbitofrontal cortex of the limbic system . . ." (Grand, 2015). Another technique touted on the internet is somatic transformation therapy that purportedly "balances the arousal and fear of recovered memories with felt experiences of self-regulation of the emotional physiological systems. Subtle gestures and movements of the body are utilized to access sensory data and result in shifts in the brain-body continuum" (Stanley, 2015). Relatedly, dance/movement therapy (Pierce, 2014) has been proposed to treat dissociation and developmental trauma via kinesthetic mirroring, body-to-body attunement, and interactional movements. The untested mechanism by which this intervention supposedly integrates traumatic memories is dubbed "right brain integration."

For those curious about whether they have repressed memories, an internet quiz purports to address this question (Pro Profs Quizzes, 2021). The quiz questions are very general and tap common experiences (e.g., "Do you have trouble identifying and expressing your emotions with people around you?"). Accordingly, a respondent with little or no psychopathology or history of trauma could be convinced that they harbor repressed memories. The website states, "it is crucial for an individual to learn and heal from these repressed memories" and ends with (if the respondent endorses any items) the statement, "Make sure to talk to a licensed therapist to connect with the repressed memories." These sorts of claims strongly suggest that respondents harbor hidden memories recoverable in psychotherapy, thus risking the formation of false memories of traumas that never occurred in reality.

In addition to potentially suggestive methods related to repressed memories and body memories, individuals can use a journal (ElleColmDesigns, 2019) independently or with a therapist to purportedly manage up to 50 DID "alters" (a person can add pages to accommodate even more alters). The personal journal is advertised to facilitate communication between "alters," create system rules, map personality systems, manage moods, and create profiles of new "alters." In addition to memory recovery and journaling, Lynn et al. (2004) have reviewed a variety of suggestive memory recovery methods including dream interpretation, guided imagery, hypnosis, and age regression.

Concerted efforts to root out dissociated or repressed memories can risk harm (e.g., Otgaar et al., 2019). For example, Rozental et al. (2016) noted that 38% of 653 patients surveyed rated the "unpleasant memories [that] surfaced" during treatment explicitly as a negative experience. Scant evidence exists that such negative experiences are compensated for by treatment gains. In fact, the opposite may be true. Fetkewicz et al. (2000) surveyed 20 patients who participated in memory recovery treatments who were ultimately diagnosed with multiple personality disorder, even though they initially sought help for suicidal ideation and suicidal attempts. Their initial symptoms often worsened as they receded from being the focus of therapy; in fact, 60% of the patients attempted suicide. The authors concluded that "the diagnosis of multiple personality and the use of memory recovery treatment are harmful" (p. 155). Similarly, Loftus (1997b) reported that among 23 patients who received financial compensation after memory recovery therapy, two-thirds reported suicidal thoughts compared with 10% of patients before memory recovery. A causal connection of suicide with treatment cannot be pinned down with confidence. Moreover, the sample was highly select and not necessarily representative. Nevertheless, memory recovery of highly negative events like abuse may play a role in symptom deterioration and perhaps the creation of iatrogenic symptoms of DID (Lilienfeld, 2007).

7.1.4 Pseudoscientific and Questionable Interventions

7.1.4.1 Exorcism

Perhaps the most egregious and outlandish interventions for DID are exorcisms, as perpetrated in the case of Nadean Cool. Bull and collaborators (1998) reviewed 47 incidents of exorcism conducted on 15 patients with DID. Using an *Exorcism Experiences Questionnaire* (Bowman, 1993), the authors classified 23 incidents as mixed experiences with exorcism, 24 as positive, and 3 as very negative experiences. Bowman's (1993) interview findings were distinctly less sanguine. He interviewed 14 female patients diagnosed with multiple personality disorder who had experienced exorcisms. Eighty percent reported negative responses, and the rituals created new "alters" that resulted in the hospitalization of nine individuals. The use of exorcism is troubling on a scientific and ethical basis, especially given the presumption that demonic possession can be the cause of dissociative symptoms.

7.1.4.2 DID-Oriented Therapy

Lilienfeld (2007) cited suggestive DID-oriented therapy as a treatment that potentially causes harm. Such therapy is epitomized in Putnam's (1989) classic treatment treatise, *Diagnosis and Treatment of Multiple Personality*. Putnam suggests that the therapist asks direct, leading questions such as, "Do you ever feel as if there is some part (side, facet, etc.) of yourself that comes out and does or says things that you would not do or say" and probes "for a name or an attribute, function, or description that I can use as a label to elicit this other part directly" (p. 90). If the "alter" avoids giving a name, Putnam recommends that the "therapist should make one up" and continues, "I will say something such as this: 'Since you are not willing to share your name with me at this time, I am going to refer to you as the one who covers her mouth with a hand when she talks'" (p. 142).

According to Putnam (1989), a key task of the therapist is to obtain a history for each "alter," which can include journals and diaries to spur memories. Moreover, Putnam states that "In some cases . . . hypnosis or a drug-facilitated interview may be useful to facilitate the emergence of an alter" (p. 91). These two methods can produce unwarranted confidence in memories regardless of their accuracy (Lynn et al., 2004).

Lynn et al. (2013) have expressed concerns about the risk of harm to patients regarding the following recommendations that Putnam (1989) advanced: (a) the therapist treating people as if they were "multiples," despite expressed resistance to the diagnosis (p. 151); (b) "assembling whole memories from fragments" that are supposedly spread across several "alters" (pp. 198–199); (c) using dream reports to "provide access to deeply hidden trauma" (p. 201); (d) age regression for memory recovery (p. 228); and (e) internal group therapy with different personalities (p. 261).

More recent DID treatment guidelines, promulgated by the ISSTD (2011), endorse the following practices: (a) directly "accessing alters" (e.g., "I need to talk to the one(s) who went to Atlantic City last night and had unsafe sex," p. 140); (b) generating an "ongoing 'map' or 'roster' of the patients' alternate identity system" (p. 140); (c) asking patients to "listen inside" to hear what other identities have to say; and (d) the clinician may suggest that identities engage in inner conversations with one another to communicate information or negotiate important issues (p. 140). The extent to which these sorts of interventions access and describe cleavages in identity that exist before therapy or whether they create or reinforce them has not been investigated systematically. Lilienfeld (2007) noted that DID-oriented therapists typically claim that the sorts of methods reviewed "reflect the discovery rather than the creation of alters"; he argued that "multiple lines of converging evidence suggest that many and most alters are the products of inadvertent therapist suggestion" (p. 60).

To their credit, the ISSTD (2011) guidelines acknowledge that "it may be helpful to discuss issues concerning the nature of 'recovered' memory and the reconstructive aspect of autobiographical memory" (p. 142). Yet, memory recovery and a focus on trauma history still play a prominent role in recommendations for treatment of DID.

7.1.4.3 Ego State Therapy

The extent to which therapists continue to use these highly directive and suggestive interventions in treating dissociation is unknown. However, such methods rely on identifying and integrating purportedly dysfunctional ego states that are roughly equivalent to personality or identity states in DID. According to Watkins's (1978; 2001) ego state therapy, psychological symptoms can be associated with "entities" that differ from the "overt personality" and exhibit origins and developmental trajectories that diverge uniquely from the primary personality. These ego states "covertly influence the behavior, thinking, and affect of the overt, conscious personality" (p. 293). Watkins (2001) further claims that ego states "seldom reveal themselves to skeptics" and "act like multiple personality alters, but seldom become manifest except under hypnosis with a trusted operator" (p. 293), raising questions about how researchers would be able to falsify their existence. Watkins contends that a preferred way to activate ego states and "minimize demand characteristics" is to ask, "Is there a separate part of Jane who knows what is causing her disturbance, but if there is no separate part that is OK"

(Watkins, 2001, p. 294), apparently unaware that asking such a question is rife with demand characteristics to report a "part."

7.1.4.4 Internal Family Systems Therapy

Eliciting and working with alleged parts/ego states are featured in other current therapies such as internal family systems (IFS) therapies (Schwartz, 1995). Such approaches are likewise devoid of scientific support from systematic controlled research and rely almost exclusively on anecdotal data and unsubstantiated claims. Central to internal family systems is the notion that the person is comprised of "parts"; an internal system of ego states that interact, cooperate, and conflict much like family members. This system is represented by a central *self* that relates to fractured vulnerable and/or controlling ego states. Included are "exile" parts that carry the painful residues of hurtful experiences, controlling and protective "manager" parts, and "firefighters" tasked with dousing the flames of emotion generated by exiles via dissociation and escapism related to drug use, for example. According to Twombly (2013), people with dissociative disorders are burdened with extreme emotions and beliefs and with "firefighters" and "managers" who are either easily overwhelmed or rigidly controlling. Expensive training workshops and certificates to practice this therapy are available on the internet. Not surprisingly, perhaps, Pignotti and Thyer (2011) noted that internal family systems therapy was the main treatment at the Castlewood Treatment Center where Lisa Nasseff, described in the case above, was treated.

7.2 Research-Supported Approaches

Unfortunately, no pharmacological or psychological treatments for dissociation have been empirically supported using randomized controlled trials, and much of the literature on the topic is based on case studies, anecdotal accounts, and methodologically flawed research (see Ganslev et al., 2020; Maxwell et al., 2018 for a review). Whatever interventions are used for DID, we suggest that they start from the position that treating the whole person is a priority and focus on the promising approaches described next (Huntjens et al., 2019; Mohajerin et al., 2020).

We are aware of no data that indicate that the interventions that concern us are more effective in treating dissociative conditions than evidence-based ones for other disorders that abstain from using memory recovery. These approaches include present-oriented exposure therapies, traditional cognitive-behavioral therapies, third-wave approaches, and transtheoretical/transdiagnostic approaches that are more oriented toward improving present-day functioning. Transtheoretical and trans-diagnostic approaches, which are used to treat a variety of emotional disorders, are particularly promising as they target mechanisms shown to be empirically related to dissociation as well as other disorders (e.g., borderline personality disorder and schizophrenia spectrum disorders; see Lynn et al., 2019). These include deficits in cognitive-behavioral-affective self-regulation, meta-cognition/alexithymia, thought suppression, and sleep disturbances (see Lynn et al., 2022). Effective, empirically supported interventions are sorely needed to vie with and supplant the numerous untested, unsupported, and potentially harmful treatments that exist in the vast psychotherapy marketplace.

7.3 Conclusion

We have reviewed numerous untested, unsupported, and potentially harmful interventions for treating dissociation. Therapies that focus on memory recovery and that reify "parts" are particularly emblematic of our concerns. We strongly recommend that therapists, and perhaps more importantly, patients, steer away from such therapies as they have the potential for creating and worsening psychological symptoms when compared to the evidence-based approaches that are used for other disorders (or even no treatment at all). We further suggest that therapists employ interventions only after obtaining a patient's informed consent. In some approaches, such consent should specifically indicate potential risks of (a) false memories, (b) suggestive procedures, and (c) reifying the existence of parts of the personality for which there is no compelling evidence.

Indeed, we believe that DID is best conceptualized as a disorder of belief and meta-cognitions regarding the self, rather than as personality parts that interact and are embroiled in internal conflict. Researchers have found no reliable evidence for inter-identity amnesia across "alters" when using objective measures (e.g., behavioral tasks, event-related potentials) of memory (see Lynn et al., 2022 for a review). These findings sharply contradict the assumption that DID "alters" harbor memories that are separated by amnesic barriers and thereby undermine the rationale for pursuing memory recovery with patients.

We suggest that informed consent procedures ideally present the relative strengths, limitations, costs, and benefits of different treatment approaches. In addition to underlining the imperative to provide patients with science-based informed consent, clinical training programs should promote a clinical science model. Students should be taught to infuse their clinical work with critical thinking and the ability to distinguish evidence-based approaches from pseudoscience, potentially harmful methods, and dubious theories that masquerade as science. We further suggest that professional organizations like the American Psychological Association and the Association for Psychological Science engage in even more active and effective efforts to advocate for scientifically grounded education for mental health professionals, judges, journalists, the media, and the public about memory and pseudoscience (Sauerland & Otgaar, 2022). Finally, researchers should not fail to evaluate the potentially harmful effects of psychotherapies, including evidence-based therapies, as research is very limited in this regard. Only when these steps are taken will the consumers of psychotherapy be better protected from false and misleading claims and interventions that can do more harm than good.

Steven Jay Lynn, PhD, is a Distinguished Professor of Psychology at Binghamton University (SUNY). He is co-editor of the book *Evidence-Based Psychotherapy: The State of the Science and Practice* (2018).

Fiona Sleight, MS, is a doctoral student in psychology at Binghamton University (SUNY).

Craig P. Polizzi, PhD, completed a doctoral degree in psychology at Binghamton University (SUNY).

Damla Aksen, MS, is a doctoral student in psychology at Binghamton University (SUNY).

Lawrence Patihis, PhD, is a Senior Lecturer of Psychology at the University of Plymouth in the United Kingdom. He is author of the book *Trauma, Memory, and Law: Enhanced Lectures on Repressed Memories, Memory Distortions, and Trauma* (2022).

Henry Otgaar, PhD, is a Professor of Psychology at Maastricht University in the Netherlands. He is co-editor of the book *Finding the Truth in the Courtroom: Dealing with Deception, Lies, and Memories* (2017).

Olivier Dodier, PhD, is a Contract Lecturer of Psychology at the University of Nîmes in France.

References

American Psychiatric Association (2022). *Diagnostic and statistical manual of mental disorders, fifth edition, text revision (DSM-5-TR)*. American Psychiatric Association.

Berntsen, D., & Rubin, D. C. (2014). Involuntary memories and dissociative amnesia: Assessing key assumptions in posttraumatic stress disorder research. *Clinical Psychological Science*, 2(2), 174–186. https://doi.org/10.1177/2167702613496241

Bowman, E. S. (1993). Clinical and spiritual effects of exorcism in fifteen patients with multiple personality disorder. *Dissociation: Progress in the Dissociative Disorders*, 6(4), 222–238.

Bull, D. L., Ellason, J. W., & Ross, C. A. (1998). Exorcism revisited: Positive outcomes with dissociative identity disorder. *Journal of Psychology and Theology*, 26(2), 188–196. https://doi.org/10.1177/009164719802600205

Caron, C. (2011). Therapist "brainwashed" woman into believing she was in a satanic cult, attorney says. ABC News. https://abcnews.go.com/US/therapist-accused-implanting-satanic-memories/story?id=15043529

Dalenberg, C. J., Brand, B. L., Gleaves, D. H., Dorahy, M. J., Loewenstein, R. J., Cardeña, E., Frewen, P. A., Carlson, E. B., & Spiegel, D. (2012). Evaluation of the evidence for the trauma and fantasy models of dissociation. *Psychological Bulletin*, 138, 550–588.

Dalenberg, C. J., Brand, B. L., Loewenstein, R. J., Gleaves, D. H., Dorahy, M. J., Cardeña, E., Frewen, P. A., Carlson, E. B., & Spiegel, D. (2014). Reality versus fantasy: Reply to Lynn et al. (2014). *Psychological Bulletin*, 140(3), 911–920. https://doi.org/10.1037/a0036685

Dr. Janov's Primal Center. What is primal therapy? Santa Monica (CA): Dr. Janov's Primal Center; 2008 [cited 2021 Dec 23]. www.primaltherapy.com/what-is-primal-therapy.php

EllieColmDesigns. (2019). *Dissociative Identity Disorder Journal*. Author.

Fetkewicz, J., Sharma, V., & Merskey, H. (2000). A note on suicidal deterioration with recovered memory treatment. *Journal of Affective Disorders*, 58(2), 155–159. https://doi.org/10.1016/S0165-0327(98)00193-1

Ganslev, C. A., Storebø, O. J., Callesen, H. E., Ruddy, R., & Søgaard, U. (2020). Psychosocial interventions for conversion and dissociative disorders in adults. *Cochrane Database of Systematic Revs*. 7: CD005331. https://doi.org/10.1002/14651858.CD005331.pub3.

Gleaves, D. H. (1996). The sociocognitive model of dissociative identity disorder: A reexamination of the evidence. *Psychological Bulletin*, 120(1), 42–59. https://doi.org/10.1037/0033-2909.120.1.42

Grand D. What is brainspotting? [cited 2015 July 31]. brainspotting.pro/page/what-brainspotting

Houben, S. T. L., Otgaar, H., Roelofs, J., Wessel, I., Patihis, L., & Merckelbach, H. (2021). Eye movement desensitization and reprocessing (EMDR) practitioners' beliefs about memory. *Psychology of Consciousness: Theory, Research, and Practice*, 8(3), 258–273. https://doi.org/10.1037/cns0000211

Huntjens, R. J., Rijkeboer, M. M., & Arntz, A. (2019). Schema therapy for Dissociative Identity Disorder (DID): Rationale and study protocol. *European Journal of Psychotraumatology*, *10*(1), 1571377. https://doi.org /10.1080/20008198.2019.1571377

International Society for the Study of Trauma and Dissociation (ISSTD). (2011). Guidelines for treating dissociative identity disorder in adults, third revision: Summary version. *Journal of Trauma & Dissociation*, *12*(2), 188–212.

Janet, P. (1973). *L'automatisme psychologique.*Société Pierre Janet (original work published 1889).

Kluft, R. P. (1991). Clinical presentations of multiple personality disorder. *Psychiatric Clinics of North America*, *14*(3), 605–629. https://doi.org/10 .1016/S0193-953X(18)30291-0

Lambert, K., & Lilienfeld, S. O. (2007). Brain stains. *Scientific American Mind*, *18* (5), 46–53. www.jstor.org/stable/24939724

Lanning, K. V. (1991). Ritual abuse: A law enforcement view or perspective. *Child Abuse & Neglect*, *15*(3), 171–173. https://doi.org/10.1016/0145-2134(91)90061-H

Lilienfeld, S. O. (2007). Psychological treatments that cause harm. *Perspectives in Psychological Science*, *2*(1), 53–70.

Lilienfeld, S. O., Lynn, S. J., Kirsch, I., Chaves, J. F., Sarbin, T. R., Ganaway, G. K., & Powell, R. A. (1999). Dissociative identity disorder and the sociocognitive model: Recalling the lessons of the past. *Psychological Bulletin*, *125*(5), 507–523.

Loftus, E. F. (1993). The reality of repressed memories. *American Psychologist*, *48*(5), 518–537.

Loftus, E. F. (1997a). Creating false memories. https://staff.washington.edu/elof tus/Articles/sciam.htm

Loftus, E. F. (1997b). Repressed memory accusations: Devastated families and devastated patients. *Applied Cognitive Psychology*, *11*(1), 25–30. https://doi .org/10.1002/(SICI)1099-0720(199702)11:1<25::AID-ACP452>3.0.CO;2-J

Lynn, S. J., Condon, L., & Colletti, G. (2013). The treatment of dissociative identity disorder: Questions and considerations. W. O'Donohue & S. O. Lilienfeld (Eds.), *Case studies in clinical psychological science: Bridging the gap from science to practice* (pp. 329–351). Oxford.

Lynn, S. J., Knox, J. A., Fassler, O., Lilienfeld, S. O., & Loftus, E. F. (2004). Memory, trauma, and dissociation. In G. M. Rosen (Ed.), *Posttraumatic stress disorder: Issues and controversies* (pp. 163–186). John Wiley & Sons. https://doi.org/10.1002/9780470713570.ch9

Lynn, S. J., Lilienfeld, S. O., Merckelbach, H., Maxwell, R., Aksen, D., Baltman, J., & Giesbrecht, T. (2019). Dissociative disorders. In J. Maddux & B. Winstead (Eds.), *Psychopathology: Foundations for a contemporary understanding*. 5th ed. Routledge.

Lynn, S. J., Lock, T., Loftus, E. F., Krackow, E., & Lilienfeld, S. O. (2003). The remembrance of things past: Problematic memory recovery techniques in psychotherapy. In S. O. Lilienfeld, S. J. Lynn, & J. M. Lohr (Eds.), *Science and pseudoscience in clinical psychology* (pp. 205–239). Guilford Press.

Lynn, S. J., Polizzi, C., Merckelbach, H., Chui-de, C., Maxwell, R., Lilienfeld, S. O., & Van-Heughten, D. (2022). Dissociation and dissociative disorders: Beyond the sociocognitive and posttraumatic models toward a transtheoretical/trans-diagnostic perspective. *Annual Review of Clinical Psychology*, *18*, 259–289.

Mack L. (2019). Trauma, body memories, and how to heal them. https://thebody isnotanapology.com/magazine/what-are-body-memories-and-how-to-heal -them/

Mangiulli, I., Otgaar, H., Jelicic, M., Merckelbach, H. (2022). A critical review of case studies on dissociative amnesia. *Clinical Psychological Science*, *10*(2), 191–211. https://doi.org/10.1177/21677026211018194

Maxwell, R., Merckelbach, H., Lilienfeld, S. O., & Lynn, S. J. (2018). The treatment of dissociation: An evaluation of effectiveness and potential mechanisms. In D. David, S. J. Lynn, G. H. Montgomery (Eds.), *Evidence-based psychotherapy: The state of the science and practice* (pp. 329–361). Wiley-Blackwell.

McNally, R. J. (2005). *Remembering trauma*. Harvard University Press.

Mohajerin, B., Lynn, S. J., Bakhtiyari, M., & Dolatshah, B. (2020). Evaluating the unified protocol in the treatment of dissociative identity disorder. *Cognitive and Behavioral Practice*, *27*(3), 270–289. https://doi.org/10.1016/j .cbpra.2019.07.012

Otgaar, H., Howe, M. L., Patihis, L., Merckelbach, H., Lynn, S. J., Lilienfeld, S. O., & Loftus, E. F. (2019). The return of the repressed: The persistent and problematic claims of long-forgotten trauma. *Perspectives on Psychological Science*, *14*(6), 1072–1095. https://doi.org/10.1177 /1745691619862306

Patihis, L., & Pendergrast, M. H. (2019). Reports of recovered memories of abuse in therapy in a large age-representative US national sample: Therapy type and decade comparisons. *Clinical Psychological Science*, *7*(1), 3–21. https:// doi.org/10.1177/2167702618773315

Patihis, L., Ho, L. Y., Tingen, I. W., Lilienfeld, S. O., & Loftus, E. F. (2014). Are the "memory wars" over? A scientist–practitioner gap in beliefs about repressed memory. *Psychological Science*, *25*(2), 519–530. https://doi.org /10.1177/0956797613510718

Pierce, L. (2014). The integrative power of dance/movement therapy: Implications for the treatment of dissociation and developmental trauma. *The Arts in Psychotherapy*, *41*(1), 7–15.

Pignotti, M., & Thyer, B. A. (2015). New age and related novel unsupported therapies in mental health practice. In S. O. Lilienfeld, S. J. Lynn, &

J. M. Lohr (Eds.), *Science and pseudoscience in clinical psychology* (2nd ed., pp. 191–209). Guilford.

Polizzi, C. P., Aksen, D. E., & Lynn, S. J. (2022). Quality of life, emotion regulation, and dissociation: Evaluating unique relations in an undergraduate sample and probable PTSD subsample. *Psychological Trauma: Theory, Research, Practice, and Policy*, *14*(1), 107–115. https://doi.org/10.1037/tra0000904

Pro Profs Quizzes. (2021). Do I have repressed memories quiz. www.proprofs.com.

Putnam, F. W. (1989). *Diagnosis and treatment of multiple personality disorder.* Guilford.

Rozental, A., Kottorp, A., Boettcher, J., Andersson, G., & Carlbring, P. (2016). Negative effects of psychological treatments: an exploratory factor analysis of the negative effects questionnaire for monitoring and reporting adverse and unwanted events. *PLoS One*, *11*(6), e0157503.

Sauerland, M. & Otgaar, M. (2022). Teaching psychology students to change (or correct) controversial beliefs about memory works. *Memory*, *30*(6), 753–762. https://doi.org/10.1080/09658211.2021.1874994

Schwartz, R. C. (1995). *Internal family systems.* Guilford.

Scoboria, A., Wade, K. A., Lindsay, D. S., Azad, T., Strange, D., Ost, J., & Hyman, I. E. (2017). A mega-analysis of memory reports from eight peer-reviewed false memory implantation studies. *Memory*, *25*(2), 146–163. https://doi.org/10.1080/09658211.2016.1260747

Spanos, N. P. (1994). Multiple identity enactments and multiple personality disorder: A sociocognitive perspective. *Psychological Bulletin*, *116*(1), 143–165.

Stanley, S. Welcome to Somatic Transformation [Internet]. Bainbridge Island (WA): Somatic Transformations; 2015 [cited 2015 July 31]. www.somatic-transformation.org/SomaticTransformation.html.

Thyer, B. A., & Pignotti, M. (2015). *Science and pseudoscience in social work practice.* Springer.

Traumatic Incident Reduction (TIR) Association. Traumatic incident reduction (TIR) [Internet]. Ann Arbor (MI): TIR Association; [year of publication unknown] [cited 2015 July 31]. www.tir.org/about-tir.html

Twombly, J. H. (2013). Integrating IFS with phase-oriented treatment of clients with dissociative disorder. In M. Sweezy & E. L. Ziskind (Eds.), *Internal family systems therapy* (pp. 100–117). Routledge.

van der Kolk, B. A. (1994). The body keeps the score: Memory and the evolving psychobiology of posttraumatic stress. *Harvard Review of Psychiatry*, *1*, 53–265.

Watkins, J. (1978). *The therapeutic self.* Human Sciences Press.

Watkins, J. G. (2001). Comment on Lynn. *American Journal of Clinical Hypnosis*, *43*(3–4), 293–295.

8

Pain

Harriet Hall

Psychotherapists often work on multidisciplinary teams with medical doctors and other professionals to alleviate pain. To help diagnose pain, the *Diagnostic and Statistical Manual of Mental Disorders* includes a section that addresses somatic symptoms and related disorders (American Psychiatric Association, 2022). For example, somatic symptom disorder is diagnosed when one or more somatic symptoms disrupt daily functioning for more than 6 months. The somatic symptoms commonly include fatigue and pain.

Pain and pseudoscience make good partners. Pain is subjective, can't be quantified, and is hard to pin down. Pseudoscience is adept at making up rationales and designing studies to convince people that treatments relieve pain when they really don't, presenting "evidence" that looks like science but isn't.

Plenty of things in medicine are objective. A rash or a swollen joint can be easily observed and confirmed by other observers. Some things can be easily measured and quantified, like body temperature to diagnose fever, blood pressure to diagnose hypertension, and blood hemoglobin levels to diagnose anemia. The instruments consistently provide the same objective measurements to all observers.

Subjective symptoms are another matter. Doctors can observe changes in behavior, but they have no way to tell how a person *feels* other than the person's self-report. Patients are often asked to rate their pain on a scale of 1 to 10. That's very problematic. Maybe it rated 8 all last night but is barely noticeable right now. Maybe it's very annoying but not exactly what you would call a pain. Maybe you're in a good mood that makes you tend to minimize your pain; maybe you're in a terrible mood and want the provider to know you're really suffering, so you rate it as 15 on a scale of 10! Are you a stoic or a habitual complainer? It's hard to decide what number to pick, and if asked again in an hour, you might decide differently and pick a different number.

The subjectivity of pain makes it particularly susceptible to dubious interventions. The next section will review some of the most egregious examples.

8.1 Pseudoscience and Questionable Ideas

8.1.1 Acupuncture: A Theatrical Placebo

Alternative medicine offers many treatments for pain, from devices to dietary supplements. Some of their offerings have never been tested or have not been adequately tested. The evidence they cite for their treatments runs the gamut; it may be pseudoscience or junk science or science that is poorly designed or poorly carried out. It may even be good science that simply isn't good enough to have earned a place in conventional medicine. If an alternative treatment were supported by good scientific evidence, it would be readily accepted as part of science-based medicine and could no longer be called "alternative."

Whenever skeptics point this out, they are often challenged by people who ask, "But what about acupuncture? Hasn't it been scientifically proven to work?"

Some people think it has, and it has become widely accepted by some mainstream doctors and institutions, but the evidence is shaky: most of the highly regarded Cochrane systematic reviews for acupuncture were inconclusive (Jiao et al., 2013).

Acupuncture is said to be effective for a long list of conditions, and it has been extensively studied. It has been used for everything from acne to dysentery to infertility to schizophrenia, but the most positive evidence is from studies of pain. Some randomized controlled trials have indeed found that acupuncture was effective for pain, but others have found that it wasn't. When studies conflict, a systematic review can usually be done to resolve the conflict; but systematic reviews of acupuncture have conflicted with each other. So Ernst and colleagues (2011) took the next logical step. They did a systematic review of systematic reviews of acupuncture for pain. They examined a total of 57 systematic reviews and found a mix of negative, positive, and inconclusive results. There were only four conditions for which more than one systematic review reached the same conclusions. For three conditions, they agreed that acupuncture didn't work and only once did they agree that it worked (for neck pain). They explain how inconsistencies, biases, conflicting conclusions, and recent high-quality studies throw doubt on even the most positive reviews. Think about it for a minute: does it make sense that a treatment would work for neck pain if it didn't work for pain anywhere else in the body?

Colquhoun and Novella (2013) also reviewed the evidence and published their findings in the journal *Anesthesia and Analgesia*. They noted that: (a) touching the skin with a toothpick seemed to work just as well as acupuncture, (b) the positive studies were questionable because of a lack of blinding and adequate controls, (c) it didn't matter where you inserted the needles or whether needles were used at all, (d) the small excess of positive trials after thousands of studies was most consistent with an inactive intervention, and (e) there was no signal but only noise. They characterized acupuncture as "a voluntary self-imposed tax on the gullible" (p. 1362). Their conclusion: "the benefits of acupuncture are likely nonexistent, or at best are too small and too transient to be of any clinical significance. It seems that acupuncture is little or no more than a theatrical placebo" (p. 1360).

8.1.2 Hypnosis: Selective Attention/Selective Inattention

Hypnosis originated with Mesmer's "animal magnetism," a decidedly pseudoscientific concept that was easily debunked by a Board of Inquiry appointed by France's King Louis XVI and headed by Benjamin Franklin (Lopez, 1993). Hypnosis persisted as a widely accepted therapy that has been used for everything from smoking cessation to retrieval of memories from past lives. But there's really no such thing as hypnosis. The name itself is a misnomer derived from the Greek word for sleep. It has nothing to do with sleep. The Scottish surgeon James Braid popularized the word, but he thought hypnosis was a mere contrivance to induce responses that were easily explained by ordinary psychological and physiological principles (Weitzenhoffer et al., 1959). There is no such thing as a hypnotic trance. There is no objective way to tell whether a person has been hypnotized. One study compared people who had been hypnotized to people who were merely instructed to pretend to be hypnotized; the two groups were indistinguishable. All the effects attributed to hypnosis have been replicated without hypnosis.

Rather than "hypnosis," it is more accurate to call it the SASI state: selective attention/selective inattention (McDonald, 1979). As such, it is only logical that some people should find it helpful in relieving pain. Relaxation, strong suggestion, the ability to focus and direct one's thoughts, distraction, and placebo effects all come into play. Suggestion works; that's why we kiss our children's scrapes and bruises to make them better. When mothers use natural childbirth they might often be considered to use a form of hypnosis: the coaching and breathing instructions are effective in helping

women give birth without anesthesia or medication. Another way of thinking about hypnosis is to consider it a learned behavior combined with
listening to a person in authority. There's certainly nothing magical about
it, and suggestion is a big factor in any medical treatment. Rather than
a stand-alone treatment for pain, suggestion would be better used as an
adjunct to enhance the response to an effective treatment.

8.1.3 Homeopathy: Delusions about Dilutions

Homeopathy is by far the most ridiculous of all alternative medicines (Hall,
2020). When properly tested, it has been shown not to work; and indeed, it
couldn't possibly work. If it could be shown to work, it would contradict all
our hard-earned knowledge about chemistry, physics, and biology.
Homeopathy was invented by a single German doctor, Samuel
Hahnemann, in 1796. His basic principle was "like cures like," the idea
that if something causes symptoms in a healthy person it will cure the same
symptoms in a person with a disease (Loudon, 2006). An example will help
to make clear just how silly homeopathy is. Coffee keeps people awake, so
dilute coffee will put them to sleep. The more dilute the coffee, the stronger
the effect. If diluted to the point that not a single molecule of coffee remains,
the solution will work even better to put people to sleep because the water
will remember the coffee was once there. Dripping the coffee-free water
onto a sugar pill will make it an even stronger sleeping pill.

In Hahnemann's day, conventional medicine used toxic remedies that
did more harm than good; so avoiding conventional medicine and using
remedies that were nothing but water appeared to produce better results,
and patients were readily convinced. As early as 1842, Oliver Wendell
Holmes thoroughly debunked homeopathy in his book *Homeopathy and
Its Kindred Delusions* (Holmes, 1842), and that should have been the end
of it, but it has persisted. Homeopathic remedies are sold in most drug-
stores today and are widely promoted on the Internet. Various highly
dilute remedies, alone or in combination, are said to be effective for pain.
Suggestion and belief may be enough to convince users that they work,
but there's no science to back them up.

8.1.4 Herbal Remedies: Nature Doesn't Provide a Plant for Every Human Ailment

Some people believe that a remedy for every human ailment can be
found in nature. There is no reason to believe that is true. Certainly, we
know of no plant that produces a herbal version of insulin capable of

treating diabetes. Some plants produce medically useful compounds, but they do it for self-protection, not to benefit humans. Herbalists claim that the ingredients in plant remedies work together synergistically to give better results, but whenever a single active ingredient has been tested against a mixture, the active ingredient alone has been shown to be more effective. Plant extracts contain other unwanted ingredients that either do nothing or may interfere with the action of an active ingredient that works. Many prescription drugs are derived from plants; but in drug development, the active ingredient is isolated, purified, and often replaced by a synthetic compound that is safer and more effective.

As an example, Rightful is a mixture of herbal ingredients that is said to: (a) be highly effective for pain relief and improved sleep, (b) be designed by integrative and conventional medical experts, (c) have the best bio-availability on the market, and (d) provide high, clinically effective, scientifically proven precise doses of each component. Are you impressed? You might be less so after you consider the ingredients as they were described on the company's website:

- Turmeric rhizome – helps reduce inflammation
- Corydalis – promotes pain relief and healthy circulation
- Curcumin – helps inhibit inflammatory responses
- Broad-spectrum hemp – promotes healthy function of the central nervous system
- Ashwagandha – supports the body's response to stress and inflammation
- California poppy – promotes restful sleep, relaxation, and mental calm
- Black pepper – enhances the absorption and effectiveness of turmeric and hemp

The evidence for these effects is pretty sketchy. For instance, the Natural Medicines Comprehensive Database rates California poppy as having "Insufficient evidence to rate effectiveness," and it says there is insufficient evidence to establish an appropriate dose. So what does Rightful mean by scientifically proven precise doses? Further, for turmeric/curcumin, the evidence is conflicting, with some studies showing no decrease in inflammatory markers (e.g., White et al., 2019). When multiple ingredients are combined like this, there's no way to predict whether the combination will enhance the effects of the individual ingredients or lessen them. The mixture itself must be tested, and the mixture in Rightful has not been adequately tested.

Most damningly, at least one of these ingredients is known to be dangerous. When The Medical Letter (2021) reviewed ashwagandha, they concluded: "There is no convincing evidence that ashwagandha supplements are effective or safe for any indication; patients should be advised not to take them. FDA-approved drugs are available for treatment of all the conditions for which these herbal supplements are being promoted." As comedian Dara Ó Briain said, "Oh, herbal medicine's been around for thousands of years. Indeed it has, and then we tested it all and the stuff that worked became medicine. And the rest of it is just a nice bowl of soup and potpourri."

8.1.5 CBD Products: Not a Substitute for Oxycontin

Cannabidiol (CBD), derived from the marijuana plant but lacking the chemical that causes euphoria, is widely used for pain in the form of oil, creams, bath salts, oral sprays, and other products. The scientific evidence is insufficient to recommend it over other pain remedies. The Federal Trade Commission (FTC) has acted to prohibit six companies from making illegal health claims about CBD (Federal Trade Commission, 2021), one of which is that it replaces the need for prescription painkillers like oxycontin.

8.1.6 Dietary Supplements: Based on a Fiction

Thanks to the ill-conceived Dietary Supplement Health and Education Act (DSHEA) of 1994, it is legal in the United States to sell dietary supplements that have not been proven safe or effective. The fiction is that they are intended to supplement a lack of something in the diet, but the reality is that they are being used as medicine. A dietary supplement may have a single ingredient, or it may be a mixture of ingredients. More is better, right? So if you throw together several ingredients that are thought to relieve pain, the mixture should work really well, right? That's a common assumption, but it's false. When you combine ingredients, there are several possibilities. The effect may be additive ($2 + 2 = 4$), may be potentiated ($0 + 2 > 2$), may be antagonistic ($6 + 4 < 10$), or may be synergistic ($2 + 2 = \gg 4$, maybe as much as 10 times greater). There's no way to predict what will happen. The only way to find out is to do proper scientific testing with appropriate controls.

Golden Revive Plus is an example of a dietary supplement mixture that claims to treat the underlying cause of pain: inflammation. It is said to be a miraculous treatment that heals achy joints and leaves them lubricated(!?). It combines curcumin, *Boswellia*, magnesium, quercetin, pepper, and bromelain. It is said to be a result of extensive medical research by experts, but no adequate research could be found that tested this particular combination of ingredients.

8.1.7 Medical Devices: Not Adequately Tested

There are many medical devices that claim to relieve pain through various modalities: heat, cold, light, magnetism, lasers, electricity, embedded frequencies, vibration, far infrared, ineffable energies, and more. New devices are constantly appearing on the market, and they are never properly tested. They are sold on the strength of testimonials. Sometimes there is a science-based rationale as to why they ought to work, but more often the rationale is pure pseudoscience. Sometimes the description is really hilarious and would not convince anyone who knows anything about science. It will be helpful to look at specific examples. Some of these qualify as pseudoscience; others are treatments that have never been adequately tested. Bad examples can be very instructive.

8.1.7.1 Mystical Patches

Taopatch is a tiny patch that combines all good things: Tao, acupuncture, lasers, "upconverting" nanocrystals, quantum dots, carbon nanotubes, and biophoton therapy, all somehow embedded in a Mylar disc. It is said to last for 2 years. It supposedly converts body heat into specific frequencies of light, photons that travel to acupoints and produce all kinds of benefits, including treating multiple sclerosis, decreasing anxiety, and relieving chronic pain. Pinches (2020) reviewed the evidence provided by TaoPatch. He found low-quality, poorly designed preliminary studies, plagiarism, and authors who apparently don't exist. He concluded that TaoPatch is a fake placebo product. He pointed out that "While biophotons *are* a known phenomena [*sic*], there is *no* evidence that these play a role in intracellular communication, or that by simply adding more similar photons that any healing effect can be achieved" (para. 6).

Luminas skin patches are said to work through a proprietary technology that:

> allows us to capture these unique electric field signatures from 100s of natural remedies used to relieve pain and inflammation. These unique signatures are then modulated onto a resonant carrier wave allowing us to transfer these unique signatures onto the patch. Once applied to the skin, the patches are activated and energy from the 200+ remedies are released to support the body's own innate, natural healing process. This activation results in fast acting, long lasting pain and

inflammation relief without any drugs, chemicals, or known side effects. (Miracle Balance, n.d., paras. 6–7).

This is energy medicine nonsense. Electric field signatures don't exist. There's no evidence that any signatures are present, that "energy is released from the patch," or that your body knows how to choose the electrons it needs (as all electrons are identical, how could it choose?). The "evidence" they offer is before-and-after thermographic images, which are notoriously unreliable, and they didn't even try to standardize their procedures or use a control group. Gorski (2018) dubbed it quantum quackery and called for a properly controlled study.

Kailo patches are also dubious. This is how I summarized them on the Science-Based Medicine website:

Kailo patches use a patented technology; an array of billions of charged nanocapacitors that act as a bioantenna designed to assist the body in clear communication and turn down the volume on your pain in seconds. The strength of the body's electrical field allows Kailo to target the pain when placed on your skin. The patch tells the brain what it needs to know to stop the pain. (Hall, 2021, para. 6)

This is all pseudoscientific nonsense.

Signal Relief patches claim to use neuro capacitive coupling technology to relieve pain by interfering with the body's electrical signals and clearing communication. Each device apparently contains billions of micro-nano capacitors. They define "capacitor" as a small particle that conducts electricity and interacts with your body's natural electricity, but the true definition of a capacitor is a passive electronic device that stores electricity using two electrical conductors separated by a dielectric medium. The technology was designed to improve reception for communication devices. However, there's no reason to expect that technology to improve communication in a biological system would relieve pain. Apparently, one Signal Relief device is all you will ever need; it keeps working forever and only the adhesive patches will need to be replaced. It needn't even touch the skin; you can just apply it to the outside of your clothes! A study of capacitive coupling found it no more effective than the control, but the authors interpreted it as a positive study because participants reduced their use of pain medication (Rossini et al., 2010). It would be interesting to compare Signal Relief patches to placebo patches manufactured without the micro-nano capacitors; but no such study will ever be done because it would reveal the product doesn't do anything but elicit a placebo response.

8.1.7.2 Cold and Heat Applications

Ice is commonly used to treat injuries like ankle sprains. It is being encouraged less because it relieves pain but slows recovery (Byrne, 2015). Although still encouraged in some situations (e.g., extreme pain), some research shows it has been traditionally overused. Heat can also relieve pain, as everyone who has ever used a heating pad can testify. It relaxes, comforts, reassures, and takes the edge off of several types of pain. In *Pain Science*, Ingraham (2020) provides an excellent overview of the evidence. Where heating lapses into pseudoscience is when it claims to penetrate more deeply into the body than research shows it does. Far infrared saunas heat but do not heal. They are said to penetrate more deeply, but Ingraham says the only evidence provided for that claim is a paper that does not support the claim, and some experts have claimed that far infrared is actually the *least* penetrative. And then there are rubefacients, which are topical creams that *feel* hot, but not because they heat. They are irritants that produce a chemical burn. They have a counter-irritant effect. Counter-irritation is real, but it is not powerful.

8.1.7.3 Infrared Light Therapy Products

Infrared light therapy is a controversial therapeutic technique supported by little or no scientific evidence. An article on Healthline explains:

> It is thought to work by producing a biochemical effect in cells that strengthens the mitochondria. The mitochondria are the power-house of the cell – it's where the cell's energy is created. The energy-carrying molecule found in the cells of all living things is called ATP (adenosine triphosphate). By increasing the function of the mito-chondria using RLT, a cell can make more ATP. With more energy, cells can function more efficiently, rejuvenate themselves, and repair damage. (Cafasso, 2020)

Some preliminary research supports an effect on mitochondria, but there's no evidence that this translates to any meaningful clinical benefit. Clinic Red claims to be "the only product out there with Tri-Spectrum Technology that includes 630, 660, and 850 wavelengths which means their device penetrates deeper with both red and infrared light." The Clinic Red website says "studies have shown that Red Phototherapy is effective ..." but they don't tell us which studies, and no studies could be found.

8.1.7.4 Handheld Neuromodulators

Solis pain relief system uses a handheld "neuromodulator" device that is pressed directly to the area of pain. It claims that sensory nerves are triggered to produce natural body pain-blocking responses, blocking neural pain signals to the brain for lasting relief of chronic pain. Its claim to surpass other pain relief solutions appears to be based only on customer testimonials.

8.1.7.5 Transcutaneous Electrical Nerve Stimulation

TENS is used to treat many painful conditions. Ingraham (2021) reviewed its evidence at Painscience.com and found that published systematic reviews were mostly negative or inconclusive. He concluded that it "probably doesn't work much better for most pain than an aspirin, and it's not much good for anything else except maybe some relaxation or gently exercising muscles in rehab" (para. 7).

8.1.7.6 Acupuncture Pens

And now we've come back full circle to acupuncture, this time in the form of a product. The Zen acupuncture pen also purports to reduce pain, boost your mood, improve your skin condition, and promote blood circulation of your skin to give you a rejuvenated, radiant, and youthful look. Acupuncture pens allegedly detox the meridians. But meridians don't exist, and detox is an alternative medicine buzzword. We don't need any help detoxing: the kidneys and liver remove toxins very efficiently.

8.2 Research-Supported Approaches

Science-based medical interventions (e.g., medication, physical therapy) are typically the first line treatments for pain. However, when these approaches do not provide sufficient relief, psychological interventions have also been used. The Society of Clinical Psychology (Division 12 of the American Psychological Association) has reviewed the literature to identify if any psychological interventions meet their criteria for well-established evidence-based treatments (EBTs). As described in Chapter 1, treatments are considered well-established when at least two well-designed randomized controlled trials (conducted by two different research teams) demonstrate the treatment is more effective than another treatment or placebo (Chambless & Hollon, 1998). According to these criteria, different variations of cognitive-behavioral therapy have been shown to be well-established evidence-based treatment for chronic pain (see Ehde et al., 2014 for a review). Cognitive-behavioral therapy for pain includes cognitive components (e.g., acceptance, cognitive restructuring) and behavioral components (e.g., relaxation training, sleep hygiene).

According to a recent Cochrane review of 35 randomized controlled trials involving psychosocial treatments for pain (excluding headaches), cognitive-behavioral therapy had statistically significant but small effects for actual pain relief (Williams et al., 2020). This pain relief occurred immediately after treatment but did not continue 6 months later. On the other hand, cognitive-behavioral therapy did have a greater effect on improving psychological outcomes associated with pain by improving mood, decreasing catastrophic thinking, and minimizing overall disability due to pain; and these psychological improvements were also evident during the 6-month follow-up period.

8.3 Conclusion

How do we know a treatment works to relieve pain? Most people think it is a simple matter of trying it to see if the pain subsides. That's why people are so impressed by testimonials. "It worked for me." Well, maybe it did, but maybe not. It's not so simple. If the pain goes away, you can't know for sure whether it went away *because of* the pill or *in spite* of it. There's a logical fallacy called "*post hoc ergo propter hoc*," Latin for "after this, because of this." It's easy to see the fallacy if someone claims that roosters must make the sun come up, because their crowing is always followed by sunrise. But most people will assume that a treatment worked for pain just because the treatment was followed by a reduction in pain. That might be true, but it might be a false assumption like the one about roosters. The only reliable way to know if a pain remedy works is science: doing a controlled clinical trial to see if more people get relief with the treatment than without. And that gives us general information for a population, but it still doesn't prove that the treatment worked for the individual in question.

What if repeating the treatment is consistently followed by pain relief? That could be a real therapeutic effect, or it could be a conditioned response. To find out if a remedy really worked for an individual, you could do a double-blind controlled test where neither the patient nor the provider knows whether the treatment was the real one or a placebo.

Symptoms can subside for a lot of different reasons. In the natural course of illness, symptoms fluctuate. Fevers go up and down. Patients with arthritis have good days and bad days. If they try a treatment when the pain is particularly bad, regression to the mean will ensure that the pain will get better afterwards; the pain was about to improve anyway, and the treatment will get the credit for something it didn't do.

Two factors that influence awareness of pain are suggestion and distraction. We all know the power of suggestion. We tell our children that a parent's kiss will make it all better, and it does. And anything that takes attention away from the pain will reduce awareness of the pain; distraction doesn't affect the pain signals, but it can reduce the experience of suffering.

How long did it take to see results? Many testimonials claim that the pain was gone immediately after they took a pill; but that's impossible, because it takes time for a pill to be absorbed and to take effect. Barry Beyerstein (1997) wrote a classic article exploring some of the reasons that intelligent people may mistakenly come to believe that a bogus therapy has worked. The disease may have been a self-limited condition that has run its course. Spontaneous remissions have occurred, even in supposedly incurable diseases. Placebo responses can be evoked through suggestion, belief, expectancy, cognitive reinterpretation, and diversion of attention. People who hedge their bets by using multiple remedies often give the wrong one the credit (for instance, they believe a change in their diet cured the cancer when it was really the surgery and chemotherapy). Temporary mood improvement may be confused with cure.

For most of human history we had no recourse but to rely on trial and error and the testimonials of others. Now we have science, a reliable way to test our ideas against reality. We know how to do good science, but sometimes we don't apply that knowledge. Pseudoscience abounds, especially in the area of pain relief, and especially in so-called "alternative" medicine.

Harriet Hall, MD, is a retired family physician. She is author of the book *Women Aren't Supposed to Fly: The Memoirs of a Female Flight Surgeon* (2008).

References

American Psychiatric Association (2022). *Diagnostic and statistical manual of mental disorders, fifth edition, text revision* (DSM-5-TR). American Psychiatric Association.

Beyerstein, B. (1997). Why bogus therapies seem to work. www.skepticalinquirer.org.

Byrne, S. (2015). Why you should avoid ice for a sprained ankle. www.consumerreports.org.

Cafasso, J. (2020). Red light therapy benefits. www.healthline.com.

Chambless, D. L., & Hollon, S. D. (1998). Defining empirically supported therapies. *Journal of Consulting and Clinical Psychology, 66*(1), 7–18.

Colquhoun, D., & Novella, S. P. (2013). Acupuncture is theatrical placebo. *Anesthesia & Analgesia, 116*(6), 1360–1363.

Ehde, D. M., Dillworth, T. M., & Turner, J. A. (2014). Cognitive-behavioral therapy for individuals with chronic pain: Efficacy, innovations, and directions for research. *American Psychologist, 69*(2), 153–166.

Ernst, E., Lee, M. S., & Choi T. Y. (2011). Acupuncture: Does it alleviate pain and are there serious risks? A review of reviews. *Pain, 152,* 755–764.

Federal Trade Commission. (2021). FTC approves final administrative consent orders against sellers of deceptively marketed CBD products. www.ftc.gov.

Gorski, D. (2018). Luminas pain relief patches: Where the words "quantum" and "energy" really mean "magic." www.respectfulinsolence.com.

Hall, H. A. (2020). Homeopathy. www.skepdoc.info.

Hall, H. A. (2021). Energy medicine pain relief patches are laughable quackery. www.sciencebasedmedicine.com.

Holmes, O. W. (1842). *Homoeopathy, and its kindred delusions: Two lectures delivered before the Boston society for the diffusion of useful knowledge.* William D. Ticknor.

Ingraham, P. (2020). Heat for pain and rehab: A detailed guide to using heat as therapy for acute and chronic pain and recovery from injury. www.painscience.com.

Ingraham, P. (2021). Zapped! Does TENS work for pain? The peculiar popularity of being gently zapped with electrical stimulation therapy. www.painscience.com.

Jiao, S., Tsutani, K., & Haga, N. (2013). Review of Cochrane reviews on acupuncture: How Chinese resources contribute to Cochrane reviews. *Journal of Alternative and Complementary Medicine, 19*(7), 613–621. https://doi.org/10.1089/acm.2012.0113

Lopez, C. A. (1993). Franklin and Mesmer: An encounter. *The Yale Journal of Biology and Medicine, 66*(4), 325–331.

Loudon, I. (2006). A brief history of homeopathy. *Journal of the Royal Society of Medicine, 99*(12), 607–610.

McDonald, R. C. (1979). Hypnosis and hypothesis: A new graphic. *Canadian Family Physician, 25,* 200–208.

Miracle Balance. (n.d.). Holographic discs. www.miraclebalance.net.

Novella, S. (2015). Whole body cryotherapy. www.sciencebasedmedicine.org.

Pinches, S. (2020). TaoPatch – Is it a scam? www.painreliefpatchreviews.com.

Rossini, M., Viapiana, O., Gatti, D., de Terlizzi, F., & Adami, S. (2010). Capacitively coupled electric field for pain relief in patients with vertebral fractures and chronic pain. *Clinical Orthopaedics and Related Research*, *468*(3), 735–740.

The Medical Letter. (2021). Ashwagandha supplements. www.medicalletter.org.

Weitzenhoffer, A. M., Gough, P. B., & Landes, J. (1959). A study of the Braid effect: Hypnosis by visual fixation. *The Journal of Psychology*, *47*(1), 67–80.

White, C. M., Pasupuleti, V., Roman, Y. M., Li, Y., & Hernandez, A. V. (2019). Oral turmeric/curcumin effects on inflammatory markers in chronic inflammatory diseases: A systematic review and meta-analysis of randomized controlled trials. *Pharmacological Research*, *146*, 104280.

de C Williams, A. C., Fisher, E., Hearn, L., & Eccleston, C. (2020). Psychological therapies for the management of chronic pain (excluding headache) in adults. *Cochrane Database of Systematic Reviews*, *8*(8), CD007407.

9

Eating Issues

Jamie M. Loor, Jennifer Battles, Brooke L. Bennett, Brooke L. Whisenhunt, and Danae L. Hudson

According to the *Diagnostic and Statistical Manual of Mental Disorders* (DSM-5-TR; American Psychiatric Association, 2022), the three primary eating disorder diagnoses include: anorexia nervosa, bulimia nervosa, and binge eating disorder. These disorders typically begin in adolescence and young adulthood, although they can also develop earlier or later in life.

Anorexia is defined as an individual having a significantly low body weight that is maintained by extreme dietary restriction. To maintain low body weight, individuals with anorexia may primarily engage in food restriction, fasting, and/or excessive exercising, while others may also engage in purging behaviors. In contrast to earlier DSM criteria, individuals may be diagnosed with anorexia regardless of endorsement of fear of weight gain or fatness as long as they engage in persistent behaviors that interfere with weight gain (e.g., food restriction, compulsive exercise). Additionally, anorexia involves altered views of one's weight or shape, overinfluence of the importance of weight or shape on self-evaluation, and lack of acknowledgment of the seriousness of low body weight.

Bulimia is characterized by a pattern of binge eating followed by compensatory behaviors, such as self-induced vomiting or medication misuse. Binge eating is defined as eating a large amount of food and feeling out of control. Next, an individual attempts to compensate for this eating by "purging" extra calories from the body through vomiting, laxative misuse, or other means. Individuals with bulimia are often in the normal weight to overweight range. Similar to those with anorexia, the self-concepts of individuals with bulimia are overly influenced by body weight or shape.

Binge eating disorder also involves a pattern of binge eating; however, this eating is not associated with compensatory behaviors. Although individuals with binge eating disorder may fall in the overweight to obese weight categories, this disorder is distinct from obesity, and most individuals with obesity do not have binge eating disorder. Binge eating episodes are often carried out alone for fear of embarrassment regarding the amount being eaten. Additionally, binge eating episodes can occur when one is not physically hungry and often involve eating foods rapidly to the point of being uncomfortably full. As with bulimia, binge eating episodes typically lead to strong negative emotions such as disgust, depression, or guilt.

Treatments for eating disorders often result in significantly improved symptoms, enhanced quality of life, and recovery. However, eating disorders can also be quite difficult to treat, with many individuals never having access to evidence-based care. Untreated or insufficiently treated eating disorders have costs ranging from personal (e.g., impact on relationships, impaired ability to succeed in education or career settings, long-term health consequences) to financial (e.g., expensive emergency hospitalizations and costs of associated medical complications resulting from chronic eating disorders). Importantly, eating disorders carry the ultimate cost of having one of the highest mortality rates among psychiatric conditions (American Psychiatric Association, 2013; Weye et al., 2020). Therefore, the importance of accessible, quality, evidence-based treatment cannot be understated. In this chapter, we review diagnostic and assessment issues as well as myths about eating disorders. Additionally, we provide brief summaries of treatments that have substantial research support and treatments with equivocal or insufficient evidence.

9.1 Pseudoscience and Questionable Ideas

9.1.1 Diagnostic and Assessment Issues and Controversies

Eating disorder assessments can be challenging for several reasons. Due to the nature of eating disorders, symptoms may be purposely hidden or denied by the individual. An individual's intersecting social identities may also influence symptom presentation. For example, there are significant differences in symptom presentation across genders, sexual orientations, and ethnic identities (Sonneville & Lipson, 2018). Men are less likely to endorse preoccupation with thinness and more likely to endorse compensatory behaviors than women (Strother et al., 2012). Men are also more likely to endorse muscle dysmorphia and accompanying disordered behaviors to achieve muscle growth such as anabolic steroid use (Strother et al., 2012). Additionally, research suggests eating disorders are more common in sexual minority adults than cisgender heterosexual adults in the United States (Nagata et al., 2020). This underscores the unique considerations needed when assessing disordered eating behaviors in gender and sexual minorities. For example, in one study, gay men were more likely to engage in unhealthy weight control behaviors than heterosexual men (Strong et al., 2000). In another study, lesbian women endorsed greater overall eating disorder pathology than heterosexual women (Jones et al., 2019).

Although research on eating disorders in populations of transgender individuals is still in its infancy, preliminary findings have highlighted the potential difficulty of using existing measures to assess risk factors such as body dissatisfaction due to the more complex rationale for altering appearance (Weber et al., 2019). For example, transgender men may be driven to reduce body fat both to achieve a more traditionally masculine appearance and also to suppress menstruation.

Additionally, there remain significant differences in prevalence rates and symptom presentation across different ethnicities. Individuals of Asian descent have been found to have an increased likelihood of engaging in unhealthy weight control behaviors (Rodgers et al., 2017), while individuals of Hispanic or Latin descent endorsed fewer exercise behaviors and less dieting than their non-Hispanic counterparts (Lee-Winn et al., 2016).

Further complicating the assessment of eating disorders is the fact that some existing measures appear less sensitive when used among ethnic minority populations, which limits their usability as screening and diagnostic tools (Rodgers et al., 2018). While some eating disorder measures appear appropriate for use across racial and ethnic groups (Belon et al., 2011; Kelly et al., 2012), other measures and subscales do not assess equivalent constructs across some groups (Belon et al., 2015; Kelly et al., 2012) or across men and women (Elosua & Hermosilla, 2013). Most current assessments of body dissatisfaction and disordered eating pathology were developed using groups that were predominantly non-Hispanic White, straight, cisgender, young, and female identifying (Lavender et al., 2017; Rodgers et al., 2018). As a result, they place an emphasis on traditionally feminine ideals and patterns of symptoms more relevant for White, young women (Lavender et al., 2017; Ochner et al., 2009). Therefore, scores on these measures should not be compared across groups and clinical "cut-off" values should differ. More research across diverse, intersecting identities is crucial for creating appropriate measures, establishing appropriate norms for eating disorder screening, and measuring eating disorder treatment progress.

9.1.2 Myths that Influence Treatment

Myths about eating disorders are often promoted in popular media. Movies and TV shows usually portray only a stereotyped and limited view of what it means to have or to recover from an eating disorder. These myths have real consequences and can be barriers to individuals being identified as having an eating disorder or receiving appropriate referrals and treatments.

9.1.2.1 Myth: Eating Disorders Are for Life

As mentioned previously, eating disorders are notoriously difficult to treat and have one of the highest mortality rates of any psychiatric condition (Arcelus et al., 2011; Weye et al., 2020). As a result, there is a myth that eating disorders are incurable or a lifelong experience. However, in direct contrast, a substantial portion of individuals with eating disorders achieve full recovery (Schaumberg et al., 2017). Ten years after eating disorder onset, approximately 70% of individuals are in recovery (Berkman et al., 2007). Additionally, for those who do not achieve full recovery, treatment often helps improve quality of life and physical symptoms (Treasure et al., 2015).

9.1.2.2 Myth: Eating Disorders Occur Only in Young, White, Upper-Class Women and Girls

This myth involves an incorrect, narrow view of who can develop eating disorders that is not only false, but also impacts treatment access for those not fitting this limited definition. Regarding age, eating disorder onset typically occurs in late adolescence to early adulthood, but eating disorder symptoms can also begin, worsen, or reemerge in adults in middle to late life (American Psychiatric Association, 2013; Mitchison et al., 2014). Additionally, while most eating disorders have similar prevalence rates across racial and ethnic groups, binge eating is reported more frequently in Hispanic and Black individuals compared to White individuals (Marques et al., 2011). Contrary to the view that eating disorders impact only those of high socioeconomic status, eating disorders exist across income brackets, and they are associated with more physical health impairment when they occur in those of lower socioeconomic status (Mitchison et al., 2014). Regarding gender, eating disorders are more common in women overall compared to men, although rates of binge eating disorder across genders are more equivalent.

Groups not typically thought to have eating disorders (men, individuals over 45 years old, those with a low socioeconomic status) have been reporting increasing rates of eating disorders across recent years (Mitchison et al., 2014). Additionally, men and ethnic or racial minority groups have the lowest rates of help-seeking (Coffino et al., 2019).

9.1.2.3 Myth: You Can Tell by Looking that Someone Has an Eating Disorder

This myth suggests that someone's physical appearance alone can be used to determine if they have an eating disorder. The stereotypical image is usually a very thin or emaciated figure. In fact, eating disorders occur across the body mass index (BMI) spectrum. For example, atypical anorexia can be diagnosed when an individual has all the features of anorexia outside of being significantly underweight. These individuals have engaged in restriction of eating and extreme weight loss behaviors, and despite not being underweight, they have all the medical complications that come along with malnourishment, such as amenorrhea (loss of menstrual period), electrolyte disturbances, and bradycardia (dangerously low heart rate; Moskowitz & Weiselberg, 2017). Similarly, those with binge eating disorder vary across the BMI spectrum. Although those in lower and higher BMI ranges report similar levels of eating pathology, depression, and impairment, those at lower BMI levels are less likely to seek and receive treatment (Dingemans & van Furth, 2012). Therefore, it is impossible to determine eating disorder status on physical appearance, and this myth can be a harmful barrier to treatment.

9.1.2.4 Myth: All Exercise Is Good Exercise

This myth claims that all types and amounts of exercise are good for everyone. In fact, compulsive or obligatory exercise involves the rigid and intense need for physical activity and has been shown to be related to eating disorder onset, maintenance, and relapse (Goodwin et al., 2011). Individuals exercising in this way continue despite injuries or other negative consequences, and when unable to exercise, experience intense negative affect. Additionally, exercise can also be used excessively by those with eating disorders as a purging or compensatory behavior to rid the body of calories ingested. In the treatment of eating disorders, therapeutic exercise may be beneficial in some cases, although it is recommended that such exercise be closely monitored by a multidisciplinary team and involve psychoeducational components to aid in recognizing when exercise becomes problematic (Cook et al., 2016).

9.1.3 Treatments with Equivocal or Insufficient Evidence

There are several treatments that have shown deleterious effects on individuals with an eating disorder. In addition, many comprehensive eating disorder programs include a variety of modalities that have not been established as effective stand-alone treatments. In fact, many of these modalities have mixed outcomes, have research support from studies with a high chance of bias (i.e., small sample size, cross-sectional, etc.), or have not been empirically investigated. Therefore, all treatments that fall in this category should only be used with the utmost caution.

9.1.3.1 Group and Inpatient Treatment for Eating Disorders

When compared to a waitlist control condition, group psychotherapy for eating disorders is significantly more effective at decreasing rates of binge eating and purging, as well as reducing related eating disorder pathology following treatment (Grenon et al., 2017). Preliminary evidence suggests group therapy may be as effective as other common treatments (Grenon et al., 2017).

However, the strengths of group therapy for eating disorders must be considered alongside its limitations; group therapy has an additional risk. Due to the cohabitation and group therapy typically involved in these programs, these programs can unintentionally create a competitive environment involving eating disorder symptom severity and become a forum for learning new maladaptive weight control behaviors (Colton & Pistrang, 2004). When patients rated an inpatient treatment center as unhelpful, one of the main factors cited was rivalry with other patients with eating disorders (de la Rie et al., 2006).

In fact, inpatient treatment, when not necessary for medical stabilization, has not been found to be more effective for treating eating disorders than outpatient treatment (Hay et al., 2019; Lock, 2010) nor more effective for facilitating weight gain than outpatient treatment or partial hospitalization (Hay et al., 2019). Lock (2010) argued that the usefulness of hospitalization is doubtful because of the separation that occurs from family and friends as a part of the process. Further, this approach is expensive – outpatient treatment costs a mere 10% of inpatient treatment (Hay et al., 2014). In one comparison of inpatient, partial hospitalization, and outpatient treatments, patients were more likely to complete treatment when randomized to outpatient care settings (Hay et al., 2019). More high-quality research is needed to further examine overall effectiveness and long-term outcomes as well as to effectively compare treatment outcomes across inpatient versus outpatient and individual versus group settings.

9.1.3.2 Yoga

Different forms of yoga, such as Kripalu and Vinyasa Yoga, are usually taught in hour-long sessions with a certified yoga instructor as part of a larger treatment program. Initial studies on yoga for eating disorders have shown promise, with some clients reporting decreased binge eating frequency (Brennan et al., 2020), reduced body image concern (Borden & Cook-Cottone, 2020), and lower negative affect before and after meals (Pacanowski et al., 2017) compared to control participants. However, the research on yoga for eating disorders is quite limited. Most studies use varying types of yoga practice, making it difficult to compare effectiveness across studies. Yoga has also never been studied as a stand-alone intervention for eating disorders, leading to questions about the unique impact of yoga on eating disorder symptoms outside of other treatment techniques (Borden & Cook-Cottone, 2020).

9.1.3.3 Complementary and Alternative Treatments

Even though the research on the utility of complementary treatments for eating disorders is extremely limited, many of these treatment approaches are included within larger eating disorder residential programs or are sought out by clients with an eating disorder. In fact, such treatments are being increasingly offered at private residential behavioral treatment programs where it is not made clear which treatments have a strong evidence base and which treatments have no documented effect of improving symptoms (Attia et al., 2016; Kaye & Bulik, 2021).

For example, a small number of clinicians argue that equine therapy may help individuals increase body awareness and encourage emotional expression; however, only case studies and theory papers have been published on the subject (Lac, 2017; Lac et al., 2013). Moreover, the suggested mechanism of change (i.e., "understanding their body") lacks plausibility.

Treatments such as massage therapy and acupuncture have also been associated with a self-reported reduction in depression and anxiety in those diagnosed with an eating disorder (Fogarty et al., 2016), but there is no research demonstrating its impact on symptoms specific to eating disorders (i.e., objective measures). Also, their positive effects on mood could be due to placebo or simply human touch. Additionally, research on arts therapies (i.e., art therapy, drama therapy, music therapy, and dance/movement therapy) is limited to mainly narrative reflections and case studies, prohibiting clear conclusions from being made about their efficacy (Fogarty et al., 2016; Frisch et al., 2006). Across all of these complementary treatment approaches, further research would be needed to establish their definitive utility.

9.1.4 Harmful Treatments

9.1.4.1 Online Self-Help

While individuals with eating disorders may often turn to online resources for help, harmful pro-eating disorder, or "pro-ED," websites may also be accessed. These websites contain strategies and advice on disordered eating behaviors such as methods for extreme weight loss and techniques for purging calories, as well as ways to conceal these behaviors from others. Individuals often report turning to these sites to receive support, and in fact many such sites claim to only be providing support and acceptance for those with eating disorders. However, these websites promote competition to be thinner among users, praise individuals for eating disorder behaviors, and post images of extremely thin figures as so-called "thinspiration" (Rouleau & von Ranson, 2011; Sowles et al., 2018). Time spent on pro-ED websites is associated with more extreme weight loss behaviors, higher body dissatisfaction, and more frequent use of weight loss techniques (Harper et al., 2008; Jett et al., 2010; Peebles et al., 2012). Although pro-recovery websites with an explicit focus on recovery from eating disorders also exist, research has shown that individuals cannot easily differentiate between these two types of sites and that they may gain new techniques for disordered eating on both (Harper et al., 2008).

9.1.4.2 Fad Diets and Extreme Calorie Restriction

New dieting approaches are often marketed aggressively directly to consumers as being effective and safe methods of losing large amounts of weight quickly. Those with eating disorders, at high risk for eating disorders, or recovering from eating disorders may be particularly vulnerable to these marketing approaches. For example, juicing or detox diets claim to "clean" or "detoxify" the body by instructing followers to cut solid foods from their diets and drink only juices or other liquid supplements for a period of time ranging from days to weeks. In fact, approaches advocating for restricting entire food groups and extreme calorie restriction are not effective over the long term (i.e., once the diet is ended the initial lost weight is regained or rebound weight gain occurs), increase the risk for developing eating disorders, and can lead to serious health complications or even death (Klein & Kiat, 2015; Stice et al., 2017).

9.1.4.3 Other Pseudoscience Approaches

Past life regression therapy involves the use of hypnosis to access memories from past lives (Weiss, 2012). This approach does not have a plausible theory behind it, and no research has shown any positive outcomes associated with this modality for eating disorders or any other conditions (Andrade, 2017). In fact, an inherent risk of this approach is the potential to implant false memories. Patients are often not informed of these inherent risks and thus cannot ethically provide informed consent to participate.

Thought field therapy (TFT) is another pseudoscientific approach that claims to correct bodily energy imbalances using finger tapping on various points in the body. It has been marketed to treat a wide variety of emotion-related disorders, including eating disorders. Similar to other pseudoscientific approaches, TFT does not have a scientifically grounded theory, peer-reviewed research is lacking, and anecdotal evidence is solely used to support claims of its efficacy (Lee & Hunsley, 2015).

A common link across these pseudoscientific approaches is that in addition to taking time, energy, and money to complete, they delay individuals from receiving efficacious treatments. In fact, patients may often opt for these types of approaches because they do not explicitly focus on eating or require behavioral changes. Research has consistently shown that early identification of eating disorders and initial behavioral change to promote weight regain or stabilization are associated with the best outcomes (Vall & Wade, 2015). Pseudoscientific treatments for eating disorders are particularly worrisome considering that eating disorders that have some of the highest rates of mortality among psychological disorders and delayed evidence-based treatment could increase the chance of a chronic and resistant course of illness.

9.2 Research-Supported Approaches

When considering the support of a particular eating disorder treatment, it is important to recognize that eating disorders consist of different disorders and symptom presentations. Therefore, many treatments focus on one specific diagnosis or symptom, making it difficult to generalize across the spectrum. To consider a treatment to have substantial research support, we focused on treatments that have significant evidence of efficacy and effectiveness across more than one diagnostic category or symptom subset.

Existing research points to enhanced cognitive-behavioral therapy (CBT-E) for eating disorders as the leading treatment. This approach is transdiagnostic because it is designed to be used for all forms of eating disorders with a focus on the common features across them. CBT-E consists of 20 sessions over the course of 5 months (Fairburn, 2008). In this treatment, patients identify unique individualized factors that maintain their eating disorder (e.g., dieting, overevaluation of shape or weight, frequent weighing, excessive exercise, body comparisons to others). In the beginning phase of treatment, patients are presented with psychoeducation about eating disorders and are taught to self-monitor eating disorder behaviors. The goals for this phase are to reduce the frequency of eating disorder behaviors, establish regular eating patterns, and gain weight as appropriate for underweight patients. Later stages involve targeting specific cognitive and behavioral patterns that maintain disordered eating (e.g., low body image, low self-esteem, perfectionism, negative mood intolerance). CBT-E has been shown to be effective in decreasing eating pathology across eating disorder diagnoses, and treatment progress is sustained post-treatment (Atwood & Friedman, 2020; Fairburn, 2017; Fairburn et al., 2015).

Another evidence-based treatment approach for eating disorders is interpersonal psychotherapy (IPT), which focuses on how interpersonal difficulties maintain eating pathology. IPT usually consists of 15–20 sessions over the course of 4–5 months (Wilfley & Eichen, 2017). In this treatment, patients identify how their disordered eating behaviors are both caused and exacerbated by interpersonal problems along with negative affect and low self-esteem. In the beginning phase of treatment, patients identify current and past connections between interpersonal functioning and eating disorder symptoms, focusing on at least one main target area such as grief, interpersonal role disputes, role transitions, or interpersonal deficits. As treatment progresses, the focus shifts to solutions for interpersonal problems. Research has demonstrated that

IPT is an effective treatment across eating disorders, with comparable outcomes to CBT-E (Miniati et al., 2018). Additionally, some studies show that IPT might be slower-acting, with similar treatment gains as CBT-E being seen over the longer term, although no research to date has found any factors that predict who will do better in which treatment (Cooper et al., 2016; Murphy et al., 2012; Wilfley & Eichen, 2017).

9.3 Conclusion

Appropriate research-supported assessment and intervention of eating disorders is essential to decrease their personal and societal costs. Currently fewer than 20% of those diagnosed with an eating disorder receive any type of treatment, and most treatment received is not evidence-based (Kazdin et al., 2017). Additionally, historically marginalized individuals with eating disorders are even less likely to receive evidence-based care (Kazdin et al., 2017). Myths held in society about who can have an eating disorder and the impossibility of recovery further inhibit effective treatments from reaching those in need. Furthermore, ineffective or harmful approaches serve as additional barriers for accessing quality care.

Eating disorders can be difficult to treat because individuals are often ambivalent about change; however, effective treatments such as CBT-E and IPT exist. Someone is most likely to benefit from these treatments when their disorder is diagnosed early (i.e., before symptoms become more entrenched and severe) and when they make more rapid initial changes to their eating in the initial stages of treatment (Vall & Wade, 2015). Most importantly, additional research is needed to find ways to make evidence-based treatments for eating disorders more effective and accessible to all people in need of care.

Jamie M. Loor, PhD, is a Postdoctoral Fellow at the University of New Mexico.

Jennifer Battles, PhD, is a Primary Care Clinical Psychologist and a member of the Eating Disorder Treatment Team at VA St. Louis Healthcare System.

Brooke L. Bennett, PhD, is a Postdoctoral Research Fellow at UConn's Rudd Center for Food Policy and Health.

Brooke L. Whisenhunt, PhD, is a Professor of Psychology at Missouri State University. She is co-author of the book *Psychological Disorders* 5e (2023).

Danae L. Hudson, PhD, is a Professor of Psychology at Missouri State University. She is co-author of the book *Revel Psychology* (2019).

References

American Psychiatric Association. (2013). *Diagnostic and statistical manual of mental disorders, fifth edition* (DSM-5). American Psychiatric Association.

American Psychiatric Association. (2022). *Diagnostic and statistical manual of mental disorders, fifth edition, text revision* (DSM-5-TR). American Psychiatric Association.

Andrade, G. (2017). Is past life regression therapy ethical? *Journal of Medical Ethics and History of Medicine, 10*(11), 1–8.

Arcelus, J., Mitchell, A. J., Wales, J., & Nielsen, S. (2011). Mortality rates in patients with anorexia nervosa and other eating disorders: a meta-analysis of 36 studies. *Archives of General Psychiatry, 68*(7), 724–731.

Attia, E., Blackwood, K. L., Guarda, A. S., Marcus, M. D., & Rothman, D. J. (2016). Marketing residential treatment programs for eating disorders: A call for transparency. *Psychiatric Services, 67*(6), 664–666.

Atwood, M. E., & Friedman, A. (2020). A systematic review of enhanced cognitive behavioral therapy (CBT-E) for eating disorders. *International Journal of Eating Disorders, 53*(3), 311–330.

Belon, K. E., McLaughlin, E. A., Smith, J. E., Bryan, A. D., Witkiewitz, K., Lash, D. N., & Winn, J. L. (2015). Testing the measurement invariance of the eating disorder inventory in nonclinical samples of Hispanic and Caucasian women. *International Journal of Eating Disorders, 48*(3), 262–270.

Belon, K. E., Smith, J. E., Bryan, A. D., Lash, D. N., Winn, J. L., & Gianini, L. M. (2011). Measurement invariance of the Eating Attitudes Test-26 in Caucasian and Hispanic women. *Eating Behaviors, 12*(4), 317–320.

Berkman, N. D., Lohr, K. N., & Bulik, C. M. (2007). Outcomes of eating disorders: A systematic review of the literature. *International Journal of Eating Disorders, 40*(4), 293–309.

Borden, A., & Cook-Cottone, C. (2020). Yoga and eating disorder prevention and treatment: A comprehensive review and meta-analysis. *Eating Disorders, 28*(4), 400–437.

Brennan, M. A., Whelton, W. J., & Sharpe, D. (2020). Benefits of yoga in the treatment of eating disorders: Results of a randomized controlled trial. *Eating Disorders, 28*(4), 438–457.

Coffino, J. A., Udo, T., & Grilo, C. M. (2019). Rates of help-seeking in US adults with lifetime DSM-5 eating disorders: Prevalence across diagnoses and differences by sex and ethnicity/race. *Mayo Clinic Proceedings, 94*(8), 1415–1426.

Colton, A., & Pistrang, N. (2004). Adolescents' experiences of inpatient treatment for anorexia nervosa. *European Eating Disorders Review, 12*(5), 307–316.

Cook, B., Wonderlich, S. A., Mitchell, J., Thompson, R., Sherman, R., & McCallum, K. (2016). Exercise in eating disorders treatment: Systematic review and proposal of guidelines. *Medicine and Science in Sports and Exercise*, *48*(7), 1408–1414.

Cooper, Z., Allen, E., Bailey-Straebler, S., Basden, S., Murphy, R., O'Connor, M. E., & Fairburn, C. G. (2016). Predictors and moderators of response to enhanced cognitive behaviour therapy and interpersonal psychotherapy for the treatment of eating disorders. *Behaviour Research and Therapy*, *84*, 9–13.

de la Rie, S., Noordenbos, G., Donker, M., & van Furth, E. (2006). Evaluating the treatment of eating disorders from the patient's perspective. *International Journal of Eating Disorders*, *39*, 667–676.

Dingemans, A. E., & van Furth, E. F. (2012). Binge eating disorder psychopathology in normal weight and obese individuals. *International Journal of Eating Disorders*, *45*(1), 135–138.

Elosua, P., & Hermosilla, D. (2013). Does body dissatisfaction have the same meaning for males and females? A measurement invariance study. *European Review of Applied Psychology*, *63*(5), 315–321.

Fairburn, C. G. (2008). *Cognitive behavior therapy and eating disorders*. Guilford.

Fairburn, C. G. (2017). Cognitive behavior therapy and eating disorders. In K. D. Brownell & B. T. Walsh (Eds.), *Eating disorders and obesity: A comprehensive handbook* (3rd ed., pp. 284–289). Guilford.

Fairburn, C. G., Bailey-Straebler, S., Basden, S., Doll, H. A., Jones, R., Murphy, R., O'Connor, M. E., & Cooper, Z. (2015). A transdiagnostic comparison of enhanced cognitive behaviour therapy (CBT-E) and interpersonal psychotherapy in the treatment of eating disorders. *Behaviour Research and Therapy*, *70*, 64–71.

Fogarty, S., Smith, C. A., & Hay, P. (2016). The role of complementary and alternative medicine in the treatment of eating disorders: A systematic review. *Eating Behaviors*, *21*, 179–188.

Frisch, M. J., Franko, D. L., & Herzog, D. B. (2006). Arts-based therapies in the treatment of eating disorders. *Eating Disorders*, *14*(2), 131–142.

Goodwin, H., Haycraft, E., Willis, A. M., & Meyer, C. (2011). Compulsive exercise: The role of personality, psychological morbidity, and disordered eating. *International Journal of Eating Disorders*, *44*(7), 655–660.

Grenon, R., Schwartze, D., Hammond, N., Ivanova, I., Mcquaid, N., Proulx, G., & Tasca, G. A. (2017). Group psychotherapy for eating disorders: A meta-analysis. *International Journal of Eating Disorders*, *50*(9), 997–1013.

Harper, K., Sperry, S., & Thompson, J. K. (2008). Viewership of pro-eating disorder websites: Association with body image and eating disturbances. *International Journal of Eating Disorders*, *41*(1), 92–95.

Hay, P., Chinn, D., Forbes, D., Madden, S., Newton, R., Sugenor, L., … Ward, W. (2014). Royal Australian and New Zealand College of

Psychiatrists clinical practice guidelines for the treatment of eating disorders. *Australian and New Zealand Journal of Psychiatry*, *48*(11), 977–1008.

Hay, P. J., Touyz, S., Claudino, A. M., Lujic, S., Smith, C. A., & Madden, S. (2019). Inpatient versus outpatient care, partial hospitalisation and waiting list for people with eating disorders. *Cochrane Database of Systematic Reviews*, 1(1), CD010827.

Jett, S., LaPorte, D. J., & Wanchisn, J. (2010). Impact of exposure to pro-eating disorder websites on eating behaviour in college women. *European Eating Disorders Review*, *18*(5), 410–416.

Jones, C. L., Fowle, J. L., Ilyumzhinova, R., Berona, J., Mbayiwa, K., Goldschmidt, A. B., Bodell, L. P., Stepp, S. D., Hipwell, A. E., & Keenan, K. E. (2019). The relationship between body mass index, body dissatisfaction, and eating pathology in sexual minority women. *International Journal of Eating Disorders*, *52*(6), 730–734.

Kaye, W. H., & Bulik, C. M. (2021). Treatment of patients with anorexia nervosa in the US – A crisis in care. *JAMA Psychiatry*, *78*(6), 591–592.

Kazdin, A. E., Fitzsimmons-Craft, E. E., & Wilfley, D. E. (2017). Addressing critical gaps in the treatment of eating disorders. *International Journal of Eating Disorders*, *50*(3), 170–189.

Kelly, N. R., Mitchell, K. S., Gow, R. W., Trace, S. E., Lydecker, J. A., Bair, C. E., & Mazzeo, S. (2012). An evaluation of the reliability and construct validity of eating disorder measures in white and black women. *Psychological Assessment*, *24*(3), 608–617.

Klein, A. V., & Kiat, H. (2015). Detox diets for toxin elimination and weight management: A critical review of the evidence. *Journal of Human Nutrition and Dietetics*, *28*(6), 675–686.

Lac, V. (2017). Amy's story: An existential-integrative equine-facilitated psychotherapy approach to anorexia nervosa. *Journal of Humanistic Psychology*, *57*(3), 301–312.

Lac, V., Marble, E., & Boie, I. (2013). Equine-assisted psychotherapy as a creative relational approach to treating clients with eating disorders. *Journal of Creativity in Mental Health*, *8*(4), 483–498.

Lavender, J. M., Brown, T. A., & Murray, S. B. (2017). Men, muscles, and eating disorders: An overview of traditional and muscularity-oriented disordered eating. *Current Psychiatry Reports*, *19*(6), 1–7.

Lee, C. M., & Hunsley, J. (2015). Evidence-based practice: Separating science from pseudoscience. *The Canadian Journal of Psychiatry*, *60*(12), 534–540.

Lee-Winn, A. E., Reinblatt, S. P., Mojtabai, R., & Mendelson, T. (2016). Gender and racial/ethnic differences in binge eating symptoms in a nationally representative sample of adolescents in the United States. *Eating Behaviors*, *22*, 27–33.

Lock, J. (2010). Controversies and questions in current evaluation, treatment, and research related to child and adolescent eating disorders. In W. S. Agras (Ed.), *The Oxford handbook of eating disorders* (pp. 51–72). Oxford University Press.

Marques, L., Alegria, M., Becker, A. E., Chen, C. N., Fang, A., Chosak, A., & Diniz, J. B. (2011). Comparative prevalence, correlates of impairment, and service utilization for eating disorders across US ethnic groups: Implications for reducing ethnic disparities in health care access for eating disorders. *International Journal of Eating Disorders, 44*(5), 412–420.

Miniati, M., Callari, A., Maglio, A., & Calugi, S. (2018). Interpersonal psychotherapy for eating disorders: Current perspectives. *Psychology Research and Behavior Management, 11*, 353–369.

Mitchison, D., Hay, P., Slewa-Younan, S., & Mond, J. (2014). The changing demographic profile of eating disorder behaviors in the community. *BMC Public Health, 14*(1), 1–9.

Moskowitz, L., & Weiselberg, E. (2017). Anorexia nervosa/atypical anorexia nervosa. *Current Problems in Pediatric and Adolescent Health Care, 47* (4), 70–84.

Murphy, R., Straebler, S., Basden, S., Cooper, Z., & Fairburn, C. G. (2012). Interpersonal psychotherapy for eating disorders. *Clinical Psychology & Psychotherapy, 19*(2), 150–158.

Nagata, J. M., Ganson, K. T., & Austin, S. B. (2020). Emerging trends in eating disorders among sexual and gender minorities. *Current Opinion in Psychiatry, 33*(6), 562–567.

Ochner, C. N., Gray, J. A., & Brickner, K. (2009). The development and initial validation of a new measure of male body dissatisfaction. *Eating Behaviors, 10*(4), 197–201.

Pacanowski, C. R., Diers, L., Crosby, R. D., & Neumark-Sztainer, D. (2017). Yoga in the treatment of eating disorders within a residential program: A randomized controlled trial. *Eating Disorders, 25*(1), 37–51.

Peebles, R., Wilson, J. L., Litt, I. F., Hardy, K. K., Lock, J. D., Mann, J. R., & Borzekowski, D. L. (2012). Disordered eating in a digital age: Eating behaviors, health, and quality of life in users of websites with pro-eating disorder content. *Journal of Medical Internet Research, 14*(5), e148.

Rodgers, R. F., Berry, R., & Franko, D. L. (2018). Eating disorders in ethnic minorities: An update. *Current Psychiatry Reports, 20*(10), 1–11.

Rodgers, R. F., Watts, A. W., Austin, S. B., Haines, J., & Neumark-Sztainer, D. (2017). Disordered eating in ethnic minority adolescents with overweight. *International Journal of Eating Disorders, 50*(6), 665–671.

Rouleau, C. R., & von Ranson, K. M. (2011). Potential risks of pro-eating disorder websites. *Clinical Psychology Review, 31*(4), 525–531.

Schaumberg, K., Welch, E., Breithaupt, L., Hübel, C., Baker, J. H., Munn-Chernoff, M. A., Yilmaz, Z., Ehrlich, S., Mustelin, L., Ghaderi, A., Hardaway, A. J., Bulik-Sullivan, E. C., Hedman, A. M., Jangmo, A., Nilsson, I. A. K., Wiklund, C., Yao, S., Seidel, M., & Bulik, C. M. (2017). The science behind the academy for eating disorders' nine truths about eating disorders. *European Eating Disorders Review*, *25* (6), 432–450.

Sonneville, K. R., & Lipson, S. K. (2018). Disparities in eating disorder diagnosis and treatment according to weight status, race/ethnicity, socioeconomic background, and sex among college students. *International Journal of Eating Disorders*, *51*(6), 518–526.

Sowles, S. J., McLeary, M., Optican, A., Cahn, E., Krauss, M. J., Fitzsimmons-Craft, E. E., Wilfley, D. E., & Cavazos-Rehg, P. A. (2018). A content analysis of an online pro-eating disorder community on Reddit. *Body Image*, *24*, 137–144.

Stice, E., Gau, J. M., Rohde, P., & Shaw, H. (2017). Risk factors that predict future onset of each DSM-5 eating disorder: Predictive specificity in high-risk adolescent females. *Journal of Abnormal Psychology*, *126*(1), 38–51.

Strong, S. M., Williamson, D. A., Netemeyer, R. G., & Geer, J. H. (2000). Eating disorder symptoms and concerns about body differ as a function of gender and sexual orientation. *Journal of Social and Clinical Psychology*, *19*(2), 240–255.

Strother, E., Lemberg, R., Stanford, S. C., & Turberville, D. (2012). Eating disorders in men: Underdiagnosed, undertreated, and misunderstood. *Eating Disorders*, *20*(5), 346–355.

Treasure, J., Stein, D., & Maguire, S. (2015). Has the time come for a staging model to map the course of eating disorders from high risk to severe enduring illness? An examination of the evidence. *Early Intervention in Psychiatry*, *9*(3), 173–184.

Vall, E., & Wade, T. D. (2015). Predictors of treatment outcome in individuals with eating disorders: A systematic review and meta-analysis. *International Journal of Eating Disorders*, *48*(7), 946–971.

Weber, A. M., Cislaghi, B., Meausoone, V., Abdalla, S., Mejía-Guevara, I., Loftus, P., Hallgren, E., Seff, I., Stark, L., Victora, C. G., Buffarini, R., Barros, A. J. D., Domingue, B. W., Bhuskan, D., Gupta, G. R., Nagata, J. M., Shakya, H. B., Richter, L. M., Norris, S. A., … Gender Equality, Norms and Health Steering Committee. (2019). Gender norms and health: Insights from global survey data. *The Lancet*, *393*(10189), 2455–2468.

Weiss, B. L. (2012). *Through time into healing: Discovering the power of regression therapy to erase trauma and transform mind, body, and relationships*. Simon and Schuster.

Weye, N., Momen, N. C., Christensen, M. K., Iburg, K. M., Dalsgaard, S., Laursen, T. M., Mortensen, P. B., Santamauro, D. F., Scott, J. G., Whiteford, H. A., McGrath, J. J., & Plana-Ripoll, O. (2020). Association of specific mental disorders with premature mortality in the Danish population using alternative measurement methods. *JAMA Network Open, 3* (6), e206646-e206646.

Wilfley, D. E., & Eichen, D. M. (2017). Interpersonal psychotherapy. In K. D. Brownell & B. T. Walsh (Eds.), *Eating disorders and obesity: A comprehensive handbook* (3rd ed., pp. 290–295). Guilford.

10

Insomnia

Colleen E. Carney, Parky H. Lau, and Samlau Kutana

For those suffering from insomnia, symptoms of sleeplessness may be compounded by misinformation about causes and treatments that delay obtaining effective help. A long history of pseudoscience persists to the present day. Pseudoscientific insomnia advice is appealing in that it sounds scientific; however, it is not supported by rigorous inquiry. In contrast, scientific knowledge is "knowledge based on the accumulation of empirical evidence" (Kazdin, 2003, p. 3). Thus, an evidence-based approach is derived from prior rigorous scientific inquiry. Unfortunately, dubious advice and information about insomnia disorder is widely disseminated. This advice is dubious because interpretations may extend beyond the results of a particular study, and interpretations may extrapolate from basic research to clinical applications without appropriate testing. The global insomnia market is over four billion US dollars annually, and the stakes are high. There are gadgets, products, herbs, and manual treatments purporting to help, costing money, time, and suffering. So how do we distinguish between science and pseudoscience? There are journals that publish pseudoscience, so how are patients and healthcare providers to know what works and what does not? In this chapter, we will critically examine questionable assessment and treatment practices.

Insomnia disorder (American Psychiatric Association, 2022) involves the chief complaints of difficulty falling asleep, trouble maintaining sleep, and/or experiencing nonrestorative sleep. Chronic insomnia is diagnosed when these difficulties occur at least half the nights of the week for a period of 3 months or more. However, the duration is often much longer; individuals with insomnia disorder often struggle for years on average, if not decades (e.g., Hughes et al., 2018; Young, 2005). On the other hand, acute insomnia, which refers to short-term (<3 months) sleep disruptions in response to stress, does not constitute a disorder. In addition to a chronic sleep complaint, there must be accompanying distress about the problem and a daytime complaint, such as effects on mood, energy, or cognition. Approximately 1 in 10 people meet diagnostic criteria for insomnia disorder (Garland et al., 2018; Roth, 2007) and nearly 1 out of 3 adults report at least one symptom of insomnia (Morin et al., 2006; Olfson et al., 2018). The annual cost for insomnia disorder in the United States is estimated to be more than $150 billion (Reynolds & Ebben, 2007); this substantial cost is the same in Canada as well (Daley et al., 2009). The high cost associated with insomnia disorder described above does not include management of disorders or conditions that resulted from, or were exacerbated by, chronic sleep disruptions. Moreover, the economic costs of insomnia due to lowered productivity, work accidents, and absences from work have been estimated at approximately 92 billion dollars per annum (Sivertsen et al., 2011).

10.1 Pseudoscience and Questionable Ideas

10.1.1 Diagnostic and Assessment Controversies

10.1.1.1 Retrospective Symptom Measures Have Limited Validity

One controversy is the use of retrospective symptom measures or proxies, such as movement or heart rate, in lieu of prospective experiential measures such as a sleep diary. Although sleep diaries take minimal time to complete each morning, some clients worry that behavioral monitoring of their sleep, activities, or food intake will reveal that they are doing something "wrong" or that the act of monitoring will somehow make the situation worse rather than better. In response to this worry, some therapists facilitate avoidance by replacing sleep diaries with measures assessing a different construct (e.g., a retrospective symptom measure or a device that assesses movement). However, such client reactions are important, as they reveal specific targets for psychotherapy that are essential to explore before returning to the self-monitoring component. Similarly, some clients worry that they will not accurately complete the diary, even after reassurances that the diary assesses their experience so they need not watch the clock but should simply use their best "guesstimate." Perfectionism is a predisposing factor for insomnia (e.g., Akram et al., 2017) and this reaction to the diary provides useful information addressed in psychotherapy before moving forward with monitoring.

Retrospective measures such as the well-validated Pittsburgh Sleep Quality Index (Buysse et al., 1989) are useful for determining a pre- to post-treatment subjective appraisal of symptoms; however, the construct of retrospective sleep quality appraisal is confounded by anxiety (e.g., Hartmann et al., 2015) and assesses symptoms of other sleep disorders in addition to insomnia. Therefore, it is not a substitute for sleep diaries despite otherwise sound psychometrics. The Insomnia Severity Index (ISI; Morin, 1993) is a recommended insomnia-specific retrospective measure. However, retrospective recall is not as accurate as daily recall, and because insomnia disorder is a subjective disorder of complaint, subjective prospective monitoring (e.g., Consensus Sleep Diary: Carney et al., 2012) is the gold standard for use throughout treatment.

Some devices purport to track "sleep" and unfortunately, are used by some providers in lieu of sleep diaries. Actigraphs or fitness devices may appeal to those wanting objective sleep measurement, but movement is not the same as sleep. Fitness trackers actually estimate sleep based on movement in bed. Those with insomnia are not necessarily moving while awake, so a tracker's sleep estimate is more accurately described as rest. Clinical grade actigraphs are not part of clinical assessment for insomnia because of limited validity in poor sleepers (e.g., Sadeh, 2011), although they remain an option for assessment of circadian rhythm disorders. Additionally, there are populations in which self-report is not possible, so clinical grade motion detectors may be acceptable proxies for estimation. Because the reliability of some select commercial sleep trackers are comparable to clinical grade actigraphs (Chinoy et al., 2021), they may be useful for some applications but perform poorly in those with poor sleep (i.e., the group with the most interest in using said devices). Paradoxically, the use of such devices is associated with increased sleep preoccupation (Baron et al., 2017).

10.1.1.2 Insomnia Symptoms Do Not Always Mean Insomnia Disorder

The characteristics of insomnia can differ depending on the duration of the disorder, leading to the distinction of acute insomnia and chronic insomnia. Whereas acute and chronic insomnia are symptomatically similar, the processes underlying the two conditions may be different. Ellis and colleagues (2012) propose that acute insomnia is a sleep continuity disturbance (i.e., difficulty initiating and/or maintaining sleep) occurring on at least 3 days per week, lasting between 1 week and 3 months. Acute insomnia is associated with a precipitating event or trigger, which can take the form of any stressful life event that results in a significant reduction of quality of life. Acute sleep disturbances are a normal response to stress and are therefore not diagnosable (Ellis et al., 2012). Chronic insomnia, on the other hand, may or may not have an identifiable stressor (Ellis et al., 2012). Temporary bouts of acute insomnia may represent an essential and nonpathological override of the sleep regulatory systems needed during times of stress (Ellis et al., 2012). Evolutionarily speaking, this override prevents sleep from occurring during times where it is unsafe to sleep, regardless of prior wakefulness or time of day. In most cases of acute insomnia, the override is short-lived and the individual is able to recover good sleep within a period of weeks to months (Perlis et al., 2020). For some individuals, however, negative coping factors may lead to the development of chronic insomnia (Spielman et al., 1987).

A recent prospective assessment of good sleepers found an annual incidence rate of 27% for acute insomnia compared with 1.8% for chronic insomnia (Perlis et al., 2020). Of those who developed acute insomnia, 72% recovered normal sleep, while 19% developed persistent poor sleep that did not meet threshold criteria for chronic insomnia (Perlis et al., 2020). Results from this study show that most episodes of acute insomnia do not develop into chronic insomnia. Whereas acute insomnia is related to hyperarousal due to a stressful precipitating event, chronic insomnia is maintained beyond the presence of a stressor by conditioned wakefulness and homeostatic dysregulation brought on by unhelpful forms of coping. Thus, rushing to intervene with a full treatment regimen may be unnecessary for those with acute symptoms.

Failure to detect other sleep disorders that resemble insomnia can also lead to questionable intervention choices. Someone presenting with a sleep complaint will likely use the term insomnia to describe their sleep difficulty, even if it does not meet the criteria for insomnia disorder or is better explained by another condition. There are several sleep disorders that are distinct in etiology from insomnia disorder, and thus may respond poorly or not at all to evidence-based intervention for insomnia. Sleep disorders that are distinct from insomnia can still feature frequent awakenings and nonrestorative sleep; however, they often require different treatment approaches.

One example of a sleep disorder with complaints of difficulty maintaining sleep or nonrestorative sleep is obstructive sleep apnea (Lurie, 2011). Obstructive sleep apnea is a diagnosis made only following an overnight sleep study to verify a blockage of airway passages during sleep accompanied by dozens of arousals or awakenings each hour (Lacedonia et al., 2016). Gold standard treatment for obstructive sleep apnea is to keep the airway open using continuous positive airway pressure through a mask. Likewise, periodic limb movement disorder includes complaints of poor sleep quality and sleepiness and requires a sleep study for diagnosis (Chesson et al., 1999; Hornyak et al., 2006). The most common treatments for periodic limb movement disorder are dopaminergic medications

(Aurora et al., 2012). Circadian rhythm disorders are another set of sleep disorders qualitatively different from insomnia and therefore requiring different treatment approaches. In individuals with a circadian rhythm disorder, the body clock has become weakened or desynchronized from the day and night cycles. Circadian dysfunction can be caused in the short term by job demands like shift work, east/west travel (i.e., jet lag), or a mismatch between one's chronotype and life demands, such as delayed sleep phase (Drake & Wright, 2011). Treatment for circadian rhythm disorders attempt to realign the body clock, and may include phototherapy, environment or lifestyle changes, and timely administration of exogenous melatonin (Bjorvatn & Pallesen, 2009; Lu & Zee, 2006). Careful assessment of these and other sleep disorders may be necessary before treating insomnia, should it also be present.

10.1.1.3 Chronic Insomnia Is Not Typically a Symptom of Another Disorder

Insomnia has traditionally been viewed as secondary to a variety of medical conditions, such as arthritis, chronic pain, liver disease, and chronic renal failure, among others (Benca et al., 1992; Cohen et al., 2000; Wijarnpreecha et al., 2017). It is also often seen as a symptom of common psychological disorders like depression (Riemann et al., 2001). If a treatment provider maintains this belief for all cases, it may delay their patients with insomnia from receiving effective treatment for their sleep problems, as well expose them to treatments that could worsen their sleep.

A study of the relationship between insomnia disorder and physical illness over 2 years found that sleep disturbance continues even when the other illness thought to be causing the insomnia has alleviated (Katz & McHorney, 1998). In major depressive disorder, insomnia often: (1) predates the onset of depressive episodes (Baglioni et al., 2011), (2) persists after depression treatment (Carney et al., 2007), and (3) leads to a suboptimal response to depression treatment (Zisook et al., 2019). Ultimately, the discourse surrounding whether insomnia precedes other mental or medical comorbidities or vice versa is unimportant, as the treatment remains the same and there is no validity for the diagnosis of insomnia due to a mental disorder (Edinger et al. 2011), which is why it was removed from the *Diagnostic and Statistical Manual for Mental Disorders, Fifth Edition*. Furthermore, insomnia uniquely predicts lower quality of life in individuals with chronic illnesses (Broström et al., 2004; Katz & McHorney, 2002) and often worsens the comorbid condition (Taylor et al., 2007).

10.1.2 Ineffective or Limited Treatments

There has been an increase in nonevidence-based practice at previously rigorous medical centers. For instance, Kent and colleagues (2020) surveyed sports physicians on their prescribing practices of complementary and alternative medicine and found that 88% prescribed at least one type over the past year. Presumably, they did so to provide patients with options they were already requesting, regardless of the fact that they are outside the realm of scientific evidence. Below we will discuss a variety of complementary and alternative medicines for insomnia disorder.

10.1.2.1 Magnesium

Magnesium is important for many processes in the body (Abbasi et al., 2012). Magnesium supplements are cheap and widely used as over-the-counter sleep aids, although little evidence supports their effectiveness for insomnia disorder. A recent review of studies investigating the effectiveness of magnesium supplements alone or in combination with melatonin, zinc, or B vitamins found little to no effect in older adults who ingested the magnesium-containing preparations compared with placebo. Additionally, the studies included in the review were determined to have moderate-to-high risk of bias and low-quality evidence supporting their outcomes (Mah & Pitre, 2021).

10.1.2.2 Melatonin

Perhaps the most common supplement taken for sleep is melatonin. Melatonin is a hormone secreted by the pineal gland in humans that plays a role in regulating circadian rhythms, including the sleep-wake cycle. Melatonin serum concentrations begin to rise at sunset, peak in the middle of the night, and gradually decrease during the second half of the night (Brzezinski, 1997). Melatonin supplements, timed appropriately, may help advance the sleep–wake phase in those with delayed sleep phase circadian rhythm disorder without changing sleep duration (Rajaratnam et al., 2004). Its mechanism of action is chronobiotic, not hypnotic. This makes melatonin, often in combination with phototherapy, a treatment choice for delayed sleep–wake phase syndrome (van Geijlswijk et al., 2010). There is weaker evidence for melatonin's effectiveness in synchronizing the sleep–wake cycle after disruptions caused by jet lag (Herxheimer & Petrie, 2002), shift work, and circadian rhythm disorder associated with blindness (Arendt et al., 1997; Sack et al., 2000). However, there exists no good evidence for melatonin for insomnia disorder. Melatonin studies of insomnia disorder are often limited by poor and inconsistent methodological quality (Low et al., 2020). Studies across age groups find that melatonin can reduce sleep onset latency by shifting the sleep window, but it does not consistently improve other sleep indices (Armour & Paton, 2004; Buscemi et al., 2005; Rikkert & Rigaud, 2001). Moreover, the medium- and long-term safety of routine melatonin use has yet to be established (Besag et al., 2019). In sum, melatonin is not effective in treating insomnia disorder (Buscemi et al., 2005) and the American Academy of Sleep Medicine specifically advocates against its use (Sateia et al., 2017).

10.1.2.3 Valerian

Another commonly used and widely available supplement for sleep difficulties is the herb valerian. The term valerian refers to a family of flowering plants comprising over 200 species. Valerian is typically prepared as a tea or found in extract form as a tablet or capsule. The herb is believed to cause sedation through inhibiting the breakdown of γ-aminobutyric acid (GABA) or GABA metabolites in the brain (Ringdahl et al., 2004). Studies into the effectiveness of valerian for treatment of sleep disorders is limited by inconsistency and heterogeneity in participant characteristics, study design and methodology, valerian preparations used, dose, and outcome measures assessed (Randall et al., 2008). Likewise, evidence into the effectiveness of chamomile teas and extracts for treating sleep disturbances is limited by the small sample sizes and variability of treatment preparations and outcome measures (Guadagna et al., 2020). Whereas some small studies show modest improvements in "sleep quality" in specific populations (e.g., Adib-Hajbaghery & Mousavi, 2017; Chang & Chen, 2016) these studies do not include those with clinical levels of insomnia. Multiple systematic reviews have concluded that while valerian may be safe for short-term use, the best clinical evidence available does not support its use for insomnia disorder (Leach & Page, 2015; Taibi et al., 2007).

10.1.2.4 Aromatherapy

Aromatherapy involves the use of aromatic substances, generally plant-based extracts and essential oils, which enter the body through inhalation or skin absorption, to improve bodily or mental health. There is no standardized treatment protocol for aromatherapy, and practitioners use many different plants, extracts, and oils in their preparations. Whereas the most common effect reported in aromatherapy trials is subjective retrospective sleep quality, this is not a recommended outcomes measure and these studies are limited by considerable hetero-geneity in both treatment preparation and route of administration, poor and inconsistent methodological rigor, small sample sizes, nonclinical samples, and publication bias (Lin et al., 2019).

10.1.2.5 Cannabidiol

In recent years, following decriminalization or legalization of marijuana in Canada and much of the United States (Abuhasira et al., 2018), considerable attention has been devoted to determining the therapeutic effects of canna-bis and cannabinoids (Fraguas-Sánchez & Torres-Suárez, 2018). Marijuana has sleep-interfering properties both in the short-term via rapid eye move-ment sleep (REM) suppression (Schierenbeck et al., 2008) and subsequent REM rebound (increased depth and intensity of REM sleep following deprivation), as well as the long-term, via slow wave sleep suppression (Freemon, 1982). The long-term negative effects of marijuana are slow to reverse, so marijuana cessation is unlikely to improve these side effects for several weeks to months (Hirvonen et al., 2012). The negative effects of marijuana may relate to tetrahydrocannabinol (THC). One compound found in marijuana known as cannabidiol (CBD), which often has lower amounts of THC, has gained popularity as a sleep aid. To date, there have been no randomized controlled trials investigating the effectiveness of CBD for insomnia disorder. Studies of CBD and other cannabinoids report mod-est improvements in some sleep parameters such as sleep quality; however, these studies are considered to be of low quality due to high risk of bias and heterogeneity of interventions (Bhagavan et al., 2020). A systematic review investigating CBD effectiveness for mental disorders found that evidence supporting its use in insomnia disorder was "weak" (Khan et al., 2020).

10.1.2.6 Weighted Blankets

Weighted blankets have seen a recent rise in popularity as a product intended to improve sleep. So-called deep touch pressure is theorized to stimulate hormones associated with relaxation, thus helping to alleviate anxiety (Mullen et al., 2008). Because weighted blankets only recently received mainstream attention, their empirical evidence is limited. A recent systematic review identified eight studies that examined the utility of weighted blankets in treating anxiety and insomnia (Eron et al., 2020). The researchers determined that while the blankets appeared to be helpful in reducing anxiety, results were generally inconclusive for their efficacy in treating insomnia. One study compared weighted blankets to light blankets and found a subjective preference for the heavier ones; however, there were no differences in subjective sleep quality or between prospective diary measures (Gringras et al., 2014). Overall, more research is needed to determine whether weighted blankets are a useful tool for sleep. That said, the use of weighted blankets should not be discouraged in the event that an individual subjectively finds the tool to be helpful in their own lives.

10.1.2.7 Specialty Mattresses

Many companies claim that their mattresses improve sleep. Mattress quality has been proposed to facilitate sleep by providing a comfortable surface (Buckle & Fernandes, 1998). Whereas some research has suggested that mattress quality can impact sleep quality (e.g., Antonino Vitale et al., 2019), other studies indicate otherwise (e.g., Gellis & Lichstein, 2009). Importantly, one positive study was conducted in adult athletes, not individuals with insomnia. Tonetti et al. (2011) compared the use of latex and spring mattresses, measuring subjective experiences of sleep as well as movement tracker-measured sleep. They found differences on the tracker only, not on the perception of sleep quality. These results suggest that mattresses factor into comfort, but do not resolve the underlying cause of sleep complaints in many cases, especially in chronic insomnia. More research is needed to examine the effects of mattresses on sleep in individuals with insomnia.

10.1.2.8 Homeopathy

Homeopathic remedies for sleep are widely marketed and easily found online. Reviews examining the efficacy of homeopathic treatments for insomnia find that most of the studies are poorly designed, and the well-designed studies do not support the use of homeopathic medicines (Cooper & Relton, 2010; Ernst, 2011). There are many other ineffective treatments, but the above are some of the most commonly used strategies that lack support.

10.2 Research-Supported Approaches

There are two evidence-based treatments of insomnia: cognitive behavioral therapy for insomnia (CBT-I) and pharmacologic intervention. Whereas CBT-I is the frontline recommended treatment (e.g., Qaseem et al., 2016), both approaches are considered efficacious (e.g., Sateia et al., 2017). Therefore, the decision-making process for which treatment option to consider ultimately depends on the informed goals of the patient.

10.2.1 Cognitive Behavioral Therapy for Insomnia

CBT-I is an efficacious, durable, and well-tolerated intervention seen as the gold standard treatment for insomnia disorder (e.g., Edinger et al., 2021). Components of CBT-I include sleep restriction, stimulus control, sleep hygiene, and cognitive therapy. CBT-I directly addresses the theorized causes of insomnia: irregular input into the circadian clock, disruptions to the build-up of pressure in the homeostatic process, and cognitive hyperarousal (Spielman et al., 1987). For example, the prescription of a regular, optimized time-in-bed window increases sleep pressure, increases the stimulus value of the bed, bedroom, and sleep window, and provides regular input to the circadian system (Maurer et al., 2018). In other words, CBT-I targets perpetuating factors underlying chronic insomnia.

Nearly 60% of individuals achieve clinically significant change with CBT-I, after only four biweekly sessions (Edinger et al., 2009). This is defined as a 50% reduction in mean values of wake after sleep onset and improvement on measures of subjective insomnia severity. Moreover, a recent meta-analysis determined that these effects are robust at least a year post-treatment (van der Zweerde et al., 2019), with one study finding that sleep gains were maintained over a period of 3 years (Blom et al., 2016). Whereas the efficacy of CBT-I can be attributed to the strong correspondence between the active treatment components and theorized causes of insomnia, the demonstrated robustness of the intervention may be due to the treatment's ability to re-instill a sense of self-confidence in producing high-quality sleep. In support of this latter point, studies have found that sleep self-efficacy increases post-treatment (Edinger et al., 2001; Lovato et al., 2016). Given these findings, CBT-I may be best suited for individuals with long-term sleep disruptions that are perpetuated by unhelpful sleep behaviors and sleep thoughts.

10.2.2 Sleep Medication

Hypnotics, such as benzodiazepines (e.g., lorazepam and alprazolam) and nonbenzodiazepines (e.g., the "z-drugs" zopiclone and zolpidem) are a class of psychoactive drugs with a primary purpose of treating insomnia symptoms. There is some evidence for doxepin for sleep maintenance insomnia and remelteon for sleep onset insomnia (Sateia et al., 2017), although ramelteon has not met the bar for approval by Health Canada (Health Canada, 2022). With respect to their efficacy, z-drugs are comparable to CBT-I at least in the short term (Smith et al., 2002). One added benefit of sleep medication is that it is fast-acting and does not require significant time and commitment to see benefits, making medication an attractive option for addressing immediate sleep concerns. However, these effective sleep medications may be limited in that they treat insomnia only at the symptom level; that is, the underlying causes of chronic sleep disturbances are not targeted as they are in CBT-I. Moreover, a number of negative sequelae are associated with prolonged use of hypnotics, including psychological dependence and tolerance, decreased daytime functioning and fatigue, as well as insomnia rebound (Edinoff et al., 2021). Insomnia rebound is a phenomenon in which insomnia symptoms worsen in the context of abrupt discontinuation of sleep medication.

Given that hypnotics do not address underlying factors of chronic insomnia and symptoms tend to return following discontinuation, they are not recommended for long-term use. Instead, sleep medications may be ideal in circumstances of acute stressors where sleep is likely to be disrupted for a short period of time and an individual is primarily interested in the quantity of sleep rather than quality (e.g., Daurat et al., 2000; Jacobs et al., 2004). Other medications commonly used off-label (e.g., trazodone or tiagabine) or over-the-counter drugs (e.g., diphenhydramine, melatonin, tryptophan) are not recommended by the American Academy of Sleep Medicine due to insufficient evidence of efficacy (Sateia et al., 2017).

10.3 Conclusion

Insomnia disorder is a serious psychological condition associated with myriad adverse consequences and comorbidities. Timely and evidence-based interventions are essential to reduce the social, psychological, physical, and financial costs of prolonged sleep disruptions. There are numerous misconceptions and alternative treatments with limited empirical evidence that are commonly proliferated, which may impact a person's ability to seek appropriate treatment or choose interventions that are ultimately unhelpful in resolving their sleep problems. This chapter addressed misconceptions about insomnia assessment and treatment while critically evaluating the empirical evidence of alternative and complementary medicines for insomnia. Evidence-based approaches will continue to emerge from the scientific landscape, but CBT-I has remained the most efficacious approach over five decades. It is possible that future research may produce newer and more robust treatments, but treatment decisions should be based on the best-available evidence. CBT-I remains the gold standard for treatment of chronic insomnia.

Colleen E. Carney, PhD, CPsych, is an Associate Professor of Psychology at Ryerson University in Canada. She is author of the book *Goodnight Mind for Teens: Skills to Help You Quiet Noisy Thoughts and Get the Sleep You Need* (2020).

Parky H. Lau, MA, is a doctoral student in the Psychology Department at Ryerson University in Canada.

Samlau Kutana, BA, is a graduate student in the Psychology Department at the Memorial University of Newfoundland in Canada.

References

Abbasi, B., Kimiagar, M., Sadeghniiat, K., Shirazi, M. M., Hedayati, M., & Rashidkhani, B. (2012). The effect of magnesium supplementation on primary insomnia in elderly: A double-blind placebo-controlled clinical trial. Journal of Research in Medical Sciences: *The Official Journal of Isfahan University of Medical Sciences, 17*(12), 1161–1169.

Abuhasira, R., Shbiro, L., & Landschaft, Y. (2018). Medical use of cannabis and cannabinoids containing products – Regulations in Europe and North America. *European Journal of Internal Medicine, 49*, 2–6. https://doi.org/10.1016/j.ejim.2018.01.001.

Adib-Hajbaghery, M., & Mousavi, S. N. (2017). The effects of chamomile extract on sleep quality among elderly people: A clinical trial. *Complementary Therapies in Medicine, 35*, 109–114. https://doi.org/10.1016/j.ctim.2017.09.010.

Akram, U., Ellis, J. G., Myachykov, A., Chapman, A. J., & Barclay, N. L. (2017). Anxiety mediates the relationship between multidimensional perfectionism and insomnia disorder. *Personality and Individual Differences, 104*, 82–86. https://doi.org/10.1016/j.paid.2016.07.042.

American Psychiatric Association. (2022). *Diagnostic and statistical manual of mental disorders, fifth edition, text revision* (DSM-5-TR). American Psychiatric Association.

Antonino Vitale, J., Devetag, F., Colnago, S., & La Torre, A. (2019). Effect of mattress on actigraphy-based sleep quality and perceived recovery in top-level athletes: A randomized, double-blind, controlled trial. *Biological Rhythm Research, 50*(5), 689–702. https://doi.org/10.1080/09291016.2018.1490864.

Arendt, J., Skene, D. J., Middleton, B., Lockley, S. W., & Deacon, S. (1997). Efficacy of melatonin treatment in jet lag, shift work, and blindness.

Journal of Biological Rhythms, *12*(6), 604–617. https://doi.org/10.1177/074873049701200616.

Armour, D., & Paton, C. (2004). Melatonin in the treatment of insomnia in children and adolescents. *Psychiatric Bulletin*, *28*(6), 222–224. https://doi.org/10.1192/pb.28.6.222.

Aurora, R. N., Kristo, D. A., Bista, S. R., Rowley, J. A., Zak, R. S., Casey, K. R., Lamm, C. I., Tracy, S. L., & Rosenberg, R. S. (2012). The treatment of restless legs syndrome and periodic limb movement disorder in adults— An update for 2012: Practice parameters with an evidence-based systematic review and meta-analyses. *Sleep*, *35*(8), 1039–1062. https://doi.org/10.5665/sleep.1988.

Baglioni, C., Battagliese, G., Feige, B., Spiegelhalder, K., Nissen, C., Voderholzer, U., Lombardo, C., & Riemann, D. (2011). Insomnia as a predictor of depression: A meta-analytic evaluation of longitudinal epidemiological studies. *Journal of Affective Disorders*, *135*(1–3), 10–19. https://doi.org/10.1016/j.jad.2011.01.011.

Baron, K. G., Abbott, S., Jao, N., Manalo, N., & Mullen, R. (2017). Orthosomnia: Are some patients taking the quantified self too far? *Journal of Clinical Sleep Medicine*, *13*(2), 351–354.

Benca, R. M., Obermeyer, W. H., Thisted, R. A., & Gillin, J. C. (1992). Sleep and psychiatric disorders: A meta-analysis. *Archives of General Psychiatry*, *49*(8), 651–668.

Besag, F. M., Vasey, M. J., Lao, K. S., & Wong, I. C. (2019). Adverse events associated with melatonin for the treatment of primary or secondary sleep disorders: A systematic review. *CNS Drugs*, *33*(12), 1167–1186. https://doi.org/10.1007/s40263-019-00680-w.

Bhagavan, C., Kung, S., Doppen, M., John, M., Vakalalabure, I., Oldfield, K., Braithwaite, I., & Newton-Howes, G. (2020). Cannabinoids in the treatment of insomnia disorder: A systematic review and meta-analysis. *CNS Drugs*, *34*(12), 1217–1228. https://doi.org/10.1007/s40263-020-00773-x.

Bjorvatn, B., & Pallesen, S. (2009). A practical approach to circadian rhythm sleep disorders. *Sleep Medicine Reviews*, *13*(1), 47–60. https://doi.org/10.1016/j.smrv.2008.04.009.

Blom, K., Jernelöv, S., Rück, C., Lindefors, N., & Kaldo, V. (2016). Three-year follow-up of insomnia and hypnotics after controlled internet treatment for insomnia. *Sleep*, *39*(6), 1267–1274. https://doi.org/10.5665/sleep.5850.

Broström, A., Strömberg, A., Dahlström, U., & Fridlund, B. (2004). Sleep difficulties, daytime sleepiness, and health-related quality of life in patients with chronic heart failure. *Journal of Cardiovascular Nursing*, *19*(4), 234–242. https://doi.org/10.1097/00005082-200407000-00003.

Brzezinski, A. (1997). Melatonin in humans. *New England Journal of Medicine*, *336*(3), 186–195. https://doi.org/10.5665/sleep.5850.

Buckle, P., & Fernandes, A. (1998). Mattress evaluation – Assessment of contact pressure, comfort and discomfort. *Applied Ergonomics*, *29*(1), 35–39. https://doi.org/10.1016/s0003-6870(97)00023-9.

Buscemi, N., Vandermeer, B., Hooton, N., Pandya, R., Tjosvold, L., Hartling, L., Baker, G., Klassen, T. P., & Vohra, S. (2005). The efficacy and safety of exogenous melatonin for primary sleep disorders. A meta-analysis. *Journal of General Internal Medicine*, *20*(12), 1151–1158. https://doi.org/10.1111/j.1525-1497.2005.0243.x.

Buysse, D. J., Reynolds 3rd, C. F., Monk, T. H., Berman, S. R., & Kupfer, D. J. (1989). The Pittsburgh Sleep Quality Index: A new instrument for psychiatric practice and research. *Psychiatry Research*, *28*(2), 193–213. https://doi.org/10.1016/0165-1781(89)90047-4.

Carney, C. E., Buysse, D. J., Ancoli-Israel, S., Edinger, J. D., Krystal, A. D., Lichstein, K. L., & Morin, C. M. (2012). The consensus sleep diary: standardizing prospective sleep self-monitoring. *Sleep*, *35*(2), 287–302. https://doi.org/10.5665/sleep.1642.

Carney, C. E., Segal, Z. V., Edinger, J. D., & Krystal, A. D. (2007). A comparison of rates of residual insomnia symptoms following pharmacotherapy or cognitive-behavioral therapy for major depressive disorder. *The Journal of Clinical Psychiatry*, *68*(2), 254–260. https://doi.org/10.4088/jcp.v68n0211.

Chang, S. M., & Chen, C. H. (2016). Effects of an intervention with drinking chamomile tea on sleep quality and depression in sleep disturbed postnatal women: A randomized controlled trial. *Journal of Advanced Nursing*, *72*(2), 306–315. https://doi.org/10.1111/jan.12836.

Chesson, A. L., Wise, M., Davila, D., Johnson, S., Littner, M., Anderson, W. M., Hartse, K., & Rafecas, J. (1999). Practice parameters for the treatment of restless legs syndrome and periodic limb movement disorder. An American Academy of Sleep Medicine Report. Standards of Practice Committee of the American Academy of Sleep Medicine. *Sleep*, *22*(7), 961–968. https://doi.org/10.1093/sleep/22.7.961.

Chinoy, E. D., Cuellar, J. A., Huwa, K. E., Jameson, J. T., Watson, C. H., Bessman, S. C., Hirsch, D. A., Cooper, A. D., Drummond, S., & Markwald, R. R. (2021). Performance of seven consumer sleep-tracking devices compared with polysomnography. *Sleep*, *44*(5), zsaa291. https://doi.org/10.1093/sleep/zsaa291.

Cohen, M., Menefee, L. A., Doghramji, K., Anderson, W. R., & Frank, E. D. (2000). Sleep in chronic pain: Problems and treatments. *International Review of Psychiatry*, *12*(2), 115–127. https://doi.org/10.1080/09540260050007435.

Cooper, K. L., & Relton, C. (2010). Homeopathy for insomnia: A systematic review of research evidence. *Sleep Medicine Reviews*, *14*(5), 329–337. https://doi.org/10.1016/j.smrv.2009.11.005.

Daley, M., Morin, C. M., LeBlanc, M., Grégoire, J. P., & Savard, J. (2009). The economic burden of insomnia: Direct and indirect costs for individuals with insomnia syndrome, insomnia symptoms, and good sleepers. *Sleep*, *32* (1), 55–64.

Daurat, A., Benoit, O., & Buguet, A. (2000). Effects of zopiclone on the rest/ activity rhythm after a westward flight across five time zones. *Psychopharmacology*, *149*(3), 241–245. https://doi.org/10.1007 /s002139900367.

Drake, C., & Wright, K. (2011). Shift work, shift-work disorder, and jet lag. In M. H. Kryger, T. Roth, & W. C. Dement (Eds.), *Principles and practice of sleep medicine*. 5th ed. (pp. 784–798). Elsevier. https://doi.org/10.1016 /B978-1-4160-6645-3.00071-2.

Edinger, J. D., Arnedt, J. T., Bertisch, S. M., Carney, C. E., Harrington, J. J., Lichstein, K. L., Sateia, M. J., Troxel, W. M., Zhou, E. S., Kazmi, U., Heald, J. L., & Martin, J. L. (2021). Behavioral and psychological treatments for chronic insomnia disorder in adults: an American Academy of Sleep Medicine clinical practice guideline. *Journal of Clinical Sleep Medicine*, *17*(2), 255–262. https://doi.org/10.5664/jcsm.8986.

Edinger, J. D., Olsen, M. K., Stechuchak, K. M., Means, M. K., Lineberger, M. D., Kirby, A., & Carney, C. E. (2009). Cognitive behavioral therapy for patients with primary insomnia or insomnia associated predominantly with mixed psychiatric disorders: A randomized clinical trial. *Sleep*, *32* (4), 499–510. https://doi.org/10.5665/sleep/32.4.499.

Edinger, J. D., Wohlgemuth, W. K., Radtke, R. A., Marsh, G. R., & Quillian, R. E. (2001). Cognitive behavioral therapy for treatment of chronic primary insomnia: A randomized controlled trial. *Journal of the American Medical Association*, *285*(14), 1856–1864. https://doi.org/10.1001 /jama.285.14.1856.

Edinger, J. D., Wyatt, J. K., Stepanski, E. J., Olsen, M. K., Stechuchak, K. M., Carney, C. E., Chiang, A., Crisostomo, M. I., Lineberger, M. D., Means, M. K., Radtke, R. A., Wohlgemuth, W. K., & Krystal, A. D. (2011). Testing the reliability and validity of DSM-IV-TR and ICSD-2 insomnia diagnoses: Results of a multitrait–multimethod analysis. *Archives of General Psychiatry*, *68*(10), 992–1002.

Edinoff, A. N., Wu, N., Ghaffar, Y. T., Prejean, R., Gremillion, R., Cogburn, M., Chami, A. A., Kaye, A. M., & Kaye, A. D. (2021). Zolpidem: Efficacy and side effects for insomnia. *Health Psychology Research*, *9* (1). https://doi.org /10.52965/001c.24927.

Ellis, J. G., Gehrman, P., Espie, C. A., Riemann, D., & Perlis, M. L. (2012). Acute insomnia: Current conceptualizations and future directions. *Sleep Medicine Reviews*, *16*(1), 5–14. https://doi.org/10.1016/j.smrv.2011.02.002.

Ernst, E. (2011). Homeopathy for insomnia and sleep-related disorders: A systematic review of randomised controlled trials. *Focus on Alternative and Complementary Therapies*, *16*(3), 195–199. https://doi.org/10.1111/j.2042-7166.2011.01083.x.

Eron, K., Kohnert, L., Watters, A., Logan, C., Weisner-Rose, M., & Mehler, P. S. (2020). Weighted blanket use: A systematic review. *American Journal of Occupational Therapy*, *74*(2), 1–14. https://doi.org/10.5014/ajot.2020.037358.

Fraguas-Sánchez, A. I., & Torres-Suárez, A. I. (2018). Medical use of cannabinoids. *Drugs*, *78*(16), 1665–1703. https://doi.org/10.1007/s40265-018-0996-1.

Freemon, F. R. (1982). The effect of chronically administered delta-9-tetrahydrocannabinol upon the polygraphically monitored sleep of normal volunteers. *Drug and Alcohol Dependence*, *10*(4), 345–353.

Garland, S. N., Rowe, H., Repa, L. M., Fowler, K., Zhou, E. S., & Grandner, M. A. (2018). A decade's difference: 10-year change in insomnia symptom prevalence in Canada depends on sociodemographics and health status. *Sleep Health*, *4*, 160–165. https://doi.org/10.1016/j.sleh.2018.01.003.

Gellis, L. A., & Lichstein, K. L. (2009). Sleep hygiene practices of good and poor sleepers in the United States: An internet-based study. *Behavior Therapy*, *40*(1), 1–9. https://doi.org/10.1016/j.beth.2008.02.001.

Gringras, P., Green, D., Wright, B., Rush, C., Sparrowhawk, M., Pratt, K., Allgar, V., Hooke, N., Moore, D., Zaiwalla, Z., & Wiggs, L. (2014). Weighted blankets and sleep in autistic children – A randomized controlled trial. *Pediatrics*, *134*(2), 298–306. https://doi.org/10.1542/peds.2013-4285.

Guadagna, S., Barattini, D. F., Rosu, S., & Ferini-Strambi, L. (2020). Plant extracts for sleep disturbances: A systematic review. *Evidence-Based Complementary and Alternative Medicine*, 2020, 3792390. https://doi.org/10.1155/2020/3792390.

Hartmann, J. A., Carney, C. E., Lachowski, A., & Edinger, J. D. (2015). Exploring the construct of subjective sleep quality in patients with insomnia. *The Journal of Clinical Psychiatry*, *76*(6), 768–773. https://doi.org/10.4088/jcp.14m09066.

Health Canada. (2022, February 24). What's new: Drug products. Health Canada. www.canada.ca/en/health-canada/services/drugs-health-products/drug-products/what-new-drug-products-health-canada.html

Herxheimer, A., & Petrie, K. J. (2002). Melatonin for the prevention and treatment of jet lag. *The Cochrane Database of Systematic Reviews*, (2), CD001520. https://doi.org/10.1002/14651858.CD001520.

Hirvonen, J., Goodwin, R. S., Li, C. T., Terry, G. E., Zoghbi, S. S., Morse, C., Pike, V. W., Volkow, N. D., Huestis, M. A., & Innis, R. (2012). Reversible and regionally selective downregulation of brain cannabinoid CB1 receptors in chronic daily cannabis smokers. *Molecular Psychiatry*, *17*(6), 642–649. https://doi.org/10.1038/mp.2011.82.

Hornyak, M., Feige, B., Riemann, D., & Voderholzer, U. (2006). Periodic leg movements in sleep and periodic limb movement disorder: Prevalence, clinical significance and treatment. *Sleep Medicine Reviews*, *10*(3), 169–177. https://doi.org/10.1016/j.smrv.2005.12.003.

Hughes, A. J., Turner, A. P., Alschuler, K. N., Atkins, D. C., Beier, M., Amtmann, D., & Ehde, D. M. (2018). Association between sleep problems and perceived cognitive dysfunction over 12 months in individuals with multiple sclerosis. *Behavioral Sleep Medicine*, *16*(1), 79–91. https://doi.org/10.1080/15402002.2016.1173553.

Jacobs, G. D., Pace-Schott, E. F., Stickgold, R., & Otto, M. W. (2004). Cognitive behavior therapy and pharmacotherapy for insomnia: A randomized controlled trial and direct comparison. *Archives of Internal Medicine*, *164*(17), 1888–1896. https://doi.org/10.1001/archinte.164.17.1888.

Katz, D. A., & McHorney, C. A. (1998). Clinical correlates of insomnia in patients with chronic illness. *Archives of Internal Medicine*, *158*(10), 1099–1107. https://doi.org/10.1001/archinte.158.10.1099.

Katz, D. A., & McHorney, C. A. (2002). The relationship between insomnia and health-related quality of life in patients with chronic illness. *Journal of Family Practice*, *51*(3), 229–234.

Kazdin, A. E. (2003). Methodology: What it is and why it is so important. In A. E. Kazdin (Ed.), *Methodological issues & strategies in clinical research* (pp. 5–22). American Psychological Association.

Kent, J. B., Tanabe, K. O., Muthusubramanian, A., Statuta, S. M., & MacKnight, J. M. (2020). Complementary and alternative medicine prescribing practices among sports medicine providers. *Alternative Therapies in Health & Medicine*, *26*(5), 28–32.

Khan, R., Naveed, S., Mian, N., Fida, A., Raafey, M. A., & Aedma, K. K. (2020). The therapeutic role of cannabidiol in mental health: A systematic review. *Journal of Cannabis Research*, *2*(1), 2. https://doi.org/10.1186/s42238-019-0012-y.

Lacedonia, D., Carpagnano, G. E., Sabato, R., Storto, M. M. L., Palmiotti, G. A., Capozzi, V., Barbaro, M. P. F., & Gallo, C. (2016). Characterization of obstructive sleep apnea–hypopnea syndrome (OSA) population by means of cluster analysis. *Journal of Sleep Research*, *25*(6), 724–730. https://doi.org/10.1111/jsr.12429.

Leach, M. J., & Page, A. T. (2015). Herbal medicine for insomnia: A systematic review and meta-analysis. *Sleep Medicine Reviews*, *24*, 1–12. https://doi.org/10.1016/j.smrv.2014.12.003.

Lin, P. C., Lee, P. H., Tseng, S. J., Lin, Y. M., Chen, S. R., & Hou, W. H. (2019). Effects of aromatherapy on sleep quality: A systematic review and meta-analysis. *Complementary Therapies in Medicine, 45*, 156–166. https://doi.org/10.1016/j.ctim.2019.06.006.

Lovato, N., Lack, L., & Kennaway, D. J. (2016). Comparing and contrasting therapeutic effects of cognitive-behavior therapy for older adults suffering from insomnia with short and long objective sleep duration. *Sleep Medicine, 22*, 4–12. https://doi.org/10.1016/j.sleep.2016.04.001.

Low, T. L., Choo, F. N., & Tan, S. M. (2020). The efficacy of melatonin and melatonin agonists in insomnia – An umbrella review. *Journal of Psychiatric Research, 121*, 10–23. https://doi.org/10.1016/j.jpsychires.2019.10.022.

Lu, B. S., & Zee, P. C. (2006). Circadian rhythm sleep disorders. *Chest, 130*(6), 1915–1923. https://doi.org/10.1378/chest.130.6.1915.

Lurie, A. (2011). Obstructive sleep apnea in adults: Epidemiology, clinical presentation, and rreatment options. *Obstructive Sleep Apnea in Adults, 46*, 1–42. https://doi.org/10.1159/000327660.

Mah, J., & Pitre, T. (2021). Oral magnesium supplementation for insomnia in older adults: A systematic review & meta-analysis. *BMC Complementary Medicine and Therapies, 21*(1), 125. https://doi.org/10.1186/s12906-021-03297-z.

Maurer, L. F., Espie, C. A., & Kyle, S. D. (2018). How does sleep restriction therapy for insomnia work? A systematic review of mechanistic evidence and the introduction of the Triple-R model. *Sleep Medicine Reviews, 42*, 127–138. https://doi.org/10.1016/j.smrv.2018.07.005.

Morin, C. M. (1993). *Insomnia: Psychological assessment and management.* Guilford.

Morin, C. M., LeBlanc, M., Daley, M., Gregoire, J. P., & Mérette, C. (2006). Epidemiology of insomnia: Prevalence, self-help treatments, consultations, and determinants of help-seeking behaviors. *Sleep Medicine, 7*(2), 123–130. https://doi.org/10.1016/j.sleep.2005.08.008.

Mullen, B., Champagne, T., Krishnamurty, S., Dickson, D., & Gao, R. X. (2008). Exploring the safety and therapeutic effects of deep pressure stimulation using a weighted blanket. *Occupational Therapy in Mental Health, 24*, 65–89. https://doi.org/10.1300/J004v24n01_05.

Olfson, M., Wall, M., Liu, S. M., Morin, C. M., & Blanco, C. (2018). Insomnia and impaired quality of life in the United States. *The Journal of Clinical Psychiatry, 79*(5), 17m12020. https://doi.org/10.4088/JCP.17m12020.

Perlis, M. L., Vargas, I., Ellis, J. G., Grandner, M. A., Morales, K. H., Gencarelli, A., Khader, W., Kloss, J. D., Gooneratne, N. S., & Thase, M. E. (2020). The natural history of insomnia: The incidence of acute insomnia and subsequent progression to chronic insomnia or recovery in good sleeper subjects. *Sleep, 43*(6), zsz299. https://doi.org/10.1093/sleep/zsz299.

Qaseem, A., Kansagara, D., Forciea, M. A., Cooke, M., Denberg, T. D., & Clinical Guidelines Committee of the American College of Physicians (2016). Management of chronic insomnia disorder in adults: A clinical practice guideline from the American College of Physicians. *Annals of Internal Medicine, 165*(2), 125–133. https://doi.org/10.7326/M15-2175.

Rajaratnam, S. M., Middleton, B., Stone, B. M., Arendt, J., & Dijk, D. J. (2004). Melatonin advances the circadian timing of EEG sleep and directly facilitates sleep without altering its duration in extended sleep opportunities in humans. *The Journal of Physiology, 561*(Pt 1), 339–351. https://doi.org/10 .1113/jphysiol.2004.073742.

Randall, S., Roehrs, T. A., & Roth, T. (2008). Over-the-counter sleep aid medications and insomnia. *Primary Psychiatry, 15*(5), 52–58.

Reynolds, S. A., & Ebben, M. R. (2017). The cost of insomnia and the benefit of increased access to evidence-based treatment: Cognitive behavioral therapy for insomnia. *Sleep Medicine Clinics, 12*(1), 39–46. https://doi.org/10 .1016/j.jsmc.2016.10.011.

Riemann, D., Berger, M., & Voderholzer, U. (2001). Sleep and depression – Results from psychobiological studies: An overview. *Biological Psychology, 57*(1–3), 67–103. https://doi.org/10.1016/s0301-0511(01)00090-4.

Rikkert, M. O., & Rigaud, A. S. (2001). Melatonin in elderly patients with insomnia. A systematic review. *Zeitschrift für Gerontologie und Geriatrie, 34*(6), 491–497. https://doi.org/10.1007/s003910170025.

Ringdahl, E. N., Pereira, S. L., & Delzell, J. E. (2004). Treatment of primary insomnia. *The Journal of the American Board of Family Medicine, 17*(3), 212–219. https://doi.org/10.3122/jabfm.17.3.212.

Roth T. (2007). Insomnia: Definition, prevalence, etiology, and consequences. *Journal of clinical sleep medicine, 3*(5 Suppl), S7–S10.

Sack, R. L., Brandes, R. W., Kendall, A. R., & Lewy, A. J. (2000). Entrainment of free-running circadian rhythms by melatonin in blind people. *New England Journal of Medicine, 343*(15), 1070–1077. https://doi.org/ 10.1056/nejm200010123431503.

Sadeh, A. (2011). The role and validity of actigraphy in sleep medicine: An update. *Sleep Medicine Reviews, 15*(4), 259–267. https://doi.org/10.1016/j. smrv.2010.10.001.

Sateia, M. J., Buysse, D. J., Krystal, A. D., Neubauer, D. N., & Heald, J. L. (2017). Clinical practice guideline for the pharmacologic treatment of chronic insomnia in adults: An American Academy of Sleep Medicine Clinical Practice Guideline. *Journal of Clinical Sleep Medicine, 13*(2), 307–349. https://doi.org/10.5664/jcsm.6470.

Schierenbeck, T., Riemann, D., Berger, M., & Hornyak, M. (2008). Effect of illicit recreational drugs upon sleep: Cocaine, ecstasy and marijuana. *Sleep Medicine Reviews, 12*(5), 381–389. https://doi.org/10.1016/j.smrv.2007.12.004.

Sivertsen, B., Lallukka, T., & Salo, P. (2011). The economic burden of insomnia at the workplace. An opportunity and time for intervention? *Sleep*, *34*(9), 1151–1152. https://doi.org/10.5665/sleep.1224.

Smith, M. T., Perlis, M. L., Park, A., Smith, M. S., Pennington, J., Giles, D. E., & Buysse, D. J. (2002). Comparative meta-analysis of pharmacotherapy and behavior therapy for persistent insomnia. *American Journal of Psychiatry*, *159*(1), 5–11. https://doi.org/10.1037/e323162004-002.

Spielman, A. J., Caruso, L. S., & Glovinsky, P. B. (1987). A behavioral perspective on insomnia treatment. *Psychiatric Clinics of North America*, *10*(4), 541–553. https://doi.org/10.1016/S0193-953X(18)30532-X.

Taibi, D. M., Landis, C. A., Petry, H., & Vitiello, M. V. (2007). A systematic review of valerian as a sleep aid: Safe but not effective. *Sleep Medicine Reviews*, *11*(3), 209–230. https://doi.org/10.1016/j.smrv.2007.03.002.

Tang, Y., Gong, M., Qin, X., Su, H., Wang, Z., & Dong, H. (2021). The therapeutic effect of aromatherapy on insomnia: A meta-analysis. *Journal of Affective Disorders*, *288*, 1–9. https://doi.org/10.1016/j.jad.2021.03.06.

Taylor, D. J., Mallory, L. J., Lichstein, K. L., Durrence, H. H., Riedel, B. W., & Bush, A. J. (2007). Comorbidity of chronic insomnia with medical problems. *Sleep*, *30*(2), 213–218. https://doi.org/10.1093/sleep/30.2.213.

Tonetti, L., Martoni, M., & Natale, V. (2011). Effects of different mattresses on sleep quality in healthy subjects: An actigraphic study. *Biological Rhythm Research*, *42*(2), 89–97. https://doi.org/10.1080/09291010903557187.

van der Zweerde, T., Bisdounis, L., Kyle, S. D., Lancee, J., & van Straten, A. (2019). Cognitive behavioral therapy for insomnia: A meta-analysis of long-term effects in controlled studies. *Sleep Medicine Reviews*, *48*, 101208. https://doi.org/10.1016/j.smrv.2019.08.002.

van Geijlswijk, I. M., Korzilius, H. P., & Smits, M. G. (2010). The use of exogenous melatonin in delayed sleep phase disorder: A meta-analysis. *Sleep*, *33*(12), 1605–1614. https://doi.org/10.1093/sleep/33.12.1605.

Wijarnpreecha, K., Thongprayoon, C., Panjawatanan, P., & Ungprasert, P. (2017). Insomnia and risk of nonalcoholic fatty liver disease: A systematic review and meta-analysis. *Journal of Postgraduate Medicine*, *63*(4), 226. https://doi.org/10.4103/jpgm.jpgm_140_17.

Young, T. B. (2005). Natural history of chronic insomnia. *Journal of Clinical Sleep Medicine*, *1*(04), e466–e467. https://doi.org/10.5664/jcsm.26392.

Zisook, S., Johnson, G. R., Tal, I., Hicks, P., Chen, P., Davis, L., Thase, M., Zhao, Y., Vertrees, J., & Mohamed, S. (2019). General predictors and moderators of depression remission: A VAST-D report. *American Journal of Psychiatry*, *176*(5), 348–357. https://doi.org/10.1176/appi.ajp.2018.18091079.

11

Sexual Issues

Caroline F. Pukall

Sexual issues are common, affecting up to two-thirds of individuals over the course of their lifetime (Angst et al., 2015). However, not all individuals with sexual issues will meet criteria for sexual dysfunction given that a proportion of sexual issues are short-lived and capable of resolving on their own. According to the fifth edition of the *Diagnostic and Statistical Manual of Mental Disorders* (DSM-5-TR; American Psychiatric Association [APA], 2022), sexual dysfunctions are characterized by disturbances in a person's ability to respond sexually or to experience sexual pleasure. Sexual dysfunctions consist of clinically significant (i.e., distressing and lasting at least 6 months) issues with sexual desire or interest, sexual arousal, orgasm, and vaginal penetration. For women, the specified sexual dysfunctions are sexual interest/arousal disorder, orgasmic disorder, and genito-pelvic pain/penetration disorder. For men, they are hypoactive sexual desire disorder, erectile disorder, premature (early) ejaculation, and delayed ejaculation. Sexual dysfunctions can be induced by substances or medications and are classified as such. Additional sexual dysfunctions can be diagnosed as "specified" (when a name is provided; for example, sexual aversion disorder) or "unspecified" (when a name is not provided). Despite the clear-cut divisions among the various categories of sexual dysfunctions listed above, it is important to note that they are often highly comorbid (McCabe et al., 2016). For example, genito-pelvic pain can potentially interfere with any or all aspects of sexual response, and orgasm difficulties may also coexist with problems in sexual desire.

As you may have noted, the DSM-5-TR (APA, 2022) sexual dysfunctions are based on sexual and gender/sex majorities and reflect the cis- and hetero-centric perspective of sexuality represented in the dominant sexual script in North America. The division of sexual dysfunctions according to binary birth-assigned sex (i.e., male or female) is highly problematic, given that the diagnoses seem to apply only to cisgender individuals (i.e., those whose birth-assigned sex is concordant with their gender identity; for example, designated female at birth and identifying as a woman) and not to intersex individuals (i.e., people who are born with sex characteristics that represent variability between the binary sex characteristics of males and females) or gender minorities (e.g., people whose sex assigned at birth is discordant with their gender). The issue related to gender minorities remains despite the brief explanation that symptoms and experiences that are not dependent on a person's gender or sex can be applied to gender minorities and that diagnoses related to reproductive anatomy should be based on current anatomy (APA, 2022). That is, certain sexual dysfunction diagnoses specify whether they can be experienced by males or females, the explanatory text for the sexual dysfunctions refers to binary genders and sexes, and the section on sex and gender-related diagnostic issues restricts diagnoses to binary genders and sexes. Even the direct applicability of the sexual dysfunction diagnoses to sexual minorities and to those engaging in same-sex sexual activity can be questioned; the DSM-5-TR notes that although the time specifier of 1 minute for premature ejaculation may be applied to individuals "engaged in nonvaginal sexual activities, specific duration criteria have not been established for these activities" (p. 502). In sum, it is therefore essential to recognize the biases inherent in the DSM-5 diagnoses of sexual dysfunctions.

Furthermore, each category of sexual dysfunction (e.g., orgasm) is assumed to represent a cohesive construct in which pleasure is integral and higher frequency is desired. For example, sexual desire is implicitly assumed to be pleasurable and wanted in terms of people's experiences, and low desire is pathologized, yet there is no formal recognition given to high levels of desire that may be distressful, unpleasant, or unwanted. This chapter will focus on these and related issues.

11.1 Pseudoscience and Questionable Ideas

11.1.1 Questionable Models and Assumptions

The DSM-5-TR captures many people's experiences with distressing sexual issues. Clinically significant low sexual desire and erectile issues are some of the most common sexual dysfunctions reported (McCabe et al., 2016). The DSM-5-TR also allows some flexibility in terms of unspecified and other specified sexual dysfunctions to be included, it includes the category of genito-pelvic pain/penetration disorder in order to account for pain experiences that may interfere with sexual response and pleasure (but only for women, which is problematic for men with genito-pelvic pain), and its sexual interest/arousal disorder diagnosis spans desire and arousal stages for women. However, the DSM-5-TR is based on models and assumptions that reflect dominant ideas about the inherent pleasurableness and desire for more frequent experiences of sexual response. This bias has made the process of formally recognizing and properly addressing certain sexual dysfunctions difficult.

11.1.1.1 Distinct Stages

The DSM-5-TR sexual dysfunctions are based on a three-stage sexual response cycle proposed by Helen Singler Kaplan in the 1970s (Kaplan, 1974; 1979). This framework has been in place since the DSM-III, which was published in 1980 (Angel, 2010). Kaplan's three-stage cycle was an adaptation of a four-stage sexual response cycle proposed by William Masters and Virginia Johnson in the 1960s consisting of the following stages: *excitement* (otherwise known as sexual arousal, i.e., signs of physiological sexual arousal such as penile erection, vulvar swelling, vaginal lubrication, and increased heart rate, blood pressure, muscle tension, and respiration), *plateau* (i.e., increased excitement response), *orgasm* (i.e., peak of sexual excitement, characterized by involuntary, rhythmic muscle contractions throughout the body and a sense of euphoria), and *resolution* (i.e., a return to a nonsexually aroused state; Masters & Johnson, 1966). These stages were based on recordings of physiological processes (e.g., heart rate, vasocongestion) during solitary and partnered sexual activity. Kaplan's three-stage cycle consisted of *sexual desire* (which represented the psychological, emotional, and cognitive aspects of sexual response, a dimension not captured in the four-stage cycle), *excitement* (which included the plateau stage, given that it was seen as an extension of the early process of excitement), and *orgasm* (Rowland & Gutierrez, 2017). Kaplan did not consider resolution a phase of sexual response, given that it represented an absence of sexual response (Kaplan, 1974; 1979).

Both of these sexual response cycles have been criticized on several grounds, including their linearity (i.e., that the "steps" occur in a predictable sequence with no flexibility in terms of cycling through, skipping one or some, or overlap among them), their assumption that sexual desire is a spontaneous and automatic experience, and their emphasis on physiological components of sexual response. In addition, the representativeness of the four-stage sexual response cycle has been questioned given that it was based on research in samples of carefully screened, healthy, sexually responsive, and predominantly white, cisgender, heterosexual individuals (Masters & Johnson, 1966). Newer models, such as Basson's (2000) circular model of sexual response, account for some of the issues with the earlier models, specifically concerns related to their linearity and assumptions related to the experience of spontaneous desire. These models can also represent the experiences of people who have sexual issues (Nowosielski et al., 2016). It is clear, however, that no single sexual response cycle can capture people's varied sexual experiences (Giraldi et al., 2015).

11.1.1.2 Deficiency-Based Perspective of Sexual Dysfunction

The DSM-5-TR appears to assume that most sexual dysfunctions exist when there is "not enough" of an aspect of sexual response. The diagnosis of hypoactive sexual desire disorder is characterized by a lack of sexual thoughts or fantasies and of the wish to engage in sexual activity. Sexual interest/arousal disorder and erectile disorder are generally defined as concerns related to the loss of subjective feelings of sexual pleasure and reduced associated physiological changes (e.g., sexual sensations, erection). Orgasmic disorder and delayed ejaculation refer to issues surrounding orgasms that are difficult or impossible to achieve. Premature ejaculation is described as not enough time before ejaculation occurs. Genito-pelvic pain/penetration disorder is characterized by pain and pain-related reactions (e.g., severe anxiety about penetration) experienced during sexual activity that prevents vaginal penetration, leading to "not enough" sexual activity. There are no sexual dysfunctions formally listed in the DSM-5-TR with explicit criteria documenting distressing increases in aspects of sexual response, such as having "too much" desire. Although there was discussion surrounding the inclusion of hypersexual disorder in the DSM-5 as a sexual desire disorder characterized by excessive sexual thoughts, fantasies, urges, and impulsivity (Kafka, 2010), it was ultimately rejected (Kafka, 2014).

Likewise, although 1–4% of individuals experience persistent, distressing sensations of genital arousal (e.g., throbbing, tingling) in the absence of sexual desire that may last for hours, days, weeks, or longer – a key characteristic of a condition called persistent genital arousal disorder/genito-pelvic dysesthesia (Goldstein et al., 2021) – this condition is not formally listed in the DSM-5-TR. A subset of those with this diagnosis also experience frequent, unpleasant orgasms without any trigger at all, or with minimal sexual (e.g., seeing a provocative image) or nonsexual stimulation (e.g., vibrations from riding in a vehicle; Goldstein et al., 2021). In persistent genital arousal disorder/genito-pelvic dysesthesia, there is a pattern of "too much" arousal and orgasm; however, the DSM-5 only provides formal diagnoses of sexual dysfunctions that are characterized by "too little" sexual response. This focus has likely impacted many patients' experiences in the health care system; indeed, a number of those with persistent genital arousal disorder/genito-pelvic dysesthesia have reported that their healthcare providers do not take their symptoms of "too much arousal" seriously and joke about how "lucky" they are to feel so turned on all the time (Jackowich et al., 2021). In addition, existing questionnaires of sexual function (e.g., the Female Sexual Function Index [FSFI] developed by Rosen and colleagues in 2000) that are also based on the DSM diagnoses of sexual dysfunctions also reflect the idea that "more is better" by establishing cut-offs for sexual dysfunction if scores fall below (but not above) a certain cut-off (Wiegel et al., 2005).

11.1.1.3 The Conflation of Pleasure and Sexual Response

It is relatively easy to understand how some sensations, like pain, can be distressing, unpleasant, and unwanted given that they are "naturally" aversive. It is also relatively easy to assume that sensations that occur during the sexual response cycle, like arousal, orgasm, and ejaculation, are "inherently" pleasurable and wanted. This assumption is prominent throughout the DSM-5-TR sexual dysfunctions, with no discussion surrounding the possible unpleasantness of any aspect of sexual response even though the definition of sexual dysfunction centers around a person's ability to respond sexually or to *experience sexual pleasure.* (Although genito-pelvic pain/penetration disorder, characterized by pain, is listed as a sexual dysfunction, pain is not part of the sexual response cycle; rather, it is seen as a condition that interferes with aspects of the sexual response cycle.) However, the conflation of sexual response with pleasure is not necessarily an accurate one.

In persistent genital arousal disorder/genito-pelvic dysesthesia, a key symptom is the experience of persistent, distressing, and unwanted sensations of genital arousal, and many affected individuals also experience distressing and unwanted orgasms (Goldstein et al., 2021). Related to this latter point, the criteria of the DSM-5-TR diagnosis of orgasmic disorder are: (1) significant delay in, infrequency of, or absence of orgasm, and (2) significantly reduced intensity of orgasmic sensations. There seems to be no possibility of having unpleasant orgasms or of having orgasms, too frequently or too intensely, experiences of which could be perceived as unpleasant, distressing, and unwanted. However, unpleasant orgasms exist in persistent genital arousal disorder/genito-pelvic dysesthesia. In addition, a condition called post-orgasmic illness syndrome, in which orgasm is associated with unpleasant flu-like and allergic symptoms for 7–10 days post-orgasm as well as negative cognitive and emotional consequences (e.g., decreased concentration, irritability), has been reported (Nguyen et al., 2018). Additionally, similar to men with premature ejaculation, reports of women with distressing "premature orgasm" have been described (Carvalho et al., 2011), and nonpleasurable (i.e., anhedonic) ejaculation has also been reported in the clinical literature (Gray et al., 2018). Nonclinical samples also report experiencing "bad" (i.e., negative, nonpositively perceived) orgasms during consensual sexual encounters (Chadwick et al., 2019), demonstrating that orgasms are not always pleasurable. None of these experiences seem to fit the framework apparent in the DSM-5-TR.

It is unfortunate that the idea that all aspects of sexual response are pleasurable has erased other possible perceptions of these sensations; indeed, questionnaires like the FSFI do not ask about distress or unwantedness of aspects of the sexual response cycle targeted in their items. This omission can lead to assumptions that someone with distressingly high levels of unwanted and unpleasant sexual desire and arousal is functioning well sexually and would not meet criteria for a sexual dysfunction. It is important to understand that all sensations can be perceived in a variety of ways. Even pain can be perceived as sexually pleasurable by some people. Thus, it is important to ask about people's perceptions of sexual sensations in order to correctly understand their experiences.

11.1.2 Diagnostic Controversies

In addition to issues related to assumptions in the DSM-5-TR about the inherent pleasurableness of sexual response and desire for more frequent experiences are several controversies around diagnoses that have and have not been included. This chapter will focus on sexual interest/arousal disorder (which was included in DSM-5-TR) and hypersexuality disorder (which was not).

11.1.2.1 The Evolution of Female Hypoactive Sexual Desire Disorder to Sexual Interest/Arousal Disorder

The sexual desire/interest dysfunctions are hypoactive sexual desire disorder for men and sexual interest/arousal disorder for women. The diagnosis of hypoactive sexual desire disorder characterizes clinically significant deficiencies of sexual thoughts or fantasies and desire for sexual activity, whereas the criteria for sexual interest/arousal disorder are absent/reduced interest in and initiation of sexual activity, and absent/reduced sexual thoughts or fantasies, pleasure, arousal, and genital and non-genital sensations. It is interesting to note that in previous versions of the DSM, parallel diagnoses of hypoactive sexual desire disorder existed for men and women; however, concerns were raised about overdiagnosing women. These concerns arose given the mismatch between women's experiences of desire and the criteria for hypoactive sexual desire disorder (Brotto, 2010a), which were found to be relevant in many men's experiences of sexual desire (reviewed in Brotto, 2010b) but erroneously assumed to be as relevant to women. For example, research has demonstrated that most women do not include sexual fantasies in their experience of desire despite the fact that they report having sexual fantasies (Brotto et al., 2009). In addition, women typically display a pattern of "responsive desire" (i.e., sexual desire that emerges from or is triggered by an arousing sexual situation) within periods of "sexual neutrality," as opposed to experiencing "spontaneous desire" (e.g., sexual desire that is present without much stimulation, usually in the form of thoughts or fantasies; Basson, 2000). Furthermore, 70% of women who were largely sexually satisfied reported that they wished to engage in sexual activity less than once per week (Cain et al., 2003).

The DSM-5 addressed these concerns by introducing the diagnosis of sexual interest/arousal disorder for women; however, this diagnosis has been met with controversy for several reasons. For example, it was not assessed for validity, reliability, or clinical utility (Balon & Clayton, 2014) before having been included in the DSM-5, and some were concerned that it would prevent diagnosis and much-needed care by making it too difficult to diagnose (Clayton et al., 2012). However, in a study comparing the hypoactive sexual desire disorder and sexual interest/arousal disorder criteria to examine frequency of diagnosis, O'Loughlin and colleagues (2018) found that nearly three-quarters of women with hypoactive sexual desire disorder also met criteria for sexual interest/arousal disorder. Those who were diagnosed with sexual interest/arousal disorder were characterized by more severe symptoms. Thus, the authors stated that the sexual interest/arousal disorder criteria may prevent those with mild and possibly transient interest and arousal symptoms from being overdiagnosed (O'Loughlin et al., 2018).

11.1.2.2 Hypersexuality

Hypersexuality, defined in the DSM-5 as "a stronger than usual urge to have sexual activity" (APA, 2013, p. 823), is listed as a feature of most of the paraphilic disorders (e.g., voyeuristic disorder, exhibitionistic disorder) but does not exist as a separate category. In 2010, Kafka proposed criteria for hypersexual disorder for inclusion in the DSM-5, defining it as a sexual desire disorder featuring increased frequency and intensity of sexual fantasies, arousal, urges, and behaviors as well as sexual impulsivity leading to adverse consequences (e.g., distress, impairment). However, hypersexual disorder was not included in the DSM-5 over concerns that it would pathologize "normal" behavior (Winters, 2010), provide justification for inappropriate behavior (Moser, 2011), and lacked sufficient scientific evidence (Kafka, 2014). With regards to the criticism that it would pathologize "normal" behavior, Winters (2010) argued that there is no clear boundary between "normal" and "too much" sexual expression. No comment was offered about the parallel lack of boundaries between "normal" and "too little" sexual expression as might be seen in cases of hypoactive sexual desire disorder (Reid & Kafka, 2014) or sexual interest/arousal disorder, which seems to reinforce the deficiency perspective of the DSM-5 described above. Indeed, hypersexuality on its own can characterize many "normal" aspects of life, such as engaging in casual sex, having multiple sexual partners, and being in new relationships (Winters, 2010). However, the impulsivity component in addition to the ensuing negative consequences differentiates hypersexual disorder from nonpathological hypersexuality (Kafka, 2014). In addition to a 6-month duration of symptoms, 80% of the criteria of hypersexual disorder needed to be met in order for the diagnosis to be made (and to prevent false diagnosis of high sexual desire, for example). Such a high standard for making a diagnosis does not appear to be characteristic of any of the other diagnoses in the previous version of the DSM (Kafka, 2014).

Aside from the issue of how much sexual expression is "too much," the idea of hypersexual disorder has been conflated with that of "sex addiction" (Karila et al., 2014), and the idea that sex can be addictive has also been highly controversial. Some argue that addictions can only be caused by external substances (e.g., alcohol, drugs), yet others recognize that behaviors such as gambling, eating, and sex can also be addictive (Phillips et al., 2015) because these behaviors can lead to changes in the brain consistent with substance dependency (Voon et al., 2014). Other studies indicate that sex addiction is not a "real" addiction based on physiological data (e.g., Prause et al., 2015). Although more research (Kraus et al., 2016) into the addictive nature of compulsive sexual behavior as well as the specific criteria for hypersexual disorder is needed, it is clear that people with functional impairment due to excessive and impulsive sexual behaviors exist (Kafka, 2014). In order to address the need for diagnosis and access to treatment, Kafka (2014) suggests the use of the diagnosis of "other specified disruptive, impulse-control, and conduct disorder" when utilizing the DSM-5. In addition, the most recent version of the *International Statistical Classification of Diseases and Related Health Problems* (World Health Organization, 2021) includes, as an impulse control disorder, compulsive sexual behavior disorder, which is characterized by a persistent pattern of failure to control intense, repetitive sexual impulses, or urges resulting in repetitive sexual behavior that lasts 6 or more months and causes significant distress or functional impairment.

Importantly, given the confusion around what might be diagnosed as "too much" sexual behavior and the conflation of pleasure and sexual response described above, some people with persistent genital arousal disorder/genito-pelvic dysesthesia have been misdiagnosed with hypersexual disorder or a related disorder (Anzellotti et al., 2010) based on their self-reported high levels of genital arousal (assumed to be pleasurable, wanted, and concordant with their subjective feelings of desire) and "excessive" sexual behavior (e.g., masturbation). However, in this case, their "excessive" sexual behavior is related to their motivation of decreasing their symptoms as opposed to being for sexual pleasure (Goldstein et al., 2021). Therefore, it is important to be aware of the complexities of experiences of sexual response and motivations for certain behaviors.

11.1.3 Ineffective Interventions

For centuries, doctors attempted to identify the causes of sexual (primarily erectile) issues with little knowledge of physiology. They looked to affected people's activities and histories, environment, and bodily and spiritual influences as potential sources of problems. For example, horseback riding, childhood trauma, stress, diet, unattractive women, fluid (humoral) imbalances, evil spells cast by witches, and curses from angry gods were considered "causes" of erection problems (Conis, 2008). Sometimes, the cures offered were benign in nature. Adding almonds, pistachios, dates, and recipes involving sesame and lentils to one's diet was believed to help (it did not). In addition, well-meaning but noneffective advice was given, including avoiding having sex after meals and in bathrooms and desisting from masturbation (Conis, 2008). Other treatments were more involved, including ground-up rhino horn that was to be ingested (Hsu, 2017), ground-up crocodile heart applied to the penis (Conis, 2008), subcutaneous animal sperm injections (Jonas, 2001), animal testicle transplants or grafts (Jonas, 2001), or rib cartilage or bone implanted into the penis (Bretan, 1989; Jonas, 2001). In addition, orgasm issues were treated in a so-called "sex box," in which people would sit to channel "orgone," a joyful life force (Louv, n.d.). These treatments were ineffective and entailed a variety of negative effects to the person who tried them, not to mention the animals involved (e.g., Hsu, 2017).

Although we may want to believe that we are long past the days in which sexual issues are being treated with ineffective methods that range from benign to harmful, unscientific and even detrimental treatments for sexual issues are still present today. Recently, numerous claims have been made about the effectiveness of jade eggs. A jade egg inserted into the vagina every day for at least a few hours is claimed to strengthen one's pelvic floor to increase orgasmic intensity and vaginal tightness during sexual activities involving vaginal penetration, decrease incontinence and premenstrual symptoms, treat uterine prolapse, and promote healing post-partum (Kassel, 2019). These effects are said to occur via "energy healers" that transform stored trauma and help connect to feminine energy (Kassel, 2019). There is no evidence for these claims; in fact, pelvic floor experts caution against the use of jade eggs because holding them in can create pelvic floor tension, which is associated with several distressing symptoms including pelvic pain, vaginal pain during sexual activity involving penetration, and pelvic floor muscle spasms (Kassel, 2019).

Likewise, numerous claims have been made about vaginal steaming procedures, in which one straddles a pot of hot herb water or tea for up to an hour to reap sexual health benefits, such as genital skin rejuvenation, increased sexual desire, toxin release from the reproductive system, and cleansing of the uterus (Kassel, 2021). Although touted by many celebrities, women's health experts have cautioned against the use of these procedures due to potential negative side effects, such as atypical vaginal discharge, unpleasant sensations of burning, stinging, or itching, burns, and infections (Kassel, 2021). In addition, there is no evidence of any sexual health benefits from this procedure.

Countless other ineffective and potentially harmful treatments for sexual issues exist, such as 24-karat gold sex toys for sexual pleasure, pharmacological or surgical options for penile enlargement, and so-called aphrodisiacs to increase sexual desire (e.g., chocolate, ginkgo). Based on anecdotal reports and exploiting people's hope to find a quick fix for sexual issues, these questionable procedures and devices are likely to come up readily in Internet searches, perhaps leading some to believe that they are helpful (and at least not harmful). However, empirically based quick fixes for complex issues like sexual dysfunctions are rare, and when they exist, they come with a host of contraindications. (For a useful article on how to separate quack medicine from science, see Myrhe & Sifris, 2020.)

11.2 Research-Supported Approaches

Both medical and psychological interventions exist for the effective treatment of sexual dysfunctions, and a combination of the two has been shown to be more successful than one type of treatment alone, at least for erectile disorder (Melnik et al., 2008). Studies examining combination versus singular therapy of other sexual dysfunctions are rare. Medical treatments tend to be specific to certain sexual dysfunctions; however, psychological interventions tend to focus on similar techniques and skills (e.g., reducing performance or sexual anxiety, enhancing pleasurable sensations and self-efficacy, increasing sexual flexibility) within the framework of second- and third-generation cognitive-behavioral therapies. For hypoactive sexual desire disorder or sexual interest/arousal disorder, sex therapy (Pukall & Bergeron, 2021) and pharmacotherapy (testosterone replacement in males who are hypogonadal [Corona et al., 2004], and although further studies are needed, flibanserin for premenopausal women and bremelanotide for women) are considered to be first-line treatments, yet it is important to note that treatment outcome has not been rigorously studied in hypoactive sexual desire disorder or sexual interest/arousal disorder overall (Pukall & Bergeron, 2021). For those with erectile disorder, first-line treatment is pharmacological (specifically, the phosphodiesterase type 5 inhibitors), with two second-line pharmacological treatment options in the form of intracavernosal injections and transurethral therapy (Shamloul & Ghanem, 2013). Nonpharmacological approaches to erectile disorder include vacuum constriction devices, penile prostheses (i.e., surgical implants), and sex/relationship therapy (for a review, see Pukall & Bergeron, 2021). Delayed ejaculation is usually treated medically if a physical etiology is found, and in addition, psychological treatment targeting areas such as performance anxiety, maximizing pleasure, and masturbation retraining is recommended and customized according to the client's experiences (Shin & Spitz, 2014). Interestingly, no pharmacological treatments for orgasmic disorder (the "female" equivalent of delayed ejaculation) seem to exist, and this condition is usually treated psychologically (Pukall & Bergeron, 2021). Premature ejaculation can be treated via a variety of medications, including tramodol and selective serotonin reuptake inhibitors, which have a common side effect of increasing ejaculatory latency time (for a review, see McMahon, 2015). In addition, psychological intervention may aid in decreasing performance anxiety and increasing latency time, among other targets. Genito-pelvic pain/penetration disorder is best treated depending on the type of pain experienced. For example, treatments for endometriosis and vulvodynia differ, but generally, psychological interventions, pelvic floor physical therapy, and some medical options have been found to be effective in (reviewed in Pukall & Bergeron, 2021).

11.3 Conclusion

Although the DSM-5-TR sexual dysfunctions are able to capture many people's experiences of distressing sexual issues associated with significant functional interference, they apply only to a small portion of the population. As a result, many experiences are disregarded, specifically, those of sexual and sex/gender minority individuals, those who engage in sexual activities outside of penile–vaginal intercourse, and those whose symptoms are inconsistent with the view of sexual response as being pleasurable, wanted, and concordant. In addition, assumptions of "low" levels of sexual response should be balanced with the acknowledgement of problematic "high" levels of sexual response when discussing sexual issues with clients. Furthermore, the treatment of sexual dysfunctions is complex and will likely involve multidisciplinary efforts.

Caroline F. Pukall, PhD, is a Professor of Psychology at Queen's University in Canada. She is editor of the book *Human Sexuality: A Contemporary Introduction, Third Edition* (2020).

References

American Psychiatric Association (2013). *Diagnostic and statistical manual of mental disorders, fifth edition* (DSM-5). American Psychiatric Association.
American Psychiatric Association (2022). *Diagnostic and statistical manual of mental disorders, fifth edition, text revision* (DSM-5-TR). American Psychiatric Association.

Angel, K. (2010). The history of "Female Sexual Dysfunction" as a mental disorder in the 20th century. *Current Opinion in Psychiatry*, *23*(6), 536–541. https://doi.org/10.1097/YCO.0b013e32833db7a1.

Angst, J., Hengartner, M. P., Rössler, W., Ajdacic-Gross, V., & Leeners, B. (2015). A Swiss longitudinal study of the prevalence of, and overlap between, sexual problems in men and women aged 20 to 50 years old. *The Journal of Sex Research*, *52*(8), 949–959. https://doi.org/10.1080/00224499.2014.1002556.

Anzellotti, F., Franciotti, R., Bonanni, L., Tamburro, G., Perrucci, M. G., Thomas, A., Pizzella, V., Romani, G. L., & Onofrj, M. (2010). Persistent genital arousal disorder associated with functional hyperconnectivity of an epileptic focus. *Neuroscience*, *167*(1), 88–96. https://doi.org/10.1016/j.neuroscience.2010.01.050.

Balon, R., & Clayton, A. H. (2014). Female sexual interest/arousal disorder: A diagnosis out of thin air. *Archives of Sexual Behavior*, *43*(7), 1227–1229. https://doi.org/10.1007/s10508-013-0247-1.

Basson, R. (2000). The female sexual response: A different model. *Journal of Sex & Marital Therapy*, *26*(1), 51–65. https://doi.org/10.1080/009262300278641.

Bretan Jr., P. (1989). History of the prosthetic treatment of impotence. *Urologic Clinics of North America*, *16*, 1–5.

Brotto L. A. (2010a). The DSM diagnostic criteria for hypoactive sexual desire disorder in women. *Archives of Sexual Behavior*, *39*(2), 221–239. https://doi.org/10.1007/s10508-009-9543-1.

Brotto L. A. (2010b). The DSM diagnostic criteria for Hypoactive Sexual Desire Disorder in men. *The Journal of Sexual Medicine*, *7*(6), 2015–2030. https://doi.org/10.1111/j.1743-6109.2010.01860.x.

Brotto, L. A., Heiman, J. R., & Tolman, D. L. (2009). Narratives of desire in mid-age women with and without arousal difficulties. *Journal of Sex Research*, *46*(5), 387–398. https://doi.org/10.1080/00224490902792624.

Cain, V. S., Johannes, C. B., Avis, N. E., Mohr, B., Schocken, M., Skurnick, J., & Ory, M. (2003). Sexual functioning and practices in a multi-ethnic study of midlife women: baseline results from SWAN. *Journal of Sex Research*, *40*(3), 266–276. https://doi.org/10.1080/00224490309552191.

Carvalho, S., Moreira, A., Rosado, M., Correia, D., Maia, D., & Pimentel, P. (2011). Female premature orgasm: Does this exist? *Sexologies: European Journal of Sexology*, *20*(4), 215–220. https://doi.org/10.1016/j.sexol.2011.08.008.

Chadwick, S. B., Francisco, M., & van Anders, S. M. (2019). When orgasms do not equal pleasure: Accounts of "bad" orgasm experiences during consensual sexual encounters. *Archives of Sexual Behavior*, *48*(8), 2435–2459. https://doi.org/10.1007/s10508-019-01527-7.

Clayton, A. H., DeRogatis, L. R., Rosen, R. C., & Pyke, R. (2012). Intended or unintended consequences? The likely implications of raising the bar for sexual dysfunction diagnosis in the proposed DSM-V revisions: 1. For women with incomplete loss of desire or sexual receptivity. *The Journal of Sexual Medicine, 9*(8), 2027–2039. https://doi.org/10.1111/j.1743-6109 .2012.02850.x.

Conis, E. (2008). Old cures were just a croc. Los Angeles Times. www .latimes.com/archives/la-xpm-2008-mar-17-he-esoterica17-story.html.

Corona, G., Petrone, L., Mannucci, E., Jannini, E. A., Mansani, R., Magini, A., Giommi, R., Forti, G., & Maggi, M. (2004). Psycho-biological correlates of rapid ejaculation in patients attending an andrologic unit for sexual dysfunctions. *European Urology, 46*(5), 615–622. https://doi.org/10.1016/j .eururo.2004.07.001.

Giraldi, A., Kristensen, E., & Sand, M. (2015). Endorsement of models describing sexual response of men and women with a sexual partner: An online survey in a population sample of Danish adults ages 20–65 years. *Journal of Sexual Medicine, 12*(1), 116–128. https://doi.org/10.1111/jsm.12720.

Goldstein, I., Komisaruk, B. R., Pukall, C. F., Kim, N. N., Goldstein, A. T., Goldstein, S. W., Hartzell-Cushanick, R., Kellogg-Spadt, S., Kim, C. W., Jackowich, R. A., Parish, S. J., Patterson, A., Peters, K. M., & Pfaus, J. G. (2021). International Society for the Study of Women's Sexual Health (ISSWSH) review of epidemiology and pathophysiology, and a consensus nomenclature and process of care for the management of Persistent Genital Arousal Disorder/Genito-Pelvic Dysesthesia (PGAD/GPD). *The Journal of Sexual Medicine, 18*(4), 665–697. https://doi.org/10 .1016/j.jsxm.2021.01.172.

Gray, M., Zillioux, J., Khourdaji, I., & Smith, R. P. (2018). Contemporary management of ejaculatory dysfunction. *Translational Andrology and Urology, 7*(4), 686–702. https://doi.org/10.21037/tau.2018.06.20.

Hsu, J. (2017). The hard truth about the rhino horn "aphrodisiac" market. Scientific American. www.scientificamerican.com/article/the-hard-truth-about-the-rhino-horn-aphrodisiac-market/.

Jackowich, R. A., Boyer, S. C., Bienias, S., Chamberlain, S., & Pukall, C. F. (2021). Healthcare experiences of individuals with Persistent Genital Arousal Disorder/Genito-Pelvic Dysesthesia. *Sexual Medicine, 9*(3), 100335. https://doi.org/10.1016/j.esxm.2021.100335.

Jonas, U. (2001). The history of erectile dysfunction management. *International Journal of Impotence Research, 13*(3), S3–S7.

Kafka, M. P. (2010). Hypersexual disorder: A proposed diagnosis for DSM-V. *Archives of Sexual Behavior, 39*(2), 377–400. https://doi.org/10.1007 /s10508-009-9574-7.

Kafka M. P. (2014). What happened to hypersexual disorder? *Archives of Sexual Behavior*, *43*(7), 1259–1261. https://doi.org/10.1007/s10508-014-0326-y.

Kaplan, H. S. (1974). *The new sex therapy: Active treatment of sexual dysfunctions*. Brunner/Mazel.

Kaplan, H. S. (1979). *Disorders of sexual desire and other new concepts and techniques in sex therapy*. Brunner/Mazel.

Karila, L., Wéry, A., Weinstein, A., Cottencin, O., Petit, A., Reynaud, M., & Billieux, J. (2014). Sexual addiction or hypersexual disorder: Different terms for the same problem? A review of the literature. *Current Pharmaceutical Design*, *20*(25), 4012–4020. https://doi.org/10.2174/13816128113199990619.

Kassel, G. (2019). You shouldn't use a jade egg – But if you want to do it anyway, read this. www.healthline.com/health/jade-egg.

Kassel, G. (2021). How to manage discharge and other side effects after yoni steaming. www.healthline.com/health/discharge-after-yoni-steam.

Kraus, S. W., Voon, V., & Potenza, M. N. (2016). Should compulsive sexual behavior be considered an addiction? *Addiction*, *111*(12), 2097–2106. https://doi.org/10.1111/add.13297.

Louv, J. (n.d.). The scientific assassination of a sexual revolutionary: How America interrupted Wilhlem Reich's orgasmic utopia. www.vice.com/en/article/mggzpn/the-american-quest-to-kill-wilhelm-reich-and-orgonomy.

Masters, W. H., & Johnson, V. E. (1966). *Human sexual response* (1st ed.). Little, Brown.

McCabe, M. P., Sharlip, I. D., Lewis, R., Atalla, E., Balon, R., Fisher, A. D., Laumann, E., Lee, S. W., & Segraves, R. T. (2016). Incidence and prevalence of sexual dysfunction in women and men: A consensus statement from the Fourth International Consultation on Sexual Medicine 2015. *Journal of Sexual Medicine*, *13*(2), 144–152. https://doi.org/10.1016/j.jsxm.2015.12.034.

McMahon C. G. (2015). Current and emerging treatments for premature ejaculation. *Sexual Medicine Reviews*, *3*(3), 183–202. https://doi.org/10.1002/smrj.49.

Melnik, T., Soares, B. G., & Nasello, A. G. (2008). The effectiveness of psychological interventions for the treatment of erectile dysfunction: Systematic review and meta-analysis, including comparisons to sildenafil treatment, intracavernosal injection, and vacuum devices. *The Journal of Sexual Medicine*, *5*(11), 2562–2574. https://doi.org/10.1111/j.1743-6109.2008.00872.x.

Moser C. (2011). Hypersexual disorder: Just more muddled thinking. *Archives of Sexual Behavior*, *40*(2), 227–232. https://doi.org/10.1007/s10508-010-9690-4.

Myrhe, J. & Sifris, D. (2020). The 5 signs of medical quackery: How to separate dodgy science from medical fact. www.verywellhealth.com/signs-of-medical-quackery-49505.

Nowosielski, K., Wróbel, B., & Kowalczyk, R. (2016). Women's endorsement of models of sexual response: Correlates and predictors. *Archives of Sexual Behavior*, *45*(2), 291–302. https://doi.org/10.1007/s10508-015-0611-4.

Nguyen, H., Bala, A., Gabrielson, A. T., & Hellstrom, W. (2018). Post-orgasmic illness syndrome: A review. *Sexual Medicine Reviews*, *6*(1), 11–15. https://doi.org/10.1016/j.sxmr.2017.08.006.

O'Loughlin, J. I., Basson, R., & Brotto, L. A. (2018). Women with hypoactive sexual desire disorder versus sexual interest/arousal disorder: An empirical test of raising the bar. *Journal of Sex Research*, *55*(6), 734–746. https://doi.org/10.1080/00224499.2017.1386764.

Phillips, B., Hajela, R., & Hilton, D. L. (2015). Sex addiction as a disease: Evidence for assessment, diagnosis, and response to critics. *Sexual Addiction & Compulsivity*, *22*(2), 167–192. https://doi.org/10.1080/10720162.2015.1036184.

Prause, N., Steele, V. R., Staley, C., Sabatinelli, D., & Hajcak, G. (2015). Modulation of late positive potentials by sexual images in problem users and controls inconsistent with "porn addiction." *Biological Psychology*, *109*, 192–199. https://doi.org/10.1016/j.biopsycho.2015.06.005.

Pukall, C. F., & Bergeron, S. (2021). Sexual dysfunctions. In L. G. Castonguay, T. F. Oltmanns, & A. Lott A (Eds.), *Psychopathology: From science to clinical practice* (2nd ed., pp. 369–397). Guilford Press.

Reid, R. C., & Kafka, M. P. (2014). Controversies about hypersexual disorder and the DSM-5. *Current Sexual Health Reports*, *6*(4), 259–264. https://doi.org/10.1007/s11930-014-0031-9.

Rosen, R., Brown, C., Heiman, J., Leiblum, S., Meston, C., Shansigh, R., Ferguson, D., & D'Agostino Jr.,R. (2000). The Female Sexual Function Index (FSFI): A multidimensional self-report instrument for the assessment of female sexual function. *Journal of Sex & Marital Therapy*, *16*, 191–208.

Rowland, D., & Gutierrez, B. R. (2017). Phases of the sexual response cycle. *Psychology Faculty Publications*, 62. https://scholar.valpo.edu/psych_fac_pub/62.

Shamloul, R., & Ghanem, H. (2013). Erectile dysfunction. *Lancet*, *381*(9861), 153–165. https://doi.org/10.1016/S0140-6736(12)60520-0.

Shin, D. H., & Spitz, A. (2014). The evaluation and treatment of Delayed Ejaculation. *Sexual Medicine Reviews*, *2*(3–4), 121–133. https://doi.org/10.1002/smrj.25.

Voon, V., Mole, T. B., Banca, P., Porter, L., Morris, L., Mitchell, S., Lapa, T. R., Karr, J., Harrison, N. A., Potenza, M. N., & Irvine, M. (2014). Neural correlates of sexual cue reactivity in individuals with and without compulsive sexual behaviours. *PLoS One*, *9*(7), e102419. https://doi.org/10.1371/journal.pone.0102419.

Wiegel, M., Meston, C., & Rosen, R. (2005). The Female Sexual Function Index (FSFI): Cross-validation and development of clinical cutoff scores. *Journal of Sex & Marital Therapy*, *31*(1), 1–20. https://doi.org/10.1080/00926230590475206.

Winters J. (2010). Hypersexual disorder: A more cautious approach. *Archives of Sexual Behavior*, *39*(3), 594–596. https://doi.org/10.1007/s10508-010-9607-2.

World Health Organization. (2021). *International classification of diseases for mortality and morbidity statistics* (11th revision). https://icd.who.int/browse11/l-m/en.

12

Substance Use and Addiction

Jonathan N. Stea, Igor Yakovenko, Hyoun S. Kim, and David C. Hodgins

Between 1880 and 1920, more than 500,000 people received Dr. Leslie Keeley's "Gold Cure" in over 200 locations in the United States and Europe at the Keeley Institutes (White, 1998). The "Gold Cure," also known as the "Keeley Cure," was a purported scientific treatment for alcohol and drug problems via injections and tonics – ironically, the formula was secretive and it's unlikely it contained gold. Suffice it to say, even during that time period, there was much controversy and debate with respect to the nature, effectiveness, and ethics of the treatment.

Fast forward to the present day, and the provision of evidence-based treatments for substance use and addiction has solidified its position as an ethical imperative of health professionals. Unfortunately, nonevidence-based and pseudoscientific treatments for addiction and mental health are still promoted and used within various healthcare systems (Hughes, 2008). Clinically, it is not uncommon for healthcare professionals to regularly encounter patients who have received such treatments to address their addiction-related concerns, which can include naturopathy, energy medicine, hypnosis therapies, chiropractic, and animal-assisted therapies, among myriad others.

Some pseudoscientific treatments lay claim to the idea that they target root causes of addictive disorders, such as pain, anxiety, depression, and trauma, while others opt to target more esoteric and controversial mechanisms, such as "the genetic deficiency of well-being neurotransmitters" (Addiction Reach Home, n.d.), "post-acute withdrawal syndrome" (Butehorn et al., 2017), or misalignments of the spine (subluxations; Elevate Rehab, 2017).

While the demarcation between science and pseudoscience has always remained fuzzy, it is in the service of ethical care to scientifically and critically appraise and identify potential pseudoscientific therapies for substance use and addiction.

In research and practice, addiction is most often diagnosed using two classification systems (Grant & Chamberlain, 2016): the *Diagnostic and*

Statistical Manual of Mental Disorders (DSM-5-TR; American Psychiatric Association [APA], 2022), and the *International Classification of Diseases, 11th Revision* (ICD-11; World Health Organization, 2019). In both the DSM-5-TR and the ICD-11, addiction is described as a reliable cluster of symptoms that manifest as a substance use or addictive disorder. Significant changes were made to the diagnostic criteria for addictive disorders in the DSM-5 (APA, 2013), compared to previous editions. For example, the distinction between alcohol or substance abuse and alcohol or substance dependence was removed in favor of a single substance use disorder diagnosis with mild, moderate, and severe specifiers (APA, 2013). This change occurred due to several factors including evidence that the addiction construct likely lies on a continuum of problem severity, the low reliability and validity of the abuse diagnosis, and the existence of diagnostic orphans (Hasin et al., 2013). Diagnostic orphans occurred when individuals met two of the dependence criteria and no abuse criteria, thus they would not meet criteria for substance abuse or substance dependence. Additional changes include the removal of the illegal acts criterion and the inclusion of craving. Furthermore, the threshold was dropped from 3 symptoms to 2 (out of 11), leading to concerns that the lowered threshold may artificially increase prevalence of addictive disorders (APA, 2013).

12.1 Pseudoscience and Questionable Ideas

12.1.1 Diagnostic Controversies

The term addiction reflects a complex construct and its precise conceptualization remains the subject of considerable debate (Frank & Nagel, 2017). The historical dichotomy between the moral versus disease model of addiction has modernized into competing learning (Lewis, 2018) versus neurobiological models (Koob & Volkow, 2016), respectively. The truth likely involves a compromise.

Perhaps the most significant change to the DSM-5 with respect to addictive disorders was the inclusion of gambling disorder, the first behavioral addiction recognized as such. Gambling disorder – previously called pathological gambling in the DSM-IV-TR (American Psychiatric Association, 2000) – was moved from the Impulse Control Disorder Not Otherwise Specified section to the newly created Substance-Related and Addictive Disorders section. Additionally, Internet Gaming Disorder, otherwise known as video game addiction, was included in Section III as an area that requires further study. The inclusion of gambling as an addictive disorder occurred following accumulating research that gambling shares significant similarities to substance use disorders with respect to etiology, phenomenology, neurobiological, natural history, and treatment implications (Mann et al., 2016; Petry et al., 2014).

Since the inclusion of gambling disorder, other putative behaviors have been proposed as addictions. For example, problematic internet use, sex addiction, compulsive shopping, work, exercise, food, and others have been proposed as behavioral addictions (Petry et al., 2018). Yet, the empirical evidence for the aforementioned behaviors as addictions is considerably lacking in comparison to gambling disorder. Indeed, criticisms have been brought forth regarding the diagnostic criteria proposed for emerging behavioral addictions. Specifically, Billieux and colleagues (2015) provided a satirical blueprint for creating new behavioral addictions, which consists of three steps. The first is to use a confirmatory approach with anecdotal evidence that conceptualizes excessive behavior as an addiction. Next, screening items are developed, borrowing heavily from the existing criteria for substance use and gambling disorder. The third and final step is to establish biopsychosocial correlates of other addictions. There are often significant correlates due to the screening items being borrowed from substance use and gambling disorder. This approach has led to the genuine proposal of a wide array of alleged behavioral addictions, such as Argentine tango (Targhetta et al., 2013), fortune telling (Skryabin, 2020), and daydreaming (Pietkiewicz et al., 2018), among others, which have been published in reputable peer-reviewed journals. It has been argued that the continued proliferation and scope of proposed behavioral addictions serves to overpathologize everyday behaviors, ultimately reducing the validity of the diagnosis of addictive disorders as a whole (Kardefelt-Winther et al., 2017).

12.1.2 Myths That Influence Treatment

The promotion of pseudoscientific therapies for addictive disorders is often aided by the existence of widespread myths related to evidence-based treatments of addiction, particularly the use of medication as a standalone intervention. Several factors have been documented in the research literature that may mediate or explain the reluctance for many individuals to engage with research-supported pharmacotherapies such as opioid agonist therapy for opioid use disorder. Factors include ideas like: addiction is a willful choice rather than a mental health problem (Wakeman & Rich, 2018); individuals who struggle with addiction have an addictive personality (Sadava, 1978); and individuals who enter the criminal justice system for drug-related offences should be punished rather than treated (Tonry & Lynch, 1996). The truth is that none of these myths are accurate. Modern psychological theories of addictive behaviors acknowledge that the reality is more complex. For example, studies examining personality and addiction have shown that certain personality characteristics such as high levels of neuroticism and low levels of conscientiousness do indeed predict addiction symptoms, but there is no overarching personality that predisposes someone to develop an addiction (Griffiths, 2017). Similarly, empirical evaluations of adding treatment for substance use disorders to prisons have demonstrated that offenders who complete such programs have a lower risk of rearrest than traditionally sentenced offenders and those who do not complete the program (Warner & Kramer, 2009).

The myths that discourage individuals with addiction and other mental health problems to accept pharmacotherapy may be largely driven by stigma at both the institutional and broader social levels (Wakeman & Rich, 2018). At the institutional level, there is evidence of widespread prejudice from healthcare professionals toward medication-assisted treatment for substance use, typically from abstinence-oriented professionals who disagree with the use of medications of any kind in addiction treatment (Madden, 2019). Even the commonly adopted language for opioid agonist therapy (an evidence-based treatment for opioid use disorder), *medication-assisted treatment*, suggests that the use of medication in substance abuse is an adjunct to some other kind of main treatment rather than an effective treatment in itself.

Such disparaging attitudes based on pseudoscientific information are also widespread in the general population, most palpably visible in recent reactions to the emergence of supervised consumption sites. Supervised consumption sites are an evidence-based harm reduction public health strategy for managing opioid use, aimed at reducing drug-related harm by legally permitting certain facilities to supervise people to inject and at times smoke illicit drugs under the supervision of trained staff (Hedrich, 2004). However, key systemic stakeholders like the police often report that they do not consider harm reduction to be a viable approach to population-level drug use, describing it as a form of enabling (Watson et al., 2012). Similarly, community perception of supervised consumption sites broadly reflects apprehension, concern regarding crime and public nuisance, and fear (Kolla et al., 2017). Yet, the empirical evidence for the efficacy of supervised consumption sites, as well as other harm reduction strategies such as pharmaceutical interventions and managed alcohol programs, is undeniable. Based on 30 systematic reviews, large sample data demonstrate that supervised consumption sites decrease overdoses and other risk behaviors and improve access to care; pharmaceutical interventions for addictive behaviors reduce mortality, morbidity, and substance use; and managed alcohol programs reduce alcohol consumption (Magwood et al., 2020). Given the prevalence of research-supported treatment myths, it is critical for researchers and clinicians to focus on combatting stigma to bolster the success of empirically supported interventions.

12.1.3 Implausible, Ineffective, and Potentially Harmful Treatments

12.1.3.1 Naturopathy

The Canadian Association of Naturopathic Doctors describes the purview of naturopathy as encompassing "diet and lifestyle changes, natural therapies including botanical medicine, clinical nutrition, hydrotherapy, homeopathy, naturopathic manipulation and traditional Chinese medicine/acupuncture" (Canadian Association of Naturopathic Doctors, n.d.). Naturopathy is therefore an umbrella term for a host of treatments that adopt a philosophy "to stimulate the healing power of the body and treat the underlying cause of disease" (Canadian Association of Naturopathic Doctors, n.d.). However, with respect to addiction (and many other health problems), the "underlying cause" is a multifaceted interaction of biological, psychological, and social factors. The precise nature of how naturopathy treats the underlying cause of addiction remains unclear and dependent upon the theoretical rationale for the particular naturopathic treatment. Unfortunately, naturopathic treatments for addiction are widely promoted (Association of Accredited Naturopathic Medical Colleges, 2019) in popular media and alternative medicine circles while high-quality evidence for effectiveness is typically sorely lacking.

12.1.3.2 Homeopathy

Homeopathy is a pseudoscience that was created in 1796 by Samuel Hahnemann and is predicated on the principle of "like cures like," meaning that diseases can be treated by substances that produce the same signs and symptoms in a healthy individual (Loudon, 2006). With respect to the treatment of addiction specifically, that principle is not problematic per se, as some of the strongest evidence-based treatments operate from the harm reduction perspective (e.g., opioid agonist thera-pies, nicotine replacement therapies). Homeopathy, however, also requires that its therapies involve a process of serial dilution, commonly to the extent that no molecules of the original substance remain. In other words, the final product is typically just distilled water and therefore any effects of homeopathy must be nonspecific placebo effects (World Health Organization, 2009). For this reason, homeopathy is widely con-sidered by medical experts to be a discredited approach to health as it violates the laws of physics and fundamental principles of pharmacology and biochemistry. Further, the practice of homeopathy by regulated health professionals is appropriately considered to be unethical. It is therefore disconcerting that the advertising of homeopathy as a treatment for addiction remains prevalent, as well as its study in low-quality, alternative medicine-based peer-reviewed journals (Butehorn, 2017).

12.1.3.3 Orthomolecular Medicine

Orthomolecular medicine is an ideology that hyperfocuses on the role of poor nutrition in the etiology of health conditions and therefore the use of supplements as treatment (Zell & Grundmann, 2012). The term "orthomolecular" was popularized by Linus Pauling in the context of treating psychiatric disorders (Hawkins & Pauling, 1973). With respect to addiction, a potentially harmful application of an unsupported therapy for opioid use disorder is the administration of high-dose vitamin C (Schauss, 2012). While it might be argued that extremely low-quality evidence exists for this treatment, it is often promoted in a way that is not proportional to the strength of its evidence (Gaby, n.d.). In the midst of an overdose crisis in North America, the professional mismanagement of opioid addiction can be life-threatening, especially if such a treatment is promoted in lieu of first-line opioid agonist therapies (Bergman et al., 2019). A similar argument can be made for the use of niacin (vitamin B3) in the treatment of alcohol use disorder (Prousky, 2014).

12.1.3.4 Acupuncture

Acupuncture – including auricular (ear) acupuncture – emerged as a treatment for addiction in the 1970s (Shin et al., 2017). It has been purported to improve health by balancing the flow of energy in the body (known as Qi or Chi), which supposedly moves through meridian points and connects organs and systems. The protocol involves inserting thin solid needles into such meridian points to relieve blockages in the flow of Qi, which is purported to target cravings and withdrawal symptoms by regulating dopamine and decreasing cortisol (Grant et al., 2016). With respect to addiction, an evidence base (Motlagh et al., 2016) exists that is riddled with methodological confounds and unconvincing evidence that acupuncture is superior to placebo (Ernst, 2002; Shin et al., 2017).

12.1.3.5 Energy Medicine

Energy medicine is a branch of alternative medicine that employs a variety of unequivocal pseudoscientific therapies called energy healing therapies, such as reiki, polarity therapy, healing touch, and craniosacral therapy (Ross, 2019). Energy healing therapies are premised on the idea that protocols can modulate energy balances in the human biofield or human energy field. The theoretical rationale of these therapies is completely divorced from the broader scientific literature. Even the National Center for Complementary and Integrative Health (2018) has noted that there is no scientific evidence supporting the existence of the human energy field; and with respect to the evidence base for reiki in particular, they note that "Reiki hasn't been clearly shown to be effective for any health-related purpose" (para. 2). Unfortunately, the scientifically unconvincing rationale and lack of evidence supporting the effectiveness of energy-healing therapies has not stopped their marketing toward the treatment of addiction (Addiction Rehab Toronto, n.d.; Recreate Life Counselling, n.d.; Schooler & Kantor, 2018).

12.1.3.6 Hypnosis Therapies

Hypnosis or hypnotherapy has enjoyed a long history as a controversial treatment for a variety of physical and psychiatric conditions. It dates back to eighteenth-century use by Austrian physician Franz Mesmer, after whom the term "mesmerize" was coined. Broadly speaking, hypnosis involves the induction of a deeply relaxed state – sometimes called a hypnotic trance – with increased suggestibility and suspension of critical faculties to the point where patients are given therapeutic suggestions to facilitate changes in behavior or relief of symptoms (Vickers et al., 2001). The theoretical rationale is that the hypnotized state provides opportunity for the conscious mind to present fewer barriers to psychotherapeutic exploration and insight. Notwithstanding debate about the hypothesized mechanism of change of hypnotherapy, the evidence base is limited with respect to its treatment for addiction. The treatment of cigarette smoking boasts the most research, whereby a recent Cochrane review of 14 studies concluded that there is no clear evidence that hypnotherapy is better than other approaches with a possible small benefit if a benefit is indeed present (Barnes et al., 2019). Unfortunately, the use of hypnosis can be hijacked as a mechanism of change for the promotion of adapted pseudoscientific therapies. For example, past life regression therapy is an unequivocally pseudoscientific therapy that is predicated on the reincarnation hypothesis and has been used to treat mental health disorders including addiction by using hypnosis to recover memories from events that an individual went through before they were born in this life (Gabor, n.d.; Swerdloff, 2017). It is unethical and potentially harmful (Andrade, 2017).

12.1.3.7 Chiropractic

Chiropractic care focuses on treating health conditions by correcting misalignments of the spine known as subluxations (Shelley et al., 2015). There is no shortage of claims that chiropractic use is an effective treatment for addiction (Laikin & Mcintyre, 2020; Press Release PR Newswire, 2019), whereby the rationale is that subluxation corrections can alter neurotransmitter functioning to the extent that it can relieve cravings (Elevate Rehab, 2017). While there is some evidence of an association between chiropractic use and lower opioid receipt among patients with spinal pain (Corcoran et al., 2020), there have been no clinical trials to our knowledge evaluating chiropractic use specifically for the treatment of addiction.

12.1.3.8 Animal-Assisted Therapy

A variety of animal-assisted therapies have been purported to be effective treatments for mental disorders as well as addiction – including, for example, dolphin-assisted therapy (Luxury Rehab, n.d.), equine-assisted therapy (Smith, 2020), and even wolf-assisted therapy (New Method Wellness, n.d.). Numerous ill-defined mechanisms of change are typically offered, such as the ability of animal-assisted therapy to facilitate "balancing internal feelings" and "banishing negative emotions" (Smith, 2020, para. 3). Research examining the effectiveness of animal-assisted therapy is plagued by threats to validity and seriously flawed data and conclusions to the extent that the current evidence base does not justify its marketing and use for mental disorders and addiction (Anestis et al., 2014). Moreover, ethical concerns have been raised from the standpoint of captive animal welfare and risk of disease spread (Marino & Lilienfeld, 2007).

12.1.3.9 Miscellaneous

It is an unfortunate reality that such a vast variety of pseudoscientific and otherwise questionable treatments for addiction exist that the space constraints of a book chapter cannot adequately accommodate their coverage. Some other honorable mentions that are not only without a systematic evidence base but in all cases are widely promoted and implausible due to a disconnect from the broader scientific addiction literature include: hyperbaric oxygen therapy (Epifanova, 1995); biosound therapy (Sylvermist, n.d.); and ideologically designed and dubious components of particular rehabilitation programs (e.g., "New Life Detoxification," "Brain Mapping," etc.; Baum, 2020). Additionally, ethically questionable and potentially harmful medical procedures have been studied with limited evidence, including ultra-rapid detoxification to treat opioid addiction (Lawental, 2000), and apneic paralysis with succinylcholine and aversion therapy to treat alcohol addiction (Madill et al., 1966).

12.1.4 The Gray Zone: Plausible and Emerging Treatments with Limited Support

12.1.4.1 12-Step Programs

12-Step-based programs are predicated on the philosophy of Alcoholics Anonymous, Narcotics Anonymous, Gamblers Anonymous, and others that view addiction as a lifelong disease and therefore promote an abstinence-based recovery approach (Wilson, 2001). They have always been controversial in the addiction community. While these programs are most commonly delivered in the community as peer-support groups in the form of unstructured and nonmanualized meetings, there are also more structured, time-limited, treatment manual approaches to 12-step programs known as 12-Step-Facilitation (Bergman et al., 2019). Many recovery residences throughout North America (sometimes referred to as "sober living" or "sober houses") are based on 12-step principles, whereby some encourage or even mandate that residents maintain abstinence.

Despite the fact that 12-step programs remain highly variable in terms of the nature and quality of programs offered in the community, more structured 12-Step-Facilitation programs have empirical support for alcohol use disorder (Kaskutas et al., 2009; Litt et al., 2016; Project MATCH Research Group, 1998; Walitzer et al., 2009) and other substance use disorders, including cannabis (Kelley et al., 2017), cocaine (Crits-Christoph et al., 1999), and other stimulant use disorders (Donovan et al., 2013).

12-Step programs can become problematic when they undermine other evidence-based treatments and pathways to recovery by promoting a rigid, abstinence-based trajectory. For example, first-line treatments for opioid use disorder are opioid agonist therapies (Bergman et al., 2019). Some recovery residences and 12-step programs may prohibit opioid agonist therapies, which can lead to stigmatization and alienation that can undermine a feeling of social connectedness, a purported mechanism of change of 12-step programs (Bergman et al., 2019). From a systematic, empirical standpoint, the effectiveness for 12-step programs in the treatment of opioid use disorder is largely unknown.

12.1.4.2 Psychedelics

The last several years have seen an emergence of research evaluations of psychedelic compounds as novel treatment approaches for mental health concerns including addiction. The majority of this work focuses on administration of psilocybin and ketamine for the treatment of anxiety (Griffiths et al., 2016), depression (Carhart-Harris et al., 2018), and addictive behaviors like alcohol use (Bogenschutz et al., 2015), and nicotine (Johnson et al., 2017). Other hallucinogens such as LSD, peyote, ibogaine, and ayahuasca have been explored as medicinal treatments for substance abuse (Winkelman, 2014). While the exact mechanisms of action vary, these compounds are thought to potentially impact mood and behavior via the serotonergic system, similar to antidepressants, and produce acute effects of euphoria, hallucinations, changes in perception, and spiritual experiences (Romeo et al., 2020).

Of all the evaluated psychedelic and hallucinogenic substances, psilocybin and ketamine have received the most empirical support in their ability to improve mental health and addiction symptoms. Recent meta-analytic evidence has provided support for large effects of psilocybin in combination with behavioral interventions for the treatment of anxiety and depression in both the general medical context (Goldberg et al., 2020) and specifically for mental health problems arising from life-threatening diseases (Vargas et al., 2020). It has also received some support in promoting long-term abstinence from cigarette smoking

(Johnson et al., 2017) and reducing craving and increasing abstinence self-efficacy in participants with alcohol use disorder (Bogenschutz et al., 2015).

Despite the initial evidence for the use of psychedelics to treat addictive behaviors and mental health problems, there appears to be a significant incongruency between the amount and quality of such evidence and the eager adoption of these agents in healthcare and social communities, particularly in North America. Mainstream outlets such as *Scientific American* (Jacobson, 2017) and the U.S. Food & Drug Administration (U.S. FDA, 2019) have touted psychedelics as "breakthroughs" and have approved them in the United States in cases of treatment-resistant depression. Similarly, premier institutions such as the Johns Hopkins University have founded centers dedicated to psychedelic and consciousness research. Yet, an examination of the existing evidence for the efficacy of psychedelics for the treatment of addiction and mental health reveals a slender amount of evidence. Reported meta-analyses are comprised of only 4–5 studies per diagnostic category, have small sample sizes (20–30 participants), and reveal a myriad of publication biases including lack of blinding and high attrition (Goldberg et al., 2020). Furthermore, when it comes to addictive behaviors, minimal recent empirical research exists to support the use of anything other than psilocybin in experimental treatments (Bogenschutz et al., 2015; Johnson et al., 2017). Consequently, widespread experimentation and approval of psychedelics for clinical application is at best premature and at worst dangerous given that many of them demonstrate high rates of dissociation and other transient side effects (Schifano et al., 2019). For now, these treatments remain firmly labeled as plausible, with some preliminary support for their use in the treatment of addiction and mental health problems, but not enough to group them alongside evidence-based treatments, such as cognitive-behavioral therapy.

12.1.4.3 Cannabis

Cannabis has been touted in popular media as a panacea for nearly all ailments, including cancer (Hodgekiss, 2014) and COVID-19 (Hill, 2020). While cannabis addiction (Zehra et al., 2018) itself is an important topic, part of the discussion has reversed in recent years as cannabis has been promoted as a treatment for other substance addictions (Marijuana Doctors, 2020), most notably opioid addiction (Kounang, 2018). The pitch is that cannabis could serve not only as a harm reduction strategy, but also as a way to treat particular addiction symptoms, such as withdrawal and cravings. Some pre-clinical studies have supported the rationale and funding of future research into cannabis treatment given the relationship of the endocannabinoid and endogenous opioid systems (Wiese & Wilson-Poe, 2018). Some state regulations in the United States (e.g., New York, Illinois) have approved medical cannabis as a treatment for opioid addiction despite critiques of these policies cautioning against the dearth of evidence to support and promote cannabis treatment (American Society for Addiction Medicine, n.d.). There is also a strong argument to be made that substituting cannabis for evidence-based opioid agonist therapies could be harmful (Humphreys & Saitz, 2019).

12.2 Research-Supported Approaches

A large number of treatments for substance use disorders have a strong empirical base, although availability and accessibility to the public varies considerably. Despite substantial research over many decades, we remain without reliable indicators of how exactly to match a person to the treatment that is likely to be most beneficial. Even at the level of outpatient versus inpatient treatment, the evidence is unreliable. In practice, individual choice – hopefully informed choice – and practical issues often guide treatment decisions. Fortunately, given a strong evidence base, it might be said that there is reason for optimism insofar as many evidence-based options are available if a first-line treatment is unsuccessful.

Psychosocial evidence-based treatments include brief interventions, which target individuals with mild to moderate addiction-related problems, often in primary care settings (Elzerbi et al., 2015). Brief interventions include a brief patient assessment and feedback followed by behavior change advice. Motivational interviewing is a variant of a brief intervention that is often delivered in one to four sessions (Miller & Rollnick, 2013). The motivational interviewing model, in contrast to brief interventions, focuses on eliciting the individual's motivations for changing their addictive behaviors and supporting their self-efficacy in achieving change. Motivational interviewing has become one of the most popular and frequently evaluated addiction treatment approaches (Magill et al., 2017) with the added benefit that it can be integrated with other treatment approaches (Miller et al., 2019). These other evidence-based treatment approaches can include branches of cognitive-behavioral therapy, such as focusing on behavioral coping skills (Kadden et al., 1992), contingency management to provide incentives for patient engagement and progress (Petry, 2012), and the community reinforcement approach to organize positive reinforcement for treatment goals (Hunt & Azrin, 1973). The community reinforcement approach includes a broader focus on family and systemic influences, which are also features of behavioral couple's therapy and various evidence-based family therapies for the treatment of addiction in adolescents. While there is much variability with respect to the nature and quality of mindfulness meditation-based therapies as an adjunct to addiction treatment, there is a growing body of randomized clinical trials that generally demonstrate positive effects (e.g., Witkiewitz et al., 2013).

Medications are playing an increasing role in addiction treatment. The strongest evidence base is for opioid agonist therapies in the treatment of opioid addiction, including methadone and buprenorphine (Bergman et al., 2019). These medications can be used alone or in conjunction with psychosocial treatment. With respect to alcohol addiction, disulfiram has a long history as a deterrent to alcohol use. While the evidence base for disulfiram is mixed, outcomes are generally positive when adherence is promoted or monitored (see reviews by Hughes & Cook, 1997; Miller & Wilbourne, 2002). Other medications with consistent support as adjuncts to psychosocial alcohol addiction treatment include naltrexone, which blocks the rewarding effects of alcohol and opioids, as well as topiramate, an antiepileptic and migraine medication (Miller et al., 2019).

It is common for people who experience addiction-related concerns to also experience concerns with mental health. The term "concurrent disorders" is used to describe the phenomenon whereby addictive disorders and mental disorders commonly co-occur. For example, a meta-analytic review found that a substance use disorder increases the likelihood of experiencing a mental health problem by 200–300% (Lai et al., 2015). It has been estimated that up to half of individuals may experience a concurrent disorder in their lifetime (McKee, 2017). Although addictive and mental disorders commonly co-occur, treatment streams delivered in the community have tended to separate the treatment of addiction and mental health in the context of either a sequential or parallel treatment model (Szerman et al., 2019), which can lead to inadequate outcomes. In a sequential treatment model, addiction and mental health concerns are addressed one after another, whereas in a parallel treatment model, addiction and mental health concerns are addressed at the same time, but by different teams of clinicians. Instead, increasing evidence supports the idea that an integrated treatment model to concurrent disorders is beneficial. In an integrated model, both addiction and mental health concerns are treated simultaneously by the same team of clinicians.

Integrated treatments have been shown to lead to improved outcomes for substance use and mental health problems (Torrens et al., 2012) as well as being more cost-effective compared to nonintegrated treatments (Karapareddy, 2019).

12.3 Conclusion

It's not uncommon for evidence-based health care professionals to encounter patients who have received pseudoscientific therapies to address their addiction-related concerns. The late and great Scott O. Lilienfeld delineated exactly why pseudoscientific therapies can be harmful: they can cause direct harm, they can indirectly drain both time and money from evidence-based treatments, and they can erode the public's trust in science (Lilienfeld et al., 2014). While researchers and clinicians must concede that the identification of pseudoscience is best achieved via a constellation of warning signs rather than a single demarcation criterion, we must remain cognizant of our ethical duty to provide the best available evidence-based care.

Jonathan N. Stea, PhD, RPsych, is an Adjunct Assistant Professor of Psychology at the University of Calgary in Canada. He is co-editor of the book *Investigating Clinical Psychology: Pseudoscience, Fringe Science, and Controversies* (2023).

Igor Yakovenko, PhD, RPsych, is an Assistant Professor of the Department of Psychology at Dalhousie University in Canada.

Hyoun S. Kim, PhD, is an Assistant Professor of Psychology at Ryerson University in Canada. He is also Director of the Addictions and Mental Health Lab.

David C. Hodgins, PhD, RPsych, FCAHS, is a Professor of Psychology at the University of Calgary in Canada. He is co-editor of the book *Research and Measurement Issues in Gambling Studies* (2007).

References

Addiction Reach Home. (n.d.). Chiropractic. www.addictionreach.com/custom-services-chiropractic.php.

Addiction Rehab Toronto. (n.d.). Reiki. https://addictionrehabtoronto.ca/reiki/.

American Psychiatric Association (2000). *Diagnostic and statistical manual of mental disorders, fourth edition, text revision* (DSM-IV-TR). American Psychiatric Association.

American Psychiatric Association. (2013). *Diagnostic and statistical manual of mental disorders* (5th ed.). https://doi.org/10.1176/appi.books.9780890 425596.

American Psychiatric Association (2022). *Diagnostic and statistical manual of mental disorders, fifth edition, text revision* (DSM-5-TR). American Psychiatric Association.

American Society of Addiction Medicine. (n.d.). American Society of Addiction Medicine. www.asam.org/asam-home-page.

Andrade, G. (2017). Is past life regression therapy ethical? *Journal of Medical Ethics and History of Medicine, 10*, 11.

Anestis, M. D., Anestis, J. C., Zawilinksi, L. L., Hopkins, T. A., & Lilienfeld, S. O. (2014). Equine-related treatments for mental disorders lack empirical support: A systematic review of empirical investigations. *Journal of Clinical Psychology, 70*(12), 1115–1132. https://doi.org/10.1002/jclp.22113.

Association of Accredited Naturopathic Medical Colleges. (2019, August 28). Can naturopathic approaches help win the battle against substance abuse? https:// aanmc.org/featured-articles/naturopathic-approaches-pain-addiction/.

Barnes, J., McRobbie, H., Dong, C. Y., Walker, N., & Hartmann-Boyce, J. (2019). Hypnotherapy for smoking cessation. *Cochrane Database for Systematic Reviews*, (6), CD001008. https://doi.org/10.1002/14651858 .CD001008.pub3.

Baum, G. (2020, February 27). Meet the controversial doctor behind the Dr. Phil empire. The Hollywood Reporter. www.hollywoodreporter.com/features/ controversial-therapist-shaping-dr-phil-1281050.

Bergman, B. G., Fallah-Sohy, N., Hoffman, L., & Kelly, J. F. (2019). Psychosocial approaches in the treatment of opioid use disorders. In J. F. Kelly & S. Wakeman (Eds.), *Treating opioid addiction* (pp. 109–138). Humana. https://doi.org/10.1007/978-3-030-16257-3_6.

Billieux, J., Schimmenti, A., Khazaal, Y., Maurage, P., & Heeren, A. (2015). Are we overpathologizing everyday life? A tenable blueprint for behavioral addiction research. *Journal of Behavioral Addictions, 4*(3), 119–123. https://doi.org/10.1556/2006.4.2015.009.

Bogenschutz, M. P., Forcehimes, A. A., Pommy, J. A., Wilcox, C. E., Barbosa, P. C. R., & Strassman, R. J. (2015). Psilocybin-assisted treatment for alcohol dependence: A proof-of-concept study. *Journal of Psychopharmacology, 29*(3), 289–299. https://doi.org/10.1177/02698811 14565144.

Butehorn, L. (2017). Post-acute withdrawal syndrome, relapse, prevention, and homeopathy. *Alternative and Complementary Therapies, 23*(6), 228–230. http://doi.org/10.1089/act.2017.29139.lbu.

Butehorn, L., Gumz, P., & Randolph L. (2017). Use of homeopathic nux vomica in reducing PAWS (post acute withdrawal syndrome) in early recovering addicted women. *International Journal of Complementary & Alternative Medicine*, 6(4). https://doi.org/10.15406/ijcam.2017.06.00197.

Canadian Association of Naturopathic Doctors. (n.d.). About naturopathic medicine. www.cand.ca/about-naturopathic-medicine/.

Carhart-Harris, R. L., Bolstridge, M., Day, C. M. J., Rucker, J., Watts, R., Erritzoe, D. E., Kaelen, M., Giribaldi, B., Bloomfield, M., Pilling, S., Rickard, J. A., Forbes, B., Feilding, A., Taylor, D., Curran, H. V., & Nutt, D. J. (2018). Psilocybin with psychological support for treatment-resistant depression: Six-month follow-up. *Psychopharmacology*, 235(2), 399–408. https://doi.org/10.1007/s00213-017-4771-x.

Corcoran, K. L., Bastian, L. A., Gunderson, C. G., Steffens, C., Brackett, A., & Lisi, A. J. (2020). Association between chiropractic use and opioid receipt among patients with spinal pain: A systematic review and meta-analysis. *Pain Medicine*, 21(2), e139–e145. https://doi.org/10.1093/pm/pnz219.

Crits-Christoph, P., Siqueland, L., Blaine, J., Frank, A., Luborsky, L., Onken, L. S., Muenz, L. R., Thase, M. E., Weiss, R. D., Gastfriend, D. R., Woody, G. E., Barber, J. P., Butler, S. F., Daley, D., Salloum, I., Bishop, S., Najavits, L. M., Lis, J., Mercer, D., . . . Beck, A. T. (1999). Psychosocial treatments for cocaine dependence: National institute on drug abuse collaborative cocaine treatment study. *Archives of General Psychiatry*, 56(6), 493–502. https://doi.org/10.1001/archpsyc.56.6.493.

Donovan, D. M., Daley, D. C., Brigham, G. S., Hodgkins, C. C., Perl, H. I., Garrett, S. B., Doyle, S. R., Floyd, A. S., Knox, P. C., Botero, C., Kelley, T. M., Killeen, T. K., Hayes, C., Baumhofer, N. K., Seamans, C., & Zammarelli, L. (2013). Stimulant abuser groups engage in 12-step: Multisite trial in the National Institute on Drug Abuse clinical trials network. *Journal of Substance Abuse Treatment*, 44(1), 103–114. https://doi.org/10.1016/j.jsat.2012.04.004.

Elevate Rehab. (2017, July 18). Chiropractic care in addiction recovery and substance abuse treatment. Elevate Addiction Services. https://elevaterehab.org/chiropractic-care-addiction-recovery-substance-abuse-treatment/.

Elzerbi, C., Donoghue, K., & Drummond, C. (2015). A comparison of the efficacy of brief interventions to reduce hazardous and harmful alcohol consumption between European and non-European countries: A systematic review and meta-analysis of randomized controlled trials. *Addiction*, 110(7), 1082–1091. https://doi.org/10.1111/add.12960.

Epifanova, N. M. (1995). Hyperbaric oxygenation in the treatment of patients with drug addiction, narcotic addiction and alcoholism in the post-intoxication and abstinence periods. *Anesteziologiia i Reanimatologiia*, (3), 34–39.

Ernst, E. (2002). Complementary therapies for addictions: Not an alternative. *Addiction, 97*(12), 1491–1492. https://doi.org/10.1046/j.1360-0443.2002.00281.x.

Frank L. E., & Nagel S. K. (2017). Addiction and moralization: The role of the underlying model of addiction. *Neuroethics, 10*(1), 129–139. https://doi.org/10.1007/s12152-017-9307-x.

Gabor, E. (n.d.). Past life regression therapy. Past Life Regression Therapy. https://drgabor.com/past-life-regression-therapy/.

Gaby, A. (n.d.). Nutritional treatments for opioid addiction. Naturopathic CE. www.naturopathicce.com/natnotes/nutritional-treatments-for-opioid-addiction/.

Goldberg, S. B., Pace, B. T., Nicholas, C. R., Raison, C. L., & Hutson, P. R. (2020). The experimental effects of psilocybin on symptoms of anxiety and depression: A meta-analysis. *Psychiatry Research, 284*, 112749. https://doi.org/10.1016/j.psychres.2020.112749.

Grant, J. E., & Chamberlain, S. R. (2016). Expanding the definition of addiction: DSM-5 vs. ICD-11. *CNS Spectrums, 21*(4), 300–303. https://doi.org/10.1017/S1092852916000183.

Grant, S., Kandrack, R., Motala, A., Shanman, R., Booth, M., Miles, J., Sorbero, M., & Hempel, S. (2016). Acupuncture for substance use disorder: A systematic review and meta-analysis. *Drug and Alcohol Dependence, 163*, 1–15. https://doi.org/10.1016/j.drugalcdep.2016.02.034.

Griffiths, M. D. (2017). The myth of 'addictive personality'. *Global Journal of Addiction & Rehabilitation Medicine (GJARM), 3*(2), 555610. https://doi.org/10.19080/GJARM.2017.03.555610.

Griffiths, R. R., Johnson, M. W., Carducci, M. A., Umbricht, A., Richards, W. A., Richards, B. D., Cosimano, M. P., & Klinedinst, M. A. (2016). Psilocybin produces substantial and sustained decreases in depression and anxiety in patients with life-threatening cancer: A randomized double-blind trial. *Journal of Psychopharmacology, 30*(12), 1181–1197. https://doi.org/10.1177/0269881116675513

Hasin, D. S., O'Brien, C. P., Auriacombe, M., Borges, G., Bucholz, K., Budney, A., Compton, W. M., Crowley, T., Ling, W., Petry, N. M., Schuckit, M., & Grant, B. F. (2013). DSM-5 criteria for substance abuse disorders: Recommendations and rationale. *The American Journal of Psychiatry, 170*(8), 834–851. https://doi.org/10.1176/appi.ajp.2013.12060782.

Hawkins, D. R., & Pauling, L. (1973). *Orthomolecular psychiatry: Treatment of schizophrenia.* W. H. Freeman.

Hedrich, D. (2004). *European report on drug consumption rooms* (p. 8). Luxembourg: Office for Official Publications of the European Communities.

Hill, K. P. (2020). Cannabinoids and the Coronavirus. *Cannabis and Cannabinoid Research*, *5*(2), 118–120. https://doi.org/10.1089/can .2020.0035.

Hodgekiss, A. (2014, July 21). Grandfather, 63, claims he cured his cancer with 'Breaking Bad' style homemade cannabis oil. Daily Mail. www.dailymail .co.uk/health/article-2699875/I-cured-cancer-CANNABIS-OIL.html.

Hughes, B. M. (2008). How should clinical psychologists approach complementary and alternative medicine? Empirical, epistemological, and ethical considerations. *Clinical Psychology Review*, *28*(4), 657–675. https://doi .org/10.1016/j.cpr.2007.09.005.

Hughes, J. C., & Cook, C. C. (1997). The efficacy of disulfiram: A review of outcome studies. *Addiction*, *92*(4), 381–395.

Humphreys, K. & Saitz, R. (2019). Should physicians recommend replacing opioids with cannabis? *Journal of the American Medical Association*, *321* (7), 639–640. https://doi.org/10.1001/jama.2019.0077.

Hunt, G. M., & Azrin, N. H. (1973). A community-reinforcement approach to alcoholism. *Behaviour Research and Therapy*, *11*(1), 91–104. https://doi.org /10.1016/0005-7967(73)90072-7.

Jacobson, R. (2017). Treating addiction with psychedelics. Scientific American. www.scientificamerican.com/article/treating-addiction-with-psychede lics/.

Johnson, M. W., Garcia-Romeu, A., & Griffiths, R. R. (2017). Long-term follow-up of psilocybin-facilitated smoking cessation. *The American Journal of Drug and Alcohol Abuse*, *43*(1), 55–60. https://doi.org/10.3109 /00952990.2016.1170135.

Kadden, R., Carroll, K., Donovan, D. M., Conney, N., Monti, P., Abrams, D. B., & Hester, R. (1992). *Cognitive-behavioral coping skills therapy manual*. National Institute on Alcohol Abuse and Alcoholism.

Karapareddy, V. (2019). A review of integrated care for concurrent disorders: Cost effectiveness and clinical outcomes. *Journal of Dual Diagnosis*, *15*(1), 56–66. https://doi.org/10.1080/15504263.2018.1518553.

Kardefelt-Winther, D., Heeren, A., Schimmenti, A., van Rooij, A., Maurage, P., Carras, M., Edman, J., Blaszczynski, A., Khazaal, Y., & Billieux, J. (2017). How can we conceptualize behavioural addiction without pathologizing common behaviours? *Addiction*, *112*(10), 1709–1715. https://doi.org/10 .1111/add.13763.

Kaskutas, L. A., Subbaraman, M. S., Witbrodt, J., & Zemore, S. E. (2009). Effectiveness of making Alcoholics Anonymous easier: A group format 12-step facilitation approach. *Journal of Substance Abuse Treatment*, *37*(3), 228–239. https://doi.org/10.1016/j.jsat.2009.01.004.

Kelley, J. F., Kaminer, Y., Kahler, C. W., Hoeppner, B., Yeterian, J., Cristello, J. V., & Timko, C. (2017). A pilot randomized clinical trial testing integrated 12-step facilitation (iTSF) treatment for adolescent substance abuse disorder. *Addiction*, *112*(12), 2155–2166. https://doi.org/10.1111/add .13920.

Kolla, G., Strike, C., Watson, T. M., Jairam, J., Fischer, B., & Bayoumi, A. M. (2017). Risk creating and risk reducing: Community perceptions of supervised consumption facilities for illicit drug use. *Health, Risk & Society*, *19*(1–2), 91–111. https://doi.org/10.1080 /13698575.2017.1291918.

Koob, G. F., & Volkow, N. D. (2016). Neurobiology of addiction: A neurocircuitry analysis. *Lancet Psychiatry*, *3*(8), 760–773. https://doi .org/10.1016/S2215-0366(16)00104-8.

Kounang, N. (2018, April 29). Getting off opioids with medical marijuana: Patients turn to pot over pills. CNN. www.cnn.com/2018/04/29/health/med ical-marijuana-opioids/index.html.

Lai, H. M. X., Cleary, M., Sitharthan, T., & Hunt, G. E. (2015). Prevalence of comorbid substance use, anxiety and mood disorders in epidemiological surveys, 1990–2014: A systematic review and meta-analysis. *Drug and Alcohol Dependence*, *154*, 1–13. https://doi.org/10.1016/j.drugalcdep .2015.05.031.

Laikin, E., & McIntyre, P. (2020, February 18). *Spinal adjustments eyed as treatment for addiction*. Long Island Press. www.longislandpress.com /2020/02/18/spinal-adjustments-eyed-as-treatment-for-addiction/.

Lawental, E. (2000). Ultra rapid opiate detoxification as compared to 30-day inpatient detoxification program – A retrospective follow-up study. *Journal of Substance Abuse*, *11*(2), 173–181. https://doi.org/10.1016 /S0899-3289(00)00019-5.

Lewis, M. (2018). Brain change in addiction as learning, not disease. *New England Journal of Medicine*, *379*(16), 1551–1560. https://doi.org/10.1056 /NEJMra1602872.

Lilienfeld, S. O., Lynn, S. J., & Lohr, J. M. (2014). *Science and pseudoscience in clinical psychology*. The Guilford Press.

Litt, M. D., Kadden, R. M., Tennen, H., & Kabela-Cormier, E. (2016). Network Support II: Randomized controlled trial of Network Support treatment and cognitive behavioral therapy for alcohol use disorder. *Drug Alcohol Dependence*, *165*, 203–212. https://doi.org/10.1016/j .drugalcdep.2016.06.010.

Loudon, I. (2006). A brief history of homeopathy. *Journal of the Royal Society of Medicine*, *99*(12), 607–610.

Luxury Rehab. (n.d.). Luxury rehab centers with dolphin therapy. https://luxur yrehabs.com/activities/dolphin-therapy/.

Madden, E. F. (2019). Intervention stigma: How medication-assisted treatment marginalizes patients and providers. *Social Science & Medicine, 232,* 324–331. https://doi.org/10.1016/j.socscimed.2019.05.027.

Madill, M. F., Campbell, D., Laverty, S. G., Sanderson, R. E., & Vandewater, S. L. (1966). Aversion treatment of alcoholics by succinylcholine-induced apneic paralysis; An analysis of early changes in drinking behavior. *Journal of Studies on Alcohol and Drugs, 27*(3), 483–509. https://doi.org/10.15288/qjsa.1966.27.483.

Magill, M., Apodaca, T. R., Borsari, B., Gaume, J., Hoadley, A., Gordon, R. E. F., Tonigan, J. S., & Moyers, T. (2017). A meta-analysis of motivational interviewing process: Technical, relational, and conditional process models of change. *Journal of Consulting and Clinical Psycholgy, 86* (2), 140–157.

Magwood, O., Salvalaggio, G., Beder, M., Kendall, C., Kpade, V., Daghmach, W., Habonimana, G., Marshall, Z., Snyder, E., O'Shea, T., Lennox, R., Hsu, H., Tugwell, P., & Pottie, K. (2020). The effectiveness of substance use interventions for homeless and vulnerably housed persons: A systematic review of systematic reviews on supervised consumption facilities, managed alcohol programs, and pharmacological agents for opioid use disorder. *PLoS One, 15*(1), e0227298. https://doi.org/10.1371/journal.pone.0227298.

Mann, K., Fauth-Bühler, M., Higuchi, S., Potenza, M. N., & Saunders, J. B. (2016). Pathological gambling: A behavioral addiction. *World Psychiatry, 15*(3), 297–298. https://doi.org/10.1002/wps.20373.

Marijuana Doctors. (2020, April 7). Medical marijuana and alcoholism. www.marijuanadoctors.com/conditions/alcoholism/.

Marino, L., & Lilienfeld, S. O. (2007). Dolphin-assisted therapy: More flawed data and more flawed conclusions. *Journal of the International Society for Anthrozoology, 20*(3), 239–249. https://doi.org/10.2752/089279307X224782.

McKee, S. A. (2017). Concurrent substance use disorders and mental illness: Bridging the gap between research and treatment. *Canadian Psychology/Psychologie Canadienne, 58*(1), 50–57. https://doi.org/10.1037/cap0000093.

Miller, W. R., Forcehimes, A., & Zweben, A. (2019). *Treating addiction: A guide for professionals* (2nd ed.). Guilford.

Miller, W. R., & Rollnick, S. (2013). *Motivational interviewing: Helping people change* (3rd ed.). Guilford.

Miller, W. R., & Wilbourne, P. L. (2002). Mesa Grande: A methodological analysis of clinical trials of treatments for alcohol use disorders. *Addiction, 97*(3), 265–277. https://doi.org/10.1046/j.1360-0443.2002.00019.x.

Motlagh, F. E., Ibrahim, F., Rashid, R. A., Seghatoleslam, T., & Habil, H. (2016). Acupuncture therapy for drug addiction. *Chinese Medicine, 11*(16). https://doi.org/10.1186/s13020-016-0088-7.

New Method Wellness. (n.d.). Wolf-assisted therapy. www.newmethodwellness.com/treatment-methods/wolf-assisted-therapy/.

Petry, N. (2012). *Contingency management for substance abuse treatment: A guide to implementing this evidence-based treatment.* Routledge.

Petry, N. M., Blanco, C., Auriacombe, M., Borges, G., Bucholz, K., Crowley, T. J., Grant, B. F., Hasin, D. S., & O'Brien, C. (2014). An overview of and rationale for changes proposed for pathological gambling in DSM-5. *Journal of Gambling Studies, 30*(2), 493–502. https://doi.org/10.1007/s10899-013-9370-0.

Petry, N. M., Zajac, K., & Ginley, M. K. (2018). Behavioral addictions as mental disorders: To be or not to be? *Annual Review of Clinical Psychology, 14*, 399–423. https://doi.org/10.1146/annurev-clinpsy-032816-045120.

Pietkiewicz, I. J., Nęcki, S., Bańbura, A., & Tomalski, R. (2018). Maladaptive daydreaming as a new form of behavioral addiction. *Journal of Behavioral Addictions, 7*(3), 838–843. https://doi.org/10.1556/2006.7.2018.95.

Press Release PR Newswire. (2019, October 14). A specific spinal adjustment is the latest development in the science of treating drug addiction. Markets Insider. https://markets.businessinsider.com/news/stocks/a-specific-spinal-adjustment-is-the-latest-development-in-the-science-of-treating-drug-addiction-1028597224.

Project MATCH Research Group. (1998). Matching alcoholism treatments to client heterogeneity: Treatment main effects and matching effects on drinking during treatment. *Journal of Studies on Alcohol and Drugs, 59*(6), 631–639. https://doi.org/10.15288/jsa.1998.59.631.

Prousky, J. E. (2014). The treatment of alcoholism with vitamin B3. *Journal of Orthomolecular Medicine, 29*(3), 123–131.

Recreate Life Counselling. (n.d.). Reiki energy healing. www.recreatelifecounseling.com/reiki-healing/.

Romeo, B., Karila, L., Martelli, C., & Benyamina, A. (2020). Efficacy of psychedelic treatments on depressive symptoms: A meta-analysis. *Journal of Psychopharmacology, 34*(10), 1079–1085. https://doi.org/10.1177/0269881120919957.

Ross, C. L. (2019). Energy medicine: Current status and future perspectives. *Global Advances in Health and Medicine, 8.* https://doi.org/10.1177/2164956119831221.

Sadava, S. W. (1978). Etiology, personality and alcoholism. *Canadian Psychological Review/Psychologie Canadienne, 19*(3), 198–214. https://doi.org/10.1037/h0081476.

Schauss, A. G. (2012). Attenuation of heroin withdrawal syndrome by the administration of high-dose vitamin C. *Journal of Orthomolecular Medicine*, 27(4), 189–197.

Schifano, F., Napoletano, F., Chiappini, S., Orsolini, L., Guirguis, A., Corkery, J. M., Bonaccorso, S., Ricciardi, A., Scherbaum, N., & Vento, A. (2019). New psychoactive substances (NPS), psychedelic experiences and dissociation: Clinical and clinical pharmacological issues. *Current Addiction Reports*, 6(2), 140–152. https://doi.org/10.1007/s40429-019-00249-z.

Schooler, D., & Kantor, I. (2018, November 1). The power of energy healing for addictive disorders. The Sober World. www.thesoberworld.com/2014/11/01/power-energy-healing-addictive-disorders/.

Shelley, J., Clark, M., & Caulfield, T. (2015). The face of chiropractic: Evidence-based? *Focus on Alternative & Complementary Therapies*, 20(1), 13–22. https://doi.org/10.1111/fct.12151.

Shin, N. Y., Lim, Y. J., Yang, C. H., & Kim, C. (2017). Acupuncture for alcohol use disorder: A meta-analysis. *Evidence-Based Complementary and Alternative Medicine*, 2017, 7823278. https://doi.org/10.1155/2017/7823278.

Skryabin, V. Y. (2020). An addiction to seeking fortune-telling services: A case report. *Journal of Addictive Diseases*, 38(2), 223–228. https://doi.org/10.1080/10550887.2020.1740637.

Smith, C. (2020, September 17). *Equine therapy*. Addiction Center. www.addictioncenter.com/treatment/equine-therapy/.

Sylvermist. (n.d.). Biosound healing therapy in Pennsylvania. Silvermist: A Premier Program by Pyramid Healthcare. www.silvermistrecovery.com/treatment/holistic-therapy/biosound-healing-therapy/.

Swerdloff, A. (2017, August 30). This woman claims remembering her past life as an Aztec cured her food addiction. Vice. www.vice.com/en_us/article/3djyx9/this-woman-claims-remembering-her-past-life-as-an-aztec-cured-her-food-addiction.

Szerman, N., Parro-Torres, C., Attas, J. D., & el-Guebaly, N. (2019). Dual disorders: Addiction and other mental health disorders. Integrating mental health. In A. Javed & K. Fountoulakis (Eds.), *Advances in psychiatry* (pp. 109–127). Springer. https://doi.org/10.1007/978-3-319-70554-5_7.

Targhetta, R., Nalpas, B., & Perney, P. (2013). Argentine tango: Another behavioral addiction? *Journal of Behavioral Addictions*, 2(3), 179–186. https://doi.org/10.1556/2006.4.2015.009.

Tonry, M., & Lynch, M. (1996). Intermediate sanctions. *Crime and Justice*, 20, 99–144. https://doi.org/10.1086/449242.

Torrens, M., Rossi, P. C., Martinez-Riera, R., Martinez-Sanvisens, D., & Bulbena, A. (2012). Psychiatric co-morbidity and substance use disorders: Treatment in parallel systems or in one integrated system? *Substance Use & Misuse, 47*(8–9), 1005–1014. https://doi.org/10.3109/10826084.2012.663296.

U.S. Food & Drug Administration (2019). FDA approves new nasal spray medication for treatment-resistant depression; available only at a certified doctor's office or clinic. www.fda.gov/news-events/press-announcements/fda-approves-new-nasal-spray-medication-treatment-resistant-depression-available-only-certified.

Vargas, A. S., Luís, Â., Barroso, M., Gallardo, E., & Pereira, L. (2020). Psilocybin as a new approach to treat depression and anxiety in the context of life-threatening diseases – A systematic review and meta-analysis of clinical trials. *Biomedicines, 8*(9), 331. https://doi.org/10.3390/biomedicines 8090331.

Vickers, A., Zollman, C., & Payne, D. K. (2001). Hypnosis and relaxation therapies. *The Western Journal of Medicine, 175*(4), 269–272. https://doi .org/10.1136/ewjm.175.4.269.

Wakeman, S. E., & Rich, J. D. (2018). Barriers to medications for addiction treatment: How stigma kills. *Substance Use & Misuse, 53*(2), 330–333. https://doi.org/10.1080/10826084.2017.1363238.

Walitzer, K. S., Dermen, K. H., & Barrick, C. (2009). Facilitating involvement in Alcoholics Anonymous during out-patient treatment: A randomized clinical trial. *Addiction, 104*(3), 391–401. https://doi.org/10.1111/j.1360-0443 .2008.02467.x.

Warner, T. D., & Kramer, J. H. (2009). Closing the revolving door? Substance abuse treatment as an alternative to traditional sentencing for drug-dependent offenders. *Criminal Justice and Behavior, 36*(1), 89–109. https://doi.org/10.1177/0093854808326743.

Watson, T. M., Bayoumi, A., Kolla, G., Penn, R., Fischer, B., Luce, J., & Strike, C. (2012). Police perceptions of supervised consumption sites (SCSs): A qualitative study. *Substance Use & Misuse, 47*(4), 364–374. https://doi.org/10.3109/10826084.2011.645104.

White, W. L. (1998). Franchising addiction treatment: The Keeley Institute. In *Slaying the dragon: The history of addiction treatment and recovery in America* (pp. 50–64). Chestnut Health Systems/Lighthouse Institute.

Wiese, B., & Wilson-Poe, A. R. (2018). Emerging evidence for cannabis' role in opioid use disorder. *Cannabis and Cannabinoid Research, 3*(1), 179–189. https://doi.org/10.1089/can.2018.0022.

Wilson, B. ("Bill W.") (2001). *Alcoholics Anonymous* (4th ed.). Alcoholics Anonymous World Services.

Winkelman, M. (2014). Psychedelics as medicines for substance abuse rehabilitation: evaluating treatments with LSD, Peyote, Ibogaine and Ayahuasca. *Current Drug Abuse Reviews, 7*(2), 101–116. https://doi.org/10.2174/ 1874473708666150107120011.

Witkiewitz, K., Lustyk, M. K. B., & Bowen, S. (2013). Retraining the addicted brain: A review of hypothesized neurobiological mechanisms of mindfulness-based relapse prevention. *Psychology of Addictive Behaviors*, *27*(2), 351–365.

World Health Organization. (2009). *Safety issues in the preparation of homeopathic medicines*. WHO Press.

World Health Organization. (2021). *International classification of diseases for mortality and morbidity statistics* (11th revision). https://icd.who.int/browse11/l-m/en.

Zehra, A., Burns, J., Liu, C. K., Manza, P., Wiers, C. E., Volkow, N. D., & Wang, G.-J. (2018). Cannabis addiction and the brain: A review. *Journal of Neuroimmune Pharmacology*, *13*, 438–452. https://doi.org/10.1007/s11481-018-9782-9.

Zell, M., & Grundmann, O. (2012). An orthomolecular approach to the prevention and treatment of psychiatric disorders. *Advances in Mind–Body Medicine*, *26*(2), 14–28.

13

Significant Cognitive Decline

Claudia Drossel and Jacqueline Pachis

Most people with major neurocognitive disorders (NCDs, formerly "dementias"; American Psychiatric Association, 2013) live at home and receive assistance from family members. Impaired thinking, reasoning, remembering, or problem-solving requires skillful scaffolding by caregivers to optimize engagement in everyday activities and prevent premature decline. For this reason, the quality of life of persons with NCD and their families hinges on caregiver skills. These skills are affected by caregiver psychological and physical health status, as well as access to supportive resources including healthcare providers with knowledge and competence in assessing and managing NCDs. As caregivers are invisible within the U.S. healthcare system, they receive little preparation to understand the heterogeneity of cognitive impairment and therefore take the steps necessary to enhance their own quality of life and that of the person they assist.

A decline in cognition can involve loss in one or across multiple repertoires that allow us to maneuver complex social and physical environments. Thus, perhaps the biggest myth related to dementia is that decline is equivalent to memory loss. Reflected by the diagnostic criteria for major NCD (DSM-5-TR; American Psychiatric Association, 2022), the term "cognitive decline" can characterize specific losses in motor speed or coordination, attention and perception, learning and memory, initiation of action, sequencing multistep tasks, problem-solving, strategizing, reasoning, and navigating social situations. When such decline occurs in adulthood, is chronic, and sufficiently severe to disrupt at minimum instrumental activities of daily living (such as managing finances or medications), then the decline meets diagnostic criteria for major NCD, provided that differential diagnostic procedures have ruled out delirium and other acute conditions or psychiatric disorders. Contrary to popular belief, the diagnostic construct of NCD spans many cognitive domains, and a person may have a diagnosis of NCD and yet preserved memory. Moving away from the highly dated and stigmatized term "dementia" and using the term "NCD" may serve to clarify the heterogeneity of the diagnostic category.

13.1 Pseudoscience and Questionable Ideas

Lack of caregiver preparation, combined with uncertainty and despair, can contribute to the perpetuation of myths and pseudoscientific approaches to major NCDs. Below is a list of *facts* that rebut pervasive myths and pseudoscience.

13.1.1 Course of Neurocognitive Disorders

13.1.1.1 Not All NCDs Are Progressive and Irreversible

Major NCD is a clinical syndrome that covers a range of chronic presentations with vastly different etiologies, including traumatic (e.g., brain injury), vascular (e.g., stroke), toxic (e.g., exposure to neurotoxins, substance use), metabolic (e.g., diabetes), infectious (e.g., meningitis), neoplastic (e.g., tumors), neurodegenerative diseases (e.g., Alzheimer's disease), or a combination of etiologies. Indeed, multiple comorbid etiologies may be the norm (Arvanitakis et al., 2019). Contrary to popular belief, a diagnosis of *major NCD not otherwise specified* is silent about prognosis. Cognitive decline may improve, stabilize, or worsen over time. For this reason, proper diagnosis by specialists is important.

As noted, the diagnosis of major NCD clusters many different underlying conditions that result in chronic cognitive impairment in adulthood. Most people, however, associate major NCDs with irreversible neurodegenerative diseases that lead to pernicious decline, that progress until assistance is needed for all activities of daily living, and that involve cessation of a person's active engagement with their surroundings. Keeping in mind that cognitive decline can have many etiologies and prognoses, the following discussion will focus exclusively on progressive and irreversible major NCDs, due to relatively common neurodegenerative diseases such as Alzheimer's disease, Lewy body disease, vascular disease, or frontotemporal lobar degeneration, itself a cluster of degenerative diseases with variants distinguished by their relative impact on behavioral, speech, and motor functioning. Examples of less frequent progressive and irreversible major NCDs are those due to Parkinson's disease, prion diseases, chronic traumatic encephalopathy, and multiple sclerosis (for details, see Arvanitakis et al., 2019). Parkinson's disease is commonly accompanied by mild cognitive difficulties; about one-third of individuals with the movement disorder develop major NCD (Saredakis et al., 2019).

13.1.1.2 Change Is Gradual, Pernicious, and Difficult to Detect

When neurodegeneration is progressive, it occurs over years and decades, with onset of subtle decline well before everyday life is affected (e.g., Wilson et al., 2011). Other than stroke, which often leads to an abrupt change in functional status, changes are gradual and initially barely noticeable. The impact of slowly narrowing repertoires on daily task performance depends on the person. Each person has unique strengths and weaknesses that reflect the person's biopsychosocial history and current circumstances. Gradual cognitive losses play out within social and medical circumstances that, in turn, affect how the person copes and how quickly decline may become nonnegligible. As familiar or routine tasks begin to seem strange and require more effort for completion, the person's coping repertoires interact with past and present contexts, including adverse childhood events, adult trauma history, and other aspects of behavioral and medical health. Often, social skills remain relatively unimpaired, leading providers and families to underestimate the cognitive deficits and misattribute changes in routines to psychiatric factors.

13.1.1.3 Behavioral and Emotional Changes Initially Overshadow Cognitive Decline

Behavioral and emotional changes associated with cognitive decline are common when the person encounters seemingly inexplicable performance failures at times. It bears repeating that the neurodegenerative decline is gradual, and the frequency of fluent performances diminishes over time. There is no off-switch that would facilitate the detection of cognitive problems, either by the person or by family or friends (Stokes et al., 2015). For this reason, family and friends might make demands that exceed the person's remaining skill set and thereby exacerbate the person's general apprehension about performance failures (for a patient view, see van Wijngaarden et al., 2019). Withdrawal from activities and avoidance of social situations are the most frequent behavioral and emotional changes associated with NCD. Family members and friends often interpret early signs of the disease – such as an emerging lack of reciprocity and engagement – as personality or emotional changes, or even as personal rejections. Attempts to argue, persuade, convince, or otherwise reengage the person in social activities without proper scaffolding can lead to prolonged conflict. Emotional or personality changes can overshadow subtle cognitive deficits, and psychiatric services or couples therapy are often initiated prior to establishing a proper neurological diagnosis (e.g., Braus et al., 2019).

Emotional and behavioral changes invariably emerge not only as a direct function of cognitive decline but from ineffective attempts to cope with decline (Fisher et al., 2007). These changes are predictors for poor clinical outcomes, including poor quality of life, caregiver burden, and institutionalization (O'Donnell et al., 1992; Spiegl et al., 2021). At the same time, emotional and behavioral changes are highly modifiable. While further cognitive decline may be unavoidable, emotional and behavioral changes can be reduced or prevented altogether with non-pharmacological interventions.

13.1.1.4 Behavioral and Emotional Changes Are Predictable

As a general principle in behavioral health, a person's feelings, thoughts, and behaviors can be understood in the context in which they occur (McCurry & Drossel, 2011). This principle applies regardless of a person's cognitive status. Yet, to this day, the Alzheimer's Association allows for aggression that "can occur suddenly, with no apparent reason [...]" (Alzheimer's Association, n.d.). This statement may reflect history. Prior to the mid-century movement to deinstitutionalize psychiatric care, many institutionalized psychiatric patients were individuals with major NCD and were viewed as unpredictable (Powell, 2019). The term "dementia" carries this institutional history and shame, and anecdotally, many individuals and their families report a fear of unpredictability or "going crazy."

Despite major advances in our understanding of NCDs, social stigma and associated fears of loss of personhood and rise of spontaneous, out-of-the-blue aggression persist. When behaviors uncharacteristic of the person like aggression occur, then pain and discomfort are often the culprits that must be ruled out (Achterberg et al., 2019). Such a rule-out may not occur when aggression is assumed to be an inevitable part of the neurodegenerative disease. Furthermore, caregivers' demands (e.g., to undress or participate in complex tasks) may overwhelm a person's skills. Caregivers of individuals with NCD typically do not learn how to break down tasks into their component parts, and how to provide appropriate cues. Consequently, social demands may create behaviors that seem aggressive yet function self-protectively (e.g., refusing to undress at the intense bidding of a perceived stranger). As made visible by the deaths within the COVID-19 pandemic, many people with NCD live in conditions that hasten decline because their uncharacteristic behaviors are taken as default symptoms of neurodegeneration, rather than signs of other serious problems the person with NCD cannot communicate (Larson & Stroud, 2021).

13.1.1.5 Specific Descriptions in Context Help Pinpoint and Categorize Difficulties

When individuals with NCD or caregivers present for behavioral health services, a thorough investigation of the problematic behavioral or emotional changes includes contextual details. For example, a caregiver might report that the person with the NCD describes events that did not happen. Queried, the caregiver endorses hallucinations. However, upon monitoring specific episodes, the caregiver notices that pressing the person with NCD for an explanation (e.g., "How did you lose your car keys") is the context for making up an explanation ("A little girl took them"). These confabulations serve to fill gaps; notably, they are very different in kind from typical hallucinations – the hearing of voices or seeing of events that nobody else can.

When hallucinations are indeed present, they tend to be a sign of altered perceptual functioning (Hamilton et al., 2012; Postuma et al., 2011). For example, people with Lewy body disease, a common form of NCD, frequently report seeing small animals, children, or fantasy creatures, and these visions tend to bother caregivers more than the person with the disorder. When persons with Lewy body disease greet these visuo-perceptual disturbances with wonder and awe rather than fear or apprehension, they do not require treatment (O'Brien et al., 2020). However, caregiver education is indicated, as caregivers' reactions may increase worry if they are not neutral or welcoming (Yumoto & Suwa, 2021) and erode the relationship with the person with Lewy body disease over time. Proper diagnosis prevents both caregivers' and providers' misattribution of visuo-perceptual disturbances to psychiatric disorders, such as primary late-onset psychosis (itself a controversial construct, see Suen et al., 2019). Importantly, proper diagnosis prevents treatment with dopaminergic (often called "antipsychotic") agents that can accelerate decline and lead to premature death due to severe neuroleptic sensitivity (McKeith et al., 2017).

13.1.2 Provider Barriers to Diagnosis and Patient Education

Early diagnosis is recommended to allow for active knowledge and skills acquisition, advance care planning, and the explicit consideration of the patient's values and preferences. However, diagnoses tend to be established when functional difficulties cannot be ignored and the person with NCD has become an unreliable reporter. Provider–patient communication during diagnostic processes is often poor, perhaps also because many providers are uncomfortable with the uncertainty that continues to surround diagnostic processes.

13.1.2.1 Diagnostic Criteria Are Evolving (and Biomarkers Are Not Used in Routine Practice)

Lack of international or cross-specialty standardizations continue to trouble researchers, providers, and consumers. Different classification systems rely on different criteria and thresholds for diagnosis. Notice, for example, that the DSM-5 (American Psychiatric Association, 2013) criteria have lowered the threshold for diagnosis by emphasizing disruptions in instrumental activities of daily living rather than disruption of social or occupational activities.

The physiological mechanisms underlying specific neurodegenerative processes are not yet well understood. Contemporary biomedical research examines disease processes from multiple perspectives (neuropathology, epidemiology, neuroimmunology, genetics, neuroradiology, behavioral neuroscience) and continuously refines classification, diagnostic guidelines, medical rule-outs, and potential biomarkers. Consider the following examples:

1. Most people have heard of plaques and tangles (see also Adelman, 1998, for the "Alzheimerization" of NCDs). Although aggregations of misfolded proteins such as tau, synuclein, beta-amyloid, and others are diagnostic markers for neurodegenerative diseases upon autopsy, the role of these aggregations is controversial. On the one hand, when cognitive loss is present, the determination of the specific proteinopathy upon autopsy classifies the neurodegenerative disease process (e.g., beta-amyloid as a marker for Alzheimer's disease [Khoury & Ghossoub, 2019]; alpha-synuclein for Parkinson's and Lewy body diseases [Erskine et al., 2021]). On the other hand, proteinopathy itself can be present without concurrent cognitive loss (Jansen et al., 2018), suggesting that the presence of proteinopathy is not sufficiently specific to indicate functional concerns. To emphasize, aggregations of

different types of misfolded proteins might present the same or very different disease mechanisms that are currently unknown. The role of genetics is similarly complex.

2. Diagnostic procedures and criteria are evolving. For example, in 2017, rapid eye movement (REM) sleep behavior disorder became one of the core clinical features necessary for the diagnosis of Lewy body disease (McKeith et al., 2017).

3. Entirely new disease classifications, such as limbic-predominant age-related TDP-43 encephalopathy (LATE; Nelson et al., 2019), add further complexity to diagnoses of presentations within the NCD clinical syndrome.

As major NCD is a quickly changing landscape, practitioners must keep up with the science, not only to provide appropriate services but also to educate patients and their caregivers. Scientific progress raises the level of complexity of major NCDs. It also demands that providers exercise caution when explaining or making attributions about cognitive loss in adulthood. At the same time, scientific efforts serve to hone clinicians' awareness of rule-outs, offer tools to better categorize and understand observed cognitive losses, closely watch them over time, and inform individuals and families.

13.1.2.2 Diagnosis Is Challenging and Takes Time

Diagnostic guidelines for Alzheimer's disease have been enhanced since 1984 (Dubois et al., 2021; McKhann et al., 1984; 2011). Because biomarkers are under development and not used in routine practice (Ahmed et al., 2014), diagnoses of major NCD are typically established by confirming significant cognitive and functional difficulties and ruling out alternatives. In the US, about 90% of major NCD diagnoses do not specify the etiology (Goodman et al., 2017).

A comprehensive workup takes time and resources. It requires individuals and families to tolerate uncertainty, but such a workup is essential to rule out reversible metabolic, toxic, inflammatory, or neoplastic conditions. To confirm the neurodegenerative nature of a condition, repeated evaluations of performance and functional status over time are sometimes indicated. Barriers to accessing diagnostic procedures consist of lack of provider training, unavailability of health services, lack of specialty providers such as geriatricians, neuropsychologists, or neurologists, and pervasive ageism – by individuals, families, and providers – that misattributes significant cognitive decline to aging-related changes. In addition, widely available cognitive screening tools, such as the Montreal Cognitive

Assessment (Nasreddine et al., 2005), do not establish diagnoses. These tools can point to vague performance difficulties in selected areas and the need for further assessment by specialty providers (for details, see Roebuck-Spencer et al., 2017). Further assessment makes sure that long-standing and preexisting cognitive difficulties due to neurodevelopmental issues or past injuries or illnesses are not misinterpreted as a recent decline. Moreover, most screeners are not designed to detect cognitive decline in all domains relevant to major NCDs, such as problems with impulsivity and navigation of social situations. To emphasize, screening is insufficient and inappropriate for diagnosis (James et al., 2020), and it does not represent the standard of care for diagnoses.

13.1.2.3 Risk Factors Are Difficult to Pinpoint

Cross-sectional, correlational studies of risk factors across NCD diagnoses (all-cause NCD) show differential risk of NCD with age, gender, and positive family history (Baumgart et al., 2015). Risk for NCDs also rises when the central nervous system is already compromised due to past traumatic brain injury or the presence of a neurodevelopmental disorder such as Down syndrome, for example. In the United States, race and ethnicity have emerged as additional risk factors. African American and Hispanic populations (hereafter, minoritized populations) carry a significantly higher risk of NCD than non-Hispanic populations of European descent. When evaluating risk factors, consider the following:

1. *Correlation is not causation.* As people age, they accumulate factors that may compromise nervous system functioning, including chronic medical conditions but also environmental exposures to neurotoxins. Increased age correlates with increased risk but is not causal to onset. Yet, the literature describes irreversible neurodegenerative diseases often as "age-associated," maintaining the myth that they invariably "go with" age. Similarly, women have a significantly greater lifetime risk of NCD than men, but here again the findings are correlational, and the mechanisms that produce greater risks are unclear.
2. *The role of genes is complex.* Genes play a large role when an NCD is due to early-onset Alzheimer's disease, but early-onset cases represent a tiny fraction of Alzheimer's disease and of NCD cases overall (Arvanitakis et al., 2019). Most Alzheimer's disease cases have a sporadic onset at age 65 or older, and the role of genes in NCDs other than early-onset Alzheimer's disease is not clear. First, a positive family history of NCD may indicate shared environments or lifestyle

patterns. Second, in addition to the involvement of many genes (also known as polygenic risk) whose physiological functions are yet to be identified, recent studies (e.g., Lourida et al., 2019) suggest that favorable lifestyles may offset polygenic risk scores.

3. *Most NCDs have mixed etiologies, often involving cardiometabolic conditions.* Notably, favorable lifestyles are defined by the reduction of cardiometabolic risk factors (i.e., nonsmoking status, regular physical activity, healthy eating patterns, and low alcohol consumption). Again, cross-sectional studies typically include NCDs of all etiologies. From a public health perspective, the implementation of population-based strategies to maintain heart health might bring about a decline in the prevalence of NCDs, even if such strategies are broad and unspecific (for a review, see Baumgart et al., 2015). It is likely that disparities in cardiovascular health and health services of women and minoritized populations contribute to the correlation of gender, race, and ethnicity with all-cause NCD (McClellan et al., 2019). Other modifiable lifestyle factors that show correlations with the onset of all-cause NCDs are sleep disturbances and substance use, including prescription benzodiazepine use.

13.1.3 Persistent Searches for the Cure and the Hype of Pharmacological Interventions

13.1.3.1 There Is No Cure

Neurodegenerative diseases are incurable and distinct from reversible NCDs that receive appropriate care for the underlying neurological conditions. Once a possible or probable diagnosis of a progressive, irreversible NCD has been established, providers initiate tertiary prevention efforts that are aimed at preventing complications and maintaining quality of life while living with NCD.

Individuals with major NCD tend to have many health conditions (i.e., comorbidities such as diabetes, hypertension, cancer). Sensory loss is also common. When these other conditions are poorly managed, the person may be more impaired than based on the probable neurodegenerative disease alone ("excess disability"; Kahn, 1965). Tertiary prevention efforts reflect the foundations of behavioral healthcare. These include managing comorbidities and pain, correcting sensory loss, scheduling regular physical activities, providing access to meaningful events (including access to the outside), promoting restful sleep, ensuring adequate nutrition and hydration, establishing bladder and bowel management, and conducting medication reviews to limit inappropriate medications and polypharmacy (Arvanitakis et al., 2019; Bernat et al., 1996).

These tertiary prevention efforts are essential because many people with NCD lose their ability to describe their own physiological status. Their self-reports of events like sensory loss or pain often wane before other communication skills do. Thus, caregivers play a pivotal role in observing the person with NCD, detecting problems that the person cannot describe, taking the necessary steps to resolve these problems, and advocating with providers to rule out sources of excess disability even when the person with NCD denies problems upon provider queries. Here, caregiver advocacy is vital to maintaining proper medical services in a fragmented healthcare system that heavily relies on patient self-report.

Recently, Hellmuth and colleagues (2019) warned of pseudomedicine in NCD. They pointed out that given the incurable nature of neurodegenerative diseases and individuals' and families' incredulity that modern medicine cannot deliver a remedy, properly licensed providers may promote treatments as scientifically supported even when the evidence base is insufficient or lacking. As a general guideline, any intervention that promises a cure and that hypothesizes unsupported etiologies for Alzheimer's disease and related neurodegenerative diseases (e.g., dietary supplements, metabolic regimens, cognitive rehabilitation, mold abatement, chelation; see also Daly et al., 2020) might attract the attention of people with NCD and their families. Providers who promote the intervention may judge it successful for multiple reasons (Lilienfeld et al., 2014), including placebo effects and personal experience. As detailed above, NCD diagnoses are often unspecified. NCD can be due to a large range of underlying etiologies, some of them reversible or improvable. Presumed anecdotal treatment successes, often based on testimonials, may represent an unspecified diagnosis and the common sociocultural misconception of NCD as Alzheimer's disease. In other words, cognitive status indeed may have improved, but the observed decline was never due to a progressive neurodegenerative disease in the first place.

Alternatively, if the person had a probable diagnosis of NCD due to Alzheimer's disease or another progressive and irreversible disease, aspects of the physical or social environment may have generated excess disability (faster decline than based on the neurodegenerative condition alone). Likely, the intervention inadvertently addressed these physical or social aspects. For example, while promoting a dietary supplement, a provider may also have introduced proper diabetes management (preventing hypoglycemic episodes that are accompanied by increased confusion), arranged for the correction of vision or hearing (Yamada et al., 2014), or reduced anticholinergic medication (e.g., diphenhydramine for allergies) known to impair cognition (American Geriatrics Society Beers Criteria® Update Expert Panel, 2019). Thus, perceiving improvement, providers stay their course, unaware that the targets upon which they intervene can be construed as tertiary prevention efforts and are not the progressive neurodegenerative diseases themselves.

13.1.3.2 No Prescription Medication Is a Curative "Medication for Dementia"

As noted earlier, individuals commonly live with major NCDs for decades. In the absence of a cure, individuals and families look for ways to slow cognitive decline, if only by a few months, thereby potentially postponing the person's increasing need for assistance. Pharmaceutical interventions, marketed directly to U.S. consumers, use aspirational drug descriptors such as "medications for memory loss" or "medications for cognition" (Alzheimer's Association, 2022). These descriptors obfuscate the complexities associated with individuals' or caregivers' medical decision-making and undermine informed consent processes.

In general, pharmacological interventions fall into three groups: disease-slowing drugs, disease-modifying drugs, and psychotropic drugs for emotional and behavioral changes (Anand et al., 2017). Individuals, surrogate decision-makers, and prescribers weigh costs (e.g., potential adverse events; expenses; the potential costs of nonintervention) and benefits in a context of urgent need and limited treatment options.

13.1.3.3 Disease-Slowing Agents Have Risks and Benefits

The most popular disease-slowing agents currently used in the US are cholinergic enhancers. They assume that cognitive difficulties arise from the depletion of one specific neurotransmitter, acetylcholine. To date, the role of the cholinergic system in Alzheimer's disease and other neurodegenerative diseases remains poorly understood (Anand et al., 2017). Overall, data from randomized clinical trials suggest that cholinergic drugs (i.e., cholinesterase inhibitors) may have small and relatively short-term benefits (Birks & Harvey, 2018).

Memantine, a drug first developed in the 1960s, works by blocking glutamate receptors. Its use is based upon the finding that excessive stimulation of glutamate receptors can result in toxic effects to brain tissue, as occurs during traumatic brain injuries or seizures. Reviews indicate small clinical benefits on cognition, activities of daily living, and emotional and behavioral changes for moderate to severe Alzheimer's disease at 6 months (McShane et al., 2019).

Both drug classes targeting Alzheimer's disease (yet used broadly across NCDs in practice) can have adverse effects. For cholinergic drugs, these commonly include gastrointestinal distress (nausea, vomiting, diarrhea, anorexia) and insomnia, but urinary incontinence may also occur (Ruangritchankul et al., 2021). Frequent adverse events related to glutamate blockers are dizziness, headache, confusion, gastrointestinal distress, and psychoactive effects (e.g., anxiety, depression, hallucinations), fatigue, sleepiness, and pain. Deprescribing guidelines are emerging (Renn et al., 2018).

13.1.3.4 There Is No Magic Bullet

In June 2021, aducanumab received approval as "the first therapy to target and affect the underlying disease process of Alzheimer's" (U.S. Food and Drug Administration, 2021). Aducanumab, administered intravenously, is a monoclonal antibody that binds to aggregated beta amyloid, reducing such plaques in the brain. Yet, the role of beta amyloid as a mechanism for cognitive decline due to Alzheimer's disease continues to be uncertain, and its clearance from the brain did not produce unequivocal stabilization, restoration, or maintenance of function (Alexander et al., 2021). The patent holder, Biogen, is expected to complete a follow-up study of the drug's effects on cognitive decline by 2030. Common adverse events are headache, diarrhea, and altered mental status, while about one-third of trial participants had cerebral edemas or microhemorrhages. Because of the severe adverse effect profile, some experts recommend that providers follow the inclusion criteria of the original clinical trials as well as ruling out prior microbleeds (Cummings et al., 2021). As of December 2021, uptake of the drug has been slow, and the manufacturer moved to significantly lower its price (Biogen, 2021).

13.1.3.5 No Medication Is Designed to Address Behavioral or Emotional Changes

Most individuals with major NCD receive drugs prescribed to change behavioral and emotional status (Brimelow et al., 2019; Joling et al., 2021). However, the majority of people with NCD and their proxy medical decision makers are not informed that the FDA has not approved any drugs for the management of behavioral and emotional changes associated with major NCD, and that psychotropic medications are prescribed off-label (Tjia et al., 2017). Contrary to individuals' and families' impressions, none of the psychotropics taken by individuals with NCD were developed or are indicated specifically to manage difficulties associated with NCD.

It should be noted that repurposing medications for other than their intended and approved use is a common and legal practice. Psychotropic drugs used with major NCD span all drug classes, including major tranquilizers (i.e., dopaminergic blockers originally developed as anesthesia drugs, often referred to as "antipsychotics") and minor tranquilizers (i.e., GABAergic anxiolytic agents associated with cognitive impairment and decline). While the former carry an FDA boxed warning about an increased risk of death for individuals with major NCD, the latter are generally not indicated for long-term use by adults aged 65 and older (American Geriatrics Society Beers Criteria® Update Expert Panel, 2019). Concerns about tranquilizers as a form of chemical restraint leading to drowsiness and inactivity, accelerated loss of repertoires, cerebrovascular events, and greater risk of falls, have led to worldwide initiatives to reduce prescription rates and improve patient outcomes (but see Rubino et al., 2020). Further, minor tranquilizers have anxiolytic properties that, when superimposed on cognitive decline, may result in impulsive, inappropriate, and uncharacteristic social behaviors that are then misattributed to the major NCD.

Lack of knowledge, placebo effects, lack of skills for implementing alternatives, convenience, lack of appropriate resources, and provider helplessness may sustain ongoing use of potentially harmful agents (Ballard & Cream, 2005). Nonpharmacological interventions are effortful, costly, and labor-intensive, while the administration of tranquilizers requires little time, minimal training, and produces immediate results. The COVID-19 pandemic highlighted how the administration of tranquilizers serves to put patches on a defunct NCD care system rather than treat problems specific to NCD. Deaths increased among adults aged 65 years and older, and lockdowns disrupted individuals' routines both in the home and in long-term service settings, severely restricting their life space (i.e., family visitation stopped, residents in long-term service settings were confined to their rooms, and day programs closed). Consequently, higher distress among caregivers as well as people with NCD, physical restriction, fewer opportunities for activities, and significant staffing problems accompanied increased prescriptions of tranquilizers (Howard et al., 2020; Larson & Stroud, 2021; Olson & Albensi, 2021). Such practices are especially problematic because deprescribing algorithms ensuring evidence-based safe and effective reduction of tranquilizers do not exist. In general, psychotropic medications should be considered medical providers' last-ditch, experimental attempts to actively intervene on behavioral and emotional changes in resource-strained environments.

13.1.3.6 Each New Symptom Should Be Treated as a Potential Adverse Event

A pervasive myth related to drug interventions is their presumed sole beneficence. This bias can result in the failure of paraprofessionals and caregivers to attribute decreases in functional status to adverse drug events (Goldberg & Ernst, 2018). As adverse events can lead to decreases in functional status and increased confusion, they may overlap with caregivers' expectations of the disease process. Adverse effects may be misclassified and misattributed to a worsening of the major NCD. Based on caregiver reports, providers may conclude that more of the drug is needed, rather than removing the offending culprit. Providers then may manage physical adverse effects with further prescriptions (referred to as a prescribing cascade), treating each new symptom as one of major NCD rather than a preventable and reversible iatrogenic event (Gill et al., 2005). If individuals or families opt to introduce drugs, then each new symptom should be treated as an adverse event.

13.1.3.7 Systematic Monitoring of Drug Effects Is Indicated (Yet Rarely Implemented)

Monitoring of existing repertoires on the one hand and adverse events on the other is indicated with each pharmacological intervention. Individuals with major NCD are in a precarious position. Reporting on one's own physiological status is a special skill that wanes even when other, everyday communications are still possible. Abrupt disruptions of repertoires (e.g., refusal to participate in activities) and uncharacteristic behaviors (e.g., self-defensiveness, refusal to be touched, yelling out) may be signs of adverse drug events. Without systematic monitoring, there is a risk of misattributing reversible adverse events to further decline.

13.2 Research-Supported Approaches

As noted above, tertiary prevention is essential for maintaining quality of life (Arvanitakis et al., 2019; Bernat et al., 1996). Nonpharmacological interventions are the first-line treatments of behavioral or emotional changes associated with cognitive decline. Some of these changes may be prodromal, initial signs of a subtle disruption of the nervous system (Singh-Manoux et al., 2017). Later emotional and behavioral changes reflect individuals' attempts to cope with cognitive decline and perceptual disturbances or alterations. Individuals may withdraw from activities, engage in safety behaviors (such as not throwing out mail if comprehension is difficult), fill gaps in recall with plausible confabulations, or reconcile seemingly disjointed or inexplicable events by blaming others (such as accusing a family member of stealing a lost wallet). Noted repeatedly throughout this chapter, emotional and behavioral changes can be understood in the context of the cognitive decline, the person's history, and the current circumstances.

In general, nonpharmacological interventions then build a prosthetic social and physical environment, aimed at scaffolding, reducing apprehension related to cognitive decline or altered perceptions, and maintaining engagement in activities that are tailored to the person's current skill set, preferences, and longstanding values (Birt et al., 2017). Because of the heterogeneity of major NCDs, the selection of specific research-supported approaches must take into consideration the treatment target (e.g., tertiary health promotion and disease prevention, improving shared decision-making, increasing in-home safety through assistive technology, reducing withdrawal, addressing sleep disturbances), the degree of impairment, and the setting (community-dwelling, hospital-based, or residential). Patient-directed multimodal interventions to stave off further decline are supported when NCD is considered mild and self-direction possible (Salzman et al., 2022). As individuals lose their ability to self-monitor and use compensatory or therapeutic strategies, caregivers are tasked with implementation. See the corresponding chapter in the companion book (Hupp & Tolin, in press) for a more detailed discussion of research-supported approaches.

Evidence-based interventions for caregivers consist of multiple components aimed at reducing caregiver stress and burden and teaching basic principles of behavior (Belle et al., 2006; Gitlin et al., 2003; Schulz et al., 2003; for a recent critique, see Scales et al., 2018). Because of the complexity of NCD diagnoses and comorbidities, individuals with NCD and their families benefit from health service models that integrate caregiver support with geriatric medical and behavioral health (Clevenger et al., 2018; Nichols et al., 2011). The problem-solving required from providers relies on sophisticated skill sets that combine knowledge of neurology and general medical conditions (to understand specific strengths and weaknesses associated with diagnoses, and to rule out excess disability) with knowledge of behavioral techniques (to assess specific behaviors in context, design and implement interventions that target social and physical factors for change, and evaluate intervention effectiveness, including caregiver barriers to implementation). At the same time, many providers are not trained in behavioral science per se, and thus are at risk at falling short of their original goal to prioritize nonpharmacological approaches. They might resort to psychotropic drugs as the default next step if problems cannot be solved immediately.

13.3 Conclusion

NCDs represent a rapidly evolving field and are prone to myths and pseudoscience, which may be viewed as growing pains – shedding relics of a troubled history and persisting uncertainty. Approaches to NCD have progressed significantly from historical marginalization and psychiatric institutionalizations to the roll-outs of general strategies for providers and caregivers. Destigmatization and demystification continue, and excess disability is addressed more often in routine care. However, emotional and behavioral aspects of NCDs that arise from complicated social histories and relationships remain poorly understood (Black et al., 2019). Moreover, psychotropic use remains common. NCD providers who have not been trained in behavioral science rely on rolled-out techniques as the first step in a stepped care model. When these techniques are ineffective, the next step should require the consultation of providers trained in behavioral science who problem-solve beyond the realm of techniques, using measurement-based care. Findings from these additional, individually tailored interventions will facilitate enhancing current models.

Claudia Drossel, PhD, is an Associate Professor of Psychology at Eastern Michigan University. She is co-editor of the book *Treating Dementia in Context* (2011).

Jacqueline Pachis, MS, BCBA, is a doctoral student of psychology at Eastern Michigan University.

References

Achterberg, W., Lautenbacher, S., Husebo, B., Erdal, A., & Herr, K. (2019). Pain in dementia. *Pain Reports*, *5*(1), e803–e803. https://doi.org/10.1097/PR9 .0000000000000803.

Adelman, R. C. (1998). The Alzheimerization of aging: A brief update. *Experimental Gerontology*, *33*(1), 155–157. https://doi.org/https://doi.org/ 10.1016/S0531-5565(97)00057-0.

Ahmed, R. M., Paterson, R. W., Warren, J. D., Zetterberg, H., O'Brien, J. T., Fox, N. C., Halliday, G. M., & Schott, J. M. (2014). Biomarkers in dementia: Clinical utility and new directions. *Journal of Neurology, Neurosurgery & Psychiatry, 85*(12), 1426–1434. https://doi.org/10.1136/jnnp-2014-307662.

Alexander, G. C., Knopman, D. S., Emerson, S. S., Ovbiagele, B., Kryscio, R. J., Perlmutter, J. S., & Kesselheim, A. S. (2021). Revisiting FDA approval of aducanumab. *The New England Journal of Medicine, 385*(9), 769–771. https://doi.org/http://dx.doi.org/10.1056/NEJMp2110468.

Alzheimer's Association. (n.d.). Stages and behaviors: Aggression and anger. www.alz.org/help-support/caregiving/stages-behaviors/agression-anger.

Alzheimer's Association. (2002). Medications for memory, cognition, and dementia-related behaviors. www.alz.org/alzheimers-dementia/treatments/medications-for-memory.

American Geriatrics Society Beers Criteria® Update Expert Panel. (2019). American Geriatrics Society 2019 updated AGS Beers Criteria® for potentially inappropriate medication use in older adults. *Journal of the American Geriatrics Society, 67*(4), 674–694. https://doi.org/10.1111/jgs.15767.

American Psychiatric Association. (2013). *Diagnostic and statistical manual of mental disorders* (5th ed.). American Psychiatric Association. https://doi.org/https://doi.org/10.1176/appi.books.9780890425596.

American Psychiatric Association. (2022). *Diagnostic and statistical manual of mental disorders, fifth edition, text revision* (DSM-5-TR). American Psychiatric Association.

Anand, A., Patience, A. A., Sharma, N., & Khurana, N. (2017). The present and future of pharmacotherapy of Alzheimer's disease: A comprehensive review. *European Journal of Pharmacology, 815*, 364–375. https://doi.org/https://doi.org/10.1016/j.ejphar.2017.09.043.

Arvanitakis, Z., Shah, R. C., & Bennett, D. A. (2019). Diagnosis and management of dementia: Review. *Journal of the American Medical Association, 322*(16), 1589–1599. https://doi.org/10.1001/jama.2019.4782.

Ballard, C., & Cream, J. (2005). Drugs used to relieve behavioral symptoms in people with dementia or an unacceptable chemical cosh? *International Psychogeriatrics, 17*(1), 4–12. https://doi.org/10.1017/S1041610205221026.

Baumgart, M., Snyder, H. M., Carrillo, M. C., Fazio, S., Kim, H., & Johns, H. (2015). Summary of the evidence on modifiable risk factors for cognitive decline and dementia: A population-based perspective. *Alzheimer's & Dementia, 11*(6), 718–726. https://doi.org/https://doi.org/10.1016/j.jalz.2015.05.016.

Belle, S. H., Burgio, L., Burns, R., Coon, D., Czaja, S. J., Gallagher-Thompson, D., Gitlin, L. N., Klinger, J., Koepke, K. M., Lee, C. C., Martindale-Adams, J., Nichols, L., Schulz, R., Stahl, S., Stevens, A., Winter, L., Zhang, S., & Resources for Enhancing Alzheimer's Caregiver Health (REACH) II Investigators. (2006). Enhancing the quality of life of dementia caregivers from different ethnic or racial groups: A randomized, controlled trial. *Annals of Internal Medicine, 145*(10), 727–738. https://doi .org/10.7326/0003-4819-145-10-200611210-00005.

Bernat, J. L., Beresford, H. R., Celesia, G. G., Cranford, R. E., McQuillen, M. P., Pellegrino, T. R., Snyder, R. D. J., Taylor, R. M., & Wichman, A. (1996). Ethical issues in the management of the demented patient: The American Academy of Neurology Ethics and Humanities Subcommittee. *Neurology, 46*(4), 1180–1183. https://doi.org/10.1212/ WNL.46.4.1180.

Biogen. (2021, December 27). Biogen announces reduced price for Aduhelm® to improve access for patients with early Alzheimer's disease. https://inves tors.biogen.com/news-releases/news-release-details/biogen-announces-reduced-price-aduhelmr-improve-access-patients.

Birks, J. S., & Harvey, R. J. (2018). Donepezil for dementia due to Alzheimer's disease. *Cochrane Database of Systematic Reviews, 6*(6), CD001190. https://doi.org/10.1002/14651858.CD001190.pub3.

Birt, L., Poland, F., Csipke, E., & Charlesworth, G. (2017). Shifting dementia discourses from deficit to active citizenship. *Sociology of Health & Illness, 39*(2), 199–211. https://doi.org/https://doi.org/10.1111/1467-9566.12530.

Black, B. S., Johnston, D., Leoutsakos, J., Reuland, M., Kelly, J., Amjad, H., Davis, K., Willink, A., Sloan, D., Lyketsos, C., & Samus, Q. M. (2019). Unmet needs in community-living persons with dementia are common, often non-medical and related to patient and caregiver characteristics. *International Psychogeriatrics, 31*(11), 1643–1654. https://doi.org/10.1017 /S1041610218002296.

Braus, B. R., Rummans, T. A., Lapid, M. I., Morgan, R. J., Sampson, S. M., Handler, E. M. & Dimsdale, J. E. (2019). Clinicians and cognitive bias: A case of frontotemporal dementia misdiagnosed as conversion disorder. *American Journal of Psychiatry, 176*(9), 690–693. https://doi.org/10.1176 /appi.ajp.2018.18050551.

Brimelow, R. E., Wollin, J. A., Byrne, G. J., & Dissanayaka, N. N. (2019). Prescribing of psychotropic drugs and indicators for use in residential aged care and residents with dementia. *International Psychogeriatrics, 31* (6), 837–847. https://doi.org/http://dx.doi.org/10.1017/S1041610218001229.

Clevenger, C. K., Cellar, J., Kovaleva, M., Medders, L., & Hepburn, K. (2018). Integrated memory care clinic: Design, implementation, and initial results. *Journal of the American Geriatrics Society, 66*(12), 2401–2407. https://doi .org/https://doi.org/10.1111/jgs.15528.

Cummings, J., Aisen, P., Apostolova, L. G., Atri, A., Salloway, S., & Weiner, M. (2021). Aducanumab: Appropriate use recommendations. *The Journal of Prevention of Alzheimer's Disease, 8*(4), 398–410. https://doi.org/10.14283 /jpad.2021.41.

Daly, T., Mastroleo, I., Gorski, D., & Epelbaum, S. (2020). The ethics of innovation for Alzheimer's disease: The risk of overstating evidence for metabolic enhancement protocols. *Theoretical Medicine and Bioethics*, *41*(5), 223–237. https://doi.org/10.1007/s11017-020-09536-7.

Dubois, B., Villain, N., Frisoni, G. B., Rabinovici, G. D., Sabbagh, M., Cappa, S., Bejanin, A., Bombois, S., Epelbaum, S., Teichmann, M., Habert, M.-O., Nordberg, A., Blennow, K., Galasko, D., Stern, Y., Rowe, C. C., Salloway, S., Schneider, L. S., Cummings, J. L., & Feldman, H. H. (2021). Clinical diagnosis of Alzheimer's disease: Recommendations of the International Working Group. *The Lancet Neurology*, *20*(6), 484–496. https://doi.org/10.1016/S1474-4422(21)00066-1.

Erskine, D., Koss, D., Korolchuk, V. I., Outeiro, T. F., Attems, J., & McKeith, I. (2021). Lipids, lysosomes and mitochondria: Insights into Lewy body formation from rare monogenic disorders. *Acta Neuropathologica*, *141*(4), 511–526. https://doi.org/10.1007/s00401-021-02266-7.

Fisher, J. E., Drossel, C., Yury, C., & Cherup, S. (2007). A contextual model of restraint-free care for persons with dementia. In P. Sturmey (Ed.), *Functional analysis in clinical treatment* (pp. 211–237). Academic Press/Elsevier.

Gill, S. S., Mamdani, M., Naglie, G., Streiner, D. L., Bronskill, S. E., Kopp, A., Shulman, K. I., Lee, P. E., & Rochon, P. A. (2005). A prescribing cascade involving cholinesterase inhibitors and anticholinergic drugs. *Archives of Internal Medicine*, *165*(7), 808–813. https://doi.org/10.1001/archinte.165.7.808.

Gitlin, L. N., Belle, S. H., Burgio, L. D., Czaja, S. J., Mahoney, D., Gallagher-Thompson, D., Burns, R., Hauck, W. W., Zhang, S., Schulz, R., & Ory, M. G. (2003). Effect of multicomponent interventions on caregiver burden and depression: The REACH multisite initiative at 6-month follow-up. *Psychology and Aging*, *18*(3), 361–374. https://doi.org/10.1037/0882-7974.18.3.361.

Goldberg, J. F., & Ernst, C. L. (2018). *Managing the side effects of psychotropic medications*. 2nd ed. American Psychiatric Association.

Goodman, R. A., Lochner, K. A., Thambisetty, M., Wingo, T. S., Posner, S. F., & Ling, S. M. (2017). Prevalence of dementia subtypes in United States Medicare fee-for-service beneficiaries, 2011–2013. *Alzheimer's & Dementia*, *13*(1), 28–37. https://doi.org/https://doi.org/10.1016/j.jalz.2016.04.002.

Hamilton, J. M., Landy, K. M., Salmon, D. P., Hansen, L. A., Masliah, E., & Galasko, D. (2012). Early visuospatial deficits predict the occurrence of visual hallucinations in autopsy-confirmed dementia with Lewy bodies. *The American Journal of Geriatric Psychiatry*, *20*(9), 773–781. https://doi.org/https://doi.org/10.1097/JGP.0b013e31823033bc.

Hellmuth, J., Rabinovici, G. D., & Miller, B. L. (2019). The rise of pseudomedicine for dementia and brain health. *Journal of the American Medical Association*, *321*(6), 543–544. https://doi.org/10.1001/jama.2018.21560.

Howard, R., Burns, A., & Schneider, L. (2020). Antipsychotic prescribing to people with dementia during COVID-19. *The Lancet Neurology*, *19*(11), 892–892. https://doi.org/10.1016/S1474-4422(20)30370-7.

Hupp, S., & Tolin, D. (in press). *Science-based therapy*. Cambridge University Press.

James, B. D., Power, M. C., Gianattasio, K. Z., Lamar, M., Oveisgharan, S., Shah, R. C., Marquez, D. X., Barnes, L. L., & Bennett, D. A. (2020). Characterizing clinical misdiagnosis of dementia using Medicare claims records linked to Rush Alzheimer's Disease Center (RADC) cohort study data. *Alzheimer's & Dementia*, *16*(S10), e044880. https://doi .org/https://doi.org/10.1002/alz.044880.

Jansen, W. J., Ossenkoppele, R., Tijms, B. M., Fagan, A. M., Hansson, O., Klunk, W. E., van der Flier, W. M., Villemagne, V. L., Frisoni, G. B., Fleisher, A. S., Lleó, A., Mintun, M. A., Wallin, A., Engelborghs, S., Na, D. L., Chételat, G., Molinuevo, J. L., Landau, S. M., Mattsson, N., ... Zetterberg, H. (2018). Association of cerebral amyloid-β aggregation with cognitive functioning in persons without dementia. *JAMA Psychiatry*, *75*(1), 84–95. https://doi.org/10.1001/jamapsy chiatry.2017.3391.

Joling, K. J., Ten Koppel, M., van Hout, H. P. J., Onwuteaka-Philipsen, B. D., Francke, A. L., Verheij, R. A., Twisk, J. W. R., & van Marum, R. J. (2021). Psychotropic drug prescription rates in primary care for people with dementia from recorded diagnosis onwards.*International Journal of Geriatric Psychiatry*, *36*(3), 443–451. https://doi.org/https://doi.org/10.1002/gps.5442.

Kahn, R. S. (1965). Comments. In M. P. Lawton, & F. G. Lawton (Eds.), *Mental impairment in the aged; Proceedings*. Philadelphia Geriatric Center.

Khoury, R., & Ghossoub, E. (2019). Diagnostic biomarkers of Alzheimer's disease: A state-of-the-art review. *Biomarkers in Neuropsychiatry*, *1*, 100005. https://doi.org/10.1016/j.bionps.2019.100005.

Larson, E. B., & Stroud, C. (2021). Meeting the challenge of caring for persons living with dementia and their care partners and caregivers: A report from the National Academies of Sciences, Engineering, and Medicine. *Journal of the American Medical Association*, *325*(18), 1831–1832. https://doi.org /10.1001/jama.2021.4928.

Lilienfeld, S. O., Ritschel, L. A., Lynn, S. J., Cautin, R. L., & Latzman, R. D. (2014). Why ineffective psychotherapies appear to work: A taxonomy of causes of spurious therapeutic effectiveness. *Perspectives on Psychological Science*, *9*(4), 355–387. https://doi.org/10.1177/1745691614535216.

Lourida, I., Hannon, E., Littlejohns, T. J., Langa, K. M., Hyppönen, E., Kuzma, E., & Llewellyn, D. J. (2019). Association of lifestyle and genetic risk with incidence of dementia. *Journal of the American Medical Association*, *322*(5), 430–437. https://doi.org/10.1001/jama.2019.9879.

estᴅ.

McClellan, M., Brown, N., Califf, R. M., & Warner, J. J. (2019). Call to action: Urgent challenges in cardiovascular disease: A presidential advisory from the American Heart Association. *Circulation, 139*(9), e44–e54. https://doi.org/doi:10.1161/CIR.0000000000000652.

McCurry, S., & Drossel, C. (2011). *Treating dementia in context: A step-by-step guide to working with individuals and families.* American Psychological Association.

McKeith, I. G., Boeve, B. F., Dickson, D. W., Halliday, G., Taylor, J.-P., Weintraub, D., Aarsland, D., Galvin, J., Attems, J., Ballard, C. G., Bayston, A., Beach, T. G., Blanc, F., Bohnen, N., Bonanni, L., Bras, J., Brundin, P., Burn, D., Chen-Plotkin, A., ... Kosaka, K. (2017). Diagnosis and management of dementia with Lewy bodies. *Fourth Consensus Report of the DLB Consortium, 89*(1), 88–100. https://doi.org/10.1212/wnl.0000000000004058.

McKhann, G., Drachman, D., Folstein, M., Katzman, R., Price, D., & Stadlan, E. M. (1984). Clinical diagnosis of Alzheimer's disease. Report of the NINCDS-ADRDA Work Group under the auspices of Department of Health and Human Services Task Force on Alzheimer's Disease. *Neurology, 34*(7), 939–939. https://doi.org/10.1212/wnl.34.7.939.

McKhann, G. M., Knopman, D. S., Chertkow, H., Hyman, B. T., Jack Jr., C. R., Kawas, C. H., Klunk, W. E., Koroshetz, W. J., Manly, J. J., Mayeux, R., Mohs, R. C., Morris, J. C., Rossor, M. N., Scheltens, P., Carrillo, M. C., Thies, B., Weintraub, S., & Phelps, C. H. (2011). The diagnosis of dementia due to Alzheimer's disease: Recommendations from the National Institute on Aging-Alzheimer's Association workgroups on diagnostic guidelines for Alzheimer's disease. *Alzheimer's & Dementia, 7*(3), 263–269. https://doi.org/10.1016/j.jalz.2011.03.005.

McShane, R., Westby, M. J., Roberts, E., Minakaran, N., Schneider, L., Farrimond, L. E., Maayan, N., Ware, J., & Debarros, J. (2019). Memantine for dementia. *Cochrane Database of Systematic Reviews, 3*(3), CD003154. https://doi.org/10.1002/14651858.CD003154.pub6.

Nasreddine, Z. S., Phillips, N. A., Bédirian, V., Charbonneau, S., Whitehead, V., Collin, I., Cummings, J. L., & Chertkow, H. (2005). The Montreal Cognitive Assessment, MoCA: A brief screening tool for mild cognitive impairment. *Journal of the American Geriatrics Society, 53*(4), 695–699. https://doi.org/https://doi.org/10.1111/j.1532-5415.2005.53221.x.

Nelson, P. T., Dickson, D. W., Trojanowski, J. Q., Jack, C. R., Boyle, P. A., Arfanakis, K., Rademakers, R., Alafuzoff, I., Attems, J., Brayne, C., Coyle-Gilchrist, I. T. S., Chui, H. C., Fardo, D. W., Flanagan, M. E., Halliday, G., Hokkanen, S. R. K., Hunter, S., Jicha, G. A., Katsumata, Y., ... Schneider, J. A. (2019). Limbic-predominant age-related TDP-43 encephalopathy (LATE): Consensus working group report. *Brain*, *142*(6), 1503–1527. https://doi.org/10.1093/brain/awz099.

Nichols, L. O., Martindale-Adams, J., Burns, R., Graney, M. J., & Zuber, J. (2011). Translation of a dementia caregiver support program in a health care system – REACH VA. *Archives of Internal Medicine*, *171*(4), 353–359. https://doi.org/10.1001/archinternmed.2010.548.

O'Brien, J., Taylor, J. P., Ballard, C., Barker, R. A., Bradley, C., Burns, A., Collerton, D., Dave, S., Dudley, R., Francis, P., Gibbons, A., Harris, K., Lawrence, V., Leroi, I., McKeith, I., Michaelides, M., Naik, C., O'Callaghan, C., Olsen, K., … Ffytche, D. (2020). Visual hallucinations in neurological and ophthalmological disease: Pathophysiology and management. *Journal of Neurology, Neurosurgery & Psychiatry*, *91*(5), 512–519. https://doi.org/10.1136/jnnp-2019-322702.

O'Donnell, B. F., Drachman, D. A., Barnes, H. J., Peterson, K. E., Swearer, J. M., & Lew, R. A. (1992). Incontinence and troublesome behaviors predict institutionalization in dementia. *Topics in geriatrics*, *5*(1), 45–52. https://doi.org/10.1177/002383099200500108.

Olson, N. L., & Albensi, B. C. (2021). Dementia-friendly "design": Impact on COVID-19 death rates in long-term care facilities around the world. *Journal of Alzheimer's Disease*, *81*, 427–450. https://doi.org/10.3233/JAD-210017.

Postuma, R. B., Gagnon, J.-F., Vendette, M., Desjardins, C., & Montplaisir, J. Y. (2011). Olfaction and color vision identify impending neurodegeneration in rapid eye movement sleep behavior disorder. *Annals of Neurology*, *69*(5), 811–818. https://doi.org/https://doi.org/10.1002/ana.22282.

Powell, T. (2019). *Dementia reimagined: Building a life of joy and dignity from beginning to end*. Avery.

Renn, B. N., Asghar-Ali, A. A., Thielke, S., Catic, A., Martini, S. R., Mitchell, B. G., & Kunik, M. E. (2018). A systematic review of practice guidelines and recommendations for discontinuation of cholinesterase inhibitors in dementia. *The American Journal of Geriatric Psychiatry*, *26*(2), 134–147. https://doi.org/https://doi.org/10.1016/j.jagp.2017.09.027.

Roebuck-Spencer, T. M., Glen, T., Puente, A. E., Denney, R. L., Ruff, R. M., Hostetter, G., & Bianchini, K. J. (2017). Cognitive screening tests versus comprehensive neuropsychological test batteries: A National Academy of Neuropsychology education paper. *Archives of Clinical Neuropsychology*, *32*(4), 491–498. https://doi.org/10.1093/arclin/acx021.

Ruangritchankul, S., Chantharit, P., Srisuma, S., & Gray, L. C. (2021). Adverse drug reactions of acetylcholinesterase inhibitors in older people living with dementia: A comprehensive literature review. *Therapeutics and Clinical Risk Management*, *17*, 927–949. https://doi.org/10.2147/TCRM.S323387.

Rubino, A., Sanon, M., Ganz, M. L., Simpson, A., Fenton, M. C., Verma, S., Hartry, A., Baker, R. A., Duffy, R. A., Gwin, K., & Fillit, H. (2020). Association of the US Food and Drug Administration antipsychotic drug boxed warning with medication use and health outcomes in elderly patients with dementia. *JAMA Network Open*, *3*(4), e203630–e203630. https://doi.org/10.1001/jamanetworkopen.2020.3630.

Salzman, T., Sarquis-Adamson, Y., Son, S., Montero-Odasso, M., & Fraser, S. (2022). Associations of multidomain interventions with improvements in cognition in mild cognitive impairment: A systematic review and meta-analysis. *JAMA Network*, *5*(5), e226744. https://doi.org/10.1001/jamanetworkopen.2022.6744.

Saredakis, D., Collins-Praino, L. E., Gutteridge, D. S., Stephan, B. C. M., & Keage, H. A. D. (2019). Conversion to MCI and dementia in Parkinson's disease: A systematic review and meta-analysis. *Parkinsonism & Related Disorders*, *65*, 20–31. https://doi.org/10.1016/j.parkreldis.2019.04.020.

Scales, K., Zimmerman, S., & Miller, S. J. (2018). Evidence-based nonpharmacological practices to address behavioral and psychological symptoms of dementia. *Gerontologist*, *58*(S1), S88–S102. https://doi.org/10.1093/geront/gnx167.

Schulz, R., Burgio, L., Burns, R., Eisdorfer, C., Gallagher-Thompson, D., Gitlin, L. N., & Mahoney, D. F. (2003). Resources for enhancing Alzheimer's caregiver health (REACH): Overview, site-specific outcomes, and future directions. *The Gerontologist*, *43*(4), 514–520. https://doi.org/10.1093/geront/43.4.514.

Singh-Manoux, A., Dugravot, A., Fournier, A., Abell, J., Ebmeier, K., Kivimäki, M., & Sabia, S. (2017). Trajectories of depressive symptoms before diagnosis of dementia: A 28-year follow-up study. *JAMA Psychiatry*, *74*(7), 712–718. https://doi.org/10.1001/jamapsychiatry.2017.0660.

Spiegl, K., Luttenberger, K., Graessel, E., Becker, L., Scheel, J., & Pendergrass, A. (2021). Predictors of institutionalization in users of day care facilities with mild cognitive impairment to moderate dementia. *BMC Health Services Research*, *21*(1), 1009. https://doi.org/10.1186/s12913-021-07017-8.

Stokes, L., Combes, H., & Stokes, G. (2015). The dementia diagnosis: A literature review of information, understanding, and attributions. *Psychogeriatrics*, *15*(3), 218–225. https://doi.org/https://doi.org/10.1111/psyg.12095.

Suen, Y. N., Wong, S. M. Y., Hui, C. L. M., Chan, S. K. W., Lee, E. H. M., Chang, W. C., & Chen, E. Y. H. (2019). Late-onset psychosis and very-late-onset-schizophrenia-like-psychosis: An updated systematic review. *International Review of Psychiatry*, *31*(5/6), 523–542. https://doi.org/10.1080/09540261.2019.1670624.

Tjia, J., Lemay, C. A., Bonner, A., Compher, C., Paice, K., Field, T., Mazor, K., Hunnicutt, J. N., Lapane, K. L., & Gurwitz, J. (2017). Informed family member involvement to improve the quality of dementia care in nursing homes. *Journal of the American Geriatrics Society, 65*(1), 59–65. https://doi.org/10.1111/jgs.14299.

U.S. Food and Drug Administration. (2021, June 7). FDA grants accelerated approval for Alzheimer's drug. www.fda.gov/news-events/press-announcements/fda-grants-accelerated-approval-alzheimers-drug.

van Wijngaarden, E., Manna, A., & Anne-Mei, T. (2019). 'The eyes of others' are what really matters: The experience of living with dementia from an insider perspective. *PLoS One, 14*(4). https://doi.org/10.1371/journal.pone.0214724.

Wilson, R. S., Leurgans, S. E., Boyle, P. A., & Bennett, D. A. (2011). Cognitive decline in prodromal Alzheimer disease and mild cognitive impairment. *Archives of Neurology, 68*(3), 351–356. https://doi.org/10.1001/archneurol.2011.31.

Yamada, Y., Vlachova, M., Richter, T., Finne-Soveri, H., Gindin, J., van der Roest, H., Denkinger, M. D., Bernabei, R., Onder, G., & Topinkova, E. (2014). Prevalence and correlates of hearing and visual impairments in European nursing homes: Results from the SHELTER study. *Journal of the American Medical Directors Association, 15*(10), 738–743. https://doi.org/https://doi.org/10.1016/j.jamda.2014.05.012.

Yumoto, A., & Suwa, S. (2021). Difficulties and associated coping methods regarding visual hallucinations caused by dementia with Lewy bodies. *Dementia, 20*(1), 291–307. https://doi.org/10.1177/1471301219879541.

14

Antisocial Behavior

Devon L. L. Polaschek

Antisocial behavior typically refers to violations of the law or of common social mores in a manner that offends, harms, or deprives another person of their rights, property or wellbeing and ultimately undermines the healthy functioning of society (Skeem & Cooke, 2010). Antisocial behavior that may not be covered by criminal codes but may still meet this definition could include abandoning one's children, gaslighting another person, or taking informal credit for another person's ideas. Antisocial behavior is common and only warrants a diagnosis when diverse forms of behavior are observed and persist over a sustained period. In adults, the most relevant diagnosis is antisocial personality disorder (ASPD). ASPD can be diagnosed only in people over the age of 18 and requires "a pervasive pattern of disregard for and violation of the rights of others, occurring since age 15 years" (American Psychiatric Association [APA], 2022, p. 748). It includes at least three of the following: behavior that is grounds for arrest, deception or lying, impulsivity, irritability, aggressiveness, recklessness or irresponsible behavior, or a failure to show remorse for those harmed.

To be diagnosed with ASPD, the person also must meet criteria for conduct disorder before the age of 15; these criteria are similar to ASPD but need only have persisted for 12 months (APA, 2022). In other words, people who pervasively break societal rules from adolescence onwards are viewed, in this way of thinking, as having a mental disorder that is referred to as ASPD. If the person does not have the necessary history to meet criteria for childhood conduct disorder as required for ASPD, the adult can instead be diagnosed with conduct disorder. Because behaviors typifying ASPD vary widely in their severity, people who have had little contact with the criminal justice system can be diagnosed with ASPD. In practice, it can be argued that the history of this diagnosis is one of attempting to produce a reliable and valid way of capturing "criminal personality" (Gurley, 2009), even though in reality the personalities of people involved in crime are quite diverse (Blackburn, 1988).

Studies of ASPD suggest that the lifetime prevalence in community samples is about 1–4%, and that compared to women, men are between 3 and 5 times as likely to meet the diagnostic criteria (Coid et al., 2006; Werner et al., 2015). Its prevalence in populations being managed in prisons is much higher. Perhaps a quarter to half of male prisoners and about a fifth of female prisoners have been diagnosed with ASPD, but figures vary widely (Fazel & Danesh, 2002; Singleton et al., 1998).

Comorbidity is common for those with ASPD, particularly with substance abuse disorders (Werner et al., 2015) and some personality disorders (e.g., borderline, narcissistic, paranoid; APA, 2022). Increased prevalence of anxiety disorders and posttraumatic stress disorder has also been noted (Goodwin & Hamilton, 2003). ASPD typically improves somewhat with age, and as individuals approach age 40, a reduction in criminal behavior, if present, often occurs (APA, 2022).

14.1 Pseudoscience and Questionable Ideas

14.1.1 Diagnostic Controversies

14.1.1.1 ASPD or Psychopathy?

Current diagnostic criteria for ASPD have historical roots in the concept of psychopathy, which was included in the first edition of the DSM published in 1952. Yet without formal diagnostic criteria, it was described in terms of key traits such as superficial charm, insincerity, irresponsibility, and absence of nervousness (Gurley, 2009). The DSM-III (APA, 1980) radically revised the diagnosis into a pattern of socially deviant or criminal behavior starting in childhood (e.g., vandalism, truancy) and persisting into adulthood (e.g., lying, stealing, aggressive behavior). Personality traits such as callousness and irresponsibility were no longer featured (Hare, 1996). Unsurprisingly, the DSM-III version of ASPD lacked utility in the criminal justice system due to its very high prevalence (Hare, 1980). As Flint-Stevens (1993, p. 1) noted, the diagnosis of ASPD in prison populations became like "looking for hay in a haystack."

The DSM-III thus parted company in important ways with the concept of psychopathy, and this gap remains to this day. ASPD is estimated to be at least three times more prevalent than psychopathy (Yoon et al., 2022). That is, many people who meet the diagnostic criteria for ASPD have low to moderate levels of psychopathy. Furthermore, ASPD is profoundly conflated with chronic criminality. Although it is a *personality* disorder, a diverse range of personality traits – not just psychopathy – underlies this pattern of chronic antisocial behavior (Poythress et al., 2010). This is just one of the issues that makes it of limited value for practical purposes. Despite this problem, ASPD is often offered as an explanation for the very behavior pattern that is used to diagnose it.

Even more confusingly, while the diagnosis is made using largely behavioral criteria, the surrounding DSM-IV text refers to personality characteristics that are central to *psychopathy*, and misleadingly implies that ASPD is equivalent to psychopathy. Similarly, the DSM-5-TR states, "This pattern has also been referred to as *psychopathy, sociopathy*, or *dissocial personality disorder*" (APA, 2022, p. 748).

The label of psychopathy is itself controversial. Especially in the criminal justice system, the most widely accepted method for identifying psychopathy is to use one of the clinician-rated Psychopathy Checklist scales developed by Hare, most often the Psychopathy Checklist – Revised (PCL-R; Hare, 1991; see also Hare, 2003). Antisocial behavior, including but not limited to criminal behavior, is central to Hare's view of psychopathy (Hare & Neumann, 2010), but so are the personality traits of psychopathy that are theorized to generate it. The Hare PCL-R contains two correlated factors, each with two facets. Factor 1 represents the key personality features of psychopathy (Hare, 1991), while Factor 2 captures characteristics of antisocial behavior and lifestyle that are found in a much wider population (Yoon et al., 2022). Although scoring cut-offs have been used to identify psychopathy with the PCL-R, the construct itself is dimensional, not categorical (Edens et al., 2006; Walters et al., 2008). Put simply, related reports should speak of people as being highly or moderately or not at all psychopathic, not as psychopaths or nonpsychopaths.

To add to the complexity, debate is ongoing within the scientific community about what psychopathy is and is not (Skeem et al., 2011). Although psychopathy is a rarer, and more narrowly defined, similar debates about ASPD exist (e.g., the extent to which the psychopathy measured by the PCL-R conflates personality characteristics with criminal behavior). Most recently, Patrick and colleagues (2009) have proposed the Triarchic Model of Psychopathy in an attempt to reconcile different measurement approaches. Debate continues about whether positive adjustment features such as lack of nervousness are part of psychopathy (Lilienfeld et al., 2016). A deficit in the ability to experience fear is considered one of the key mechanisms underlying psychopathy. Yet people with high PCL-R scores, like people with ASPD, can show significant problems with anxiety, fear, and other negative emotions (Poythress et al., 2010; see also discussions of secondary psychopathy such as Hicks & Drislane, 2018). Because both ASPD and psychopathy are important concepts for understanding psychotherapy for antisocial behavior, they are the main areas of focus for this chapter. However, the term "antisocial propensity" is used to refer to people with extensive histories of antisocial behavior and associated characteristics, whether or not they meet particular diagnostic criteria.

14.1.1.2 What Is the Value of Diagnosing ASPD?

One of the benefits of a diagnostic system is to create categories with known etiologies and established treatment approaches. But as yet, these benefits have not been realized for ASPD. Numerous issues with the validity and utility of the diagnosis have been documented (Gurley, 2009). The etiology of ASPD remains unclear, with a variety of environmental (e.g., child abuse) and genetic factors (e.g., temperament) proposed to come together to create the characteristics underlying pervasive antisocial behavior (DeLisi, et al., 2019). Following on from this lack of clarity, there is a lack of evidence that typical methods of treatment for mental health disorders (e.g., psychotropic medications) have any useful effects (Black, 2017) and other forms of treatment (e.g., psychotherapy) are also described either as ineffective, or at least underresearched (Black, 2017; Hatchett, 2015; van den Bosch et al., 2018). To date, the case remains to be made that psychopathologizing antisocial propensity has been in any way helpful and some argue that it may be harmful (Polaschek, 2010). Although a significant proportion of people with ASPD may have little or no involvement with the criminal justice system (Robins et al., 1991), many do. Perhaps due to a lack of effective treatment responses for these patients, professionals in forensic and general mental health services often have stigmatizing and pejorative attitudes to people who are chronically antisocial (Duggan & Kane, 2010). People with ASPD may be intentionally excluded (van den Bosch et al., 2018), thus denying them treatment for other mental health disorders from which they may benefit (Black, 2017; Hatchett, 2015).

In parallel with this situation, over the last 50 years the fields of developmental criminology and criminal psychology have emerged. Both now have established bodies of empirical research on important causal factors in criminal behavior that would be helpful to health professionals seeking to develop a coherent clinical picture of a person presenting with antisocial behavior and their needs. Criminal psychology, building initially on the era of functional analysis and behavior therapy techniques, has developed approaches to intervention with highly antisocial people that significantly reduce future criminal convictions. Whether these treatments reduce noncriminal characteristics of ASPD remains to be fully investigated, because this field is not concerned with diagnosis per se, making it unclear whether there are differential outcomes for those who meet or do not meet ASPD criteria. Nevertheless, this work is not necessarily very familiar to health professionals because of the way that knowledge can become siloed across different settings. The effect of this siloing on the development of effective treatments for people with mental health disorders who commit crime has been acknowledged and documented in recent years (Bonta et al., 2014; Howells et al., 2004; Skeem et al., 2015), but not specifically with respect to people whose diagnosis is primarily ASPD.

14.1.2 Questionable Assessment Practices

14.1.2.1 Unreliability of Diagnosis

People with chronic patterns of antisocial behavior can engender strong negative reactions in clinicians, making the use of reliable and valid diagnostic assessment instruments particularly important. Although the inclusion of behavioral criteria in the DSM-III was intended to increase diagnostic reliability, the DSM-5 field trials for ASPD revealed questionable inter-rater reliability (Freedman et al., 2013). That said, the PCL-R certainly *can* be scored reliably, but as with any measure requiring skill or discretion, that does not mean it will be. Scoring conducted for research purposes, for example, may differ quite substantially from scoring in routine practice. Several studies suggest that PCL-R scoring in the field is unacceptably unreliable (Olver et al., 2020; see also Polaschek, 2022 for a review). Allegiance effects – systematic differences in scoring based on whether the assessment is conducted for the defense or the prosecution – have been found, but so have stable interrater differences that are independent of who commissioned the report (Olver et al., 2020). Stable differences between raters may account for as much as 30% of variance in scores, which when compared to the estimated 45% of variance attributed to actual differences in the people being assessed (Boccaccini et al., 2008) suggests this may be a noteworthy problem.

14.1.2.2 Use of ASPD Diagnosis for Psycho-Legal Outcomes

Compared to psychopathy, there is much less evidence on both the reliability and predictive validity of an ASPD diagnosis, as well as its use for important psycho-legal decisions. However, the existing evidence suggests that a well-validated risk assessment instrument is preferable to making a diagnosis. Along with the low diagnostic reliability noted earlier, there are concerns that clinicians may overweigh discrete and distinctive events rather than testing for more chronic patterns of behavior in making a diagnosis (Cunningham & Reidy, 1998). Consequently, a diagnosis of ASPD should not be used to decide significant outcomes, such as capital sentencing or indefinite commitment for people with a history of sexual offending (Edens et al., 2018). A recent study confirmed that a diagnosis of ASPD did not predict sexual recidivism, although it did predict general and violent recidivism in a sexual offender sample (Yoon et al., 2022). Finally, in a section on various questionable assessment practices relating to the PCL-R, Hare (1998) noted the particularly concerning practice of diagnosing ASPD and then misleadingly using research on psychopathy to infer future implications of the ASPD diagnosis.

14.1.2.3 *Using the PCL-R to Decide Important Psycho-Legal Outcomes*

The lack of reliability in psychopathy scoring is particularly concerning because of two related assessment issues: the uses to which scores are put, and the stigma of the psychopathy label. The PCL-R was not designed as a risk assessment instrument, but it is widely used to predict various criminal behavior outcomes, including reconvictions for violent or sexual crimes, intimate partner violence, and violence inside institutions (i.e., prisons, secure hospitals; DeMatteo & Olver, 2022).

However, the PCL-R scales do not predict these outcomes with greater accuracy than instruments designed specifically for risk prediction: instruments that when used do not also imply that the person may have psychopathy. In fact, the part of the PCL-R that contains the core psychopathic traits (e.g., glibness, lack of remorse, pathological lying), has been found not to predict violence at all (Yang et al., 2010). Potentially more accurate purpose-designed instruments (see Yang et al., 2010) provide much more relevant useful information for less assessment time, compared to the PCL-R, without conflating the assessment of risk of violence with the diagnosis of psychopathy.

Despite these observations, a survey of more than 2000 violence risk assessors across numerous countries reported that over their career, the PCL-R was the second-most commonly used instrument in their assessments, and the most commonly used in the United States (Singh et al., 2014). It is commonly used to inform decisions about the most serious of criminal justice outcomes. For example, the PCL-R is required in some U.S. states when determining capital sentencing (i.e., the death penalty; DeMatteo et al., 2020; Olver et al., 2020). It is also used to determine treatability in youth to decide whether they are to be tried in adult court, where they may become eligible for capital sentencing. Actually, it is *required* in some states for these assessments (e.g., Texas), although this practice is also not well supported by evidence (DeMatteo et al., 2014).

14.1.2.4 Potential Prejudicial Consequences of Assessing and Identifying Psychopathy

The popularity of identifying psychopathy when the task at hand is actually to assess risk is made all the more baffling given the potential for misunderstanding its use creates for decision-makers. Myths about psychopathy are widely held (see the next section). To the extent that triers of fact – judges, juries, and perhaps even the assessors themselves – also hold these myths, it is likely that "psychopathy" labels masquerading as a risk assessment will bring these biases into the decision-making process. Kelley and colleagues' (2019) meta-analysis of jury simulation research found that even jurors' *perceptions* of the presence of the prototypical core psychopathic traits – in cases where the expert witness did not actually use the label – were related to ratings of how evil and dangerous defendants were, and to longer sentencing recommendations and more recommendations for the death penalty. It is not surprising, then, that DeMatteo and Olver recently concluded that "it is inappropriate to use the PCL-R to make life or death recommendations about an individual for ethical, humanitarian, and psychometric reasons" (2022, p. 4).

14.1.3 Myths that Influence Treatment

Erroneous or unsupported beliefs about the etiology of ASPD and psychopathy directly and indirectly undermine perceptions of treatability. People high on psychopathy measures are often described as innately evil and somehow distinct from the rest of us (Kelley et al., 2019). For example, Taylor (2013) noted that innate badness or evil is at the root of how our criminal justice system is used. The hallmark of evil is often seen as a deficit in empathy, a trait common in people with psychopathic personalities. Alongside the concept of evil, the idea that psychopathy is innate – with the implication that it is a stable entity – pops up frequently in popular media. For example, Duignan (n.d., para. 6) wrote "it is generally agreed that psychopathy is chiefly a genetic or inherited condition."

Psychopathy is often thought to be largely biological in origin because its prevalence has been stable across the ages (Walsh & Wu, 2008), yet this proposition is without scientific foundation. Sociopathy, on the other hand, has been attributed to psychosocial variables such as poverty and childhood adversity (Walsh & Wu, 2008), suggesting it is more a function of nurture than nature. This distinction is interesting, yet it is not based in evidence. Although there appear to be significant genetic and environmental contributions to psychopathy, ASPD, and antisocial rule-breaking in general (Waldman et al., 2018; Werner et al., 2015), modern understandings of gene–environment interactions and epigenetics suggest it is neither possible nor meaningful to disconnect what people are "made of" at conception from their environment and its influence over the course of development. Therefore, ASPD is neither born nor made, but a complex mix of both.

More recently, the etiology discourse has shifted more from discussions of evil or genetic predisposition to the brain. Research over the last decade has found structural and functional differences in the brains of people with histories of chronic criminality, ASPD, and psychopathy (Raine, 2018; Werner et al., 2015). In the book *The Psychopath Whisperer*, Kiehl reported that when brain abnormalities were first discovered in U.S. adult prisoners "it was truly amazing ... I had not even fantasized about such a dramatic result. I was blown away ... Psychopaths' brains were abnormal; we had solid proof" (Kiehl, 2015, p. 212). Kiehl went on to scan the brains of young people with high psychopathy scores and found they showed similar patterns of atrophy, especially in the paralimbic system. Others have found evidence in antisocial samples for reduced thickness in various parts of the cortex and in specific brain structures, and a number of functional differences have also been documented (Gao, 2019).

The idea that distinct neurodevelopmental pathways are associated with chronic antisocial behavior is far from new. For example, Moffitt (1993) proposed that factors leading to neuropsychological impairments very early in life are predictive of later antisociality. Early evidence showed that poorer performance in motor and cognitive skills at 3 and 5 years, respectively, predicted adult criminal behavior in the Dunedin longitudinal health and development study. However, it was only when the cohort members reached age 45 that MRI imaging was used, and it showed reduced cortical thickness and surface area. However, we can't conclude from this result that there were also cortical differences in childhood, because no studies have yet mapped brain structure and function from early childhood alongside the observed cognitive and motor features that predict antisocial behavior (Carlisi et al., 2020). This would be the first step of several in establishing potential causality for brain structural and functional features.

In the case of the Dunedin findings, it is unlikely that such findings, even in adulthood, are an indicator of ASPD or psychopathy, because it is unlikely that there is a distinct antisocial or psychopathic brain. Similar results to the Dunedin study are being found for many types of psychopathology, and if anything, the trend in findings is away from distinct patterns being associated with distinct disorders (Romer et al., 2021). For example, based on their own data showing reduced neocortical thickness, Romer and colleagues (2021) recently concluded that "the continued pursuit of such specific correlates may limit progress toward more effective strategies for etiological understanding, prevention, and intervention" (p. 1).

It is important to remain skeptical about what this growing body of findings does, and especially what it does *not* tell us; its practical value remains to be established. With regard to etiology, antisocial behavior is not indicated to be innate, as people often assume, nor is it unchangeable. Those with ASPD commonly experienced abuse, neglect, attachment failure, or family adversity, all of which have a demonstrated ability to negatively impact brain development (Raine, 2018). Antisocial behavior in adults is linked to a variety of factors and associated with several diagnoses. This considerable heterogeneity likely reflects multiple relevant mechanisms and pathways. Although equally relevant to ASPD, Fowles (2018) said with respect to psychopathy: "specific psychopathic features can result from different etiological processes and pathways, and causal processes or risk factors will show only a probability relationship with the development of psychopathy – due to the interplay with other variables" (p. 95). Additionally, erroneously labelling a disorder as an innate manifestation of evil tends to demotivate efforts to assist such individuals. With regard to neural substrates, many disorders that are routinely treated, albeit with varying success, can be understood in neurodevelopmental terms (Raine, 2018). Notwithstanding the excitement of finding MRI abnormalities in prisoners, Kiehl's (2015) book included evidence from a program in Wisconsin that showed reductions in psychopathic symptoms alongside reductions in antisocial behavior (Caldwell et al., 2012): acknowledging that biology is not destiny.

14.1.4 Dubious Treatments

14.1.4.1 Implausible, Untested, and/or Ineffective Treatments

Effective treatment requires both a theory of the condition to be treated and a theory of how change will be affected. Few conditions have elicited as many novel and ineffective treatments as chronic antisociality. Many treatments have no plausible underlying theory and may even be driven by disdain of scientific knowledge; some are based on anecdotal experiences, and some represent outright quackery. Latessa and colleagues (2020) have been cataloging such interventions for at least two decades, including stress reduction programs, efforts to improve self-esteem and happiness, dance programs, art and creativity-oriented therapies, acupuncture, gardening, wilderness programs, drama, heart mapping, and dressing people in diapers.

While some other treatments may be anchored in theory, they nevertheless fail because they focus on changing factors that are not empirically linked to antisociality or they utilize ineffective strategies. For example, some forms of traditional psychotherapy that may be valued for use with some clients tend not to be effective in reducing antisociality. People with long-term entrenched patterns of antisocial behavior are often restless and energetic, action-oriented, impulsive, and have poor attentional control. They have often dropped out of formal schooling after successive failure experiences. They may be mistrustful and take time to form meaningful therapeutic relationships. They may also have repeated head injuries or cognitive impairment due to alcohol and drug use. They do not tend to respond well to treatment oriented at generating insight, in supporting people in self-reflection, or in telling them rather than showing them how to behave more skillfully. Consequently, psychodynamic, humanistic, and most psychoeducational approaches have not been associated with reduced subsequent criminal behavior (Bonta & Andrews, 2016). Some psychoanalytic approaches that target deficits in mentalization related to attachment do have a plausible underlying theory (Yakeley, 2012), but they have not yet been tested for effectiveness in either symptom reduction or antisocial behavior (Gibbon et al., 2020).

14.1.4.2 Potentially Harmful Approaches

Although largely unused since the experimental heyday of the 1960s, psychedelic drugs such as LSD are again being evaluated in mental health treatment, including with forensic patients (see Holoyda, 2020).

One early intervention using LSD appears to have caused significant harm (Harris et al., 1994), although the specific contribution played by LSD has not been isolated from other treatment elements. During the 1960s, and informed by investigations into the effects of brainwashing during the Korean war, the Oak Ridge Social Therapy unit at Penetanguishene Hospital in Canada opened a highly experimental residential program that featured a patient-led community approach. It was based on the premise that people could be psychically torn down and rebuilt to improve their psychological health (Rice et al., 1992). Patients were committed involuntarily after a conviction or court finding of not guilty by reason of insanity, resided continuously with other patients, and received very little input from staff. Instead, they were confined together, naked, in a sealed room, fed through wall-mounted tubes and invited to administer doses of various drugs including LSD and methedrine to one another (Rice & Harris, 1992).

Years later, Rice and colleagues (1992) retrospectively used their records to score these patients using the PCL-R. Patients above the cut-off score for psychopathy showed higher rates of reconviction for violence than their matched prison controls. The researchers interpreted this finding to indicate that people with psychopathy should not be treated because it made them more dangerous (Harris et al., 1994). For some years, reports of any form of treatment for people with psychopathy virtually dried up. However, with the benefit of hindsight, the Oak Ridge intervention should be viewed not as a psychological treatment, but as an unethical, state-sanctioned form of abuse, which may well have selectively harmed people high on psychopathy (see Polaschek, 2014; Polaschek & Skeem, 2018).

Punishment-based interventions in general do seem to be harmful, *increasing* recidivism by a small amount compared to other types of responses (Bonta & Andrews, 2016). Some sanctions in this category are simply ineffective, such as military-style boot camps, which are mainly used with young people (Latessa et al., 2020). Based on the notion that instilling discipline is effective in reducing antisociality, attendees simply become more fit yet none the wiser about how to behave prosocially. Still other punishment interventions for antisocial behavior are less benign. It is not difficult to believe that being in prison entrenches antisociality and may increase rather than decrease symptoms of ASPD. Incarceration in and of itself increases the likelihood of returning to prison, especially when individuals are subject to highly vigilant post-prison supervision, often leading to a return to custody on minor technical violations of parole conditions having nothing to do with antisocial behavior (Harding et al., 2017). Prison has also been shown to lead to greater recidivism than much less intrusive sanctions like community service (Wermink et al., 2010). In fact, all other things being equal, any contact with the criminal justice system may promote antisocial behavior compared to no contact (Motz et al., 2020).

14.2 Research-Supported Approaches

The most significant progress made in reducing the propensity for antisocial behavior comes from interventions guided by empirically determined principles collectively referred to as the Risk–Need–Responsivity (RNR) model. An array of meta-analyses of the RNR-based intervention literature (Wormith & Zidenberg, 2018) and even more on general offender rehabilitation (McGuire, 2002) reveal a series of components associated with improved outcomes. Initially researchers categorized outcome studies based on their "brand name" (e.g., Acceptance and Commitment Therapy, Dialectical Behavior Therapy, Family Systems Therapy). But actually, programs with common labels often differ from each other in important ways that make it hard to interpret the results. A key breakthrough was the move to much more specific coding, by examining referral criteria, treatment targets, change processes, and therapist characteristics from inside each treatment as it was provided in each specific study. The results are too detailed and complex to review here (see Bonta & Andrews, 2016), but in brief, this is essentially a transdiagnostic approach where common symptoms with empirical links to recidivism are the targets for treatment. They are known variously as dynamic risk factors or criminogenic needs: relatively stable "symptoms" that result from development in people who have entrenched antisocial behavior.

Along with basing treatment on the right targets, effective therapies and interventions use evidence-based methods to change behavior (Bonta & Andrews, 2016). Insight development is often the first step. Then, individuals are explicitly taught appropriate cognitions and practical skills that offer prosocial alternatives to antisocial behavior. Effective interventions use cognitive, behavioral, and social-learning strategies alongside core therapist approaches to developing a strong relationship (e.g., firm but fair approach, interpersonal warmth, use of motivational interviewing techniques) and a delivery style that matches clients' responsivity difficulties (e.g., negative attitudes to learning, traumatic brain injury, entitlement, hostility, short attention span and active learning preferences; Polaschek, 2014). Although there is limited research that links changes in these factors to changes in expected recidivism outcomes, it is well-established that the factors themselves are correlated with reduced recidivism (Bonta & Andrews, 2016). Of course, recidivism evaluations of correctional programs are a proxy for the treatment of DSM-5-TR ASPD symptoms, but they provide a promising place to start for psychotherapists working in the health sector with clients who have extensive antisocial behavior. Additionally, they are most effective with people who are at such high risk of new offending they might seldom be considered suitable for or capable of responding to treatment in mainstream health services.

14.3 Conclusion

The DSM-5-TR primarily attempts to capture chronically antisocial behavior within the ASPD diagnosis. The extent to which having such a diagnosis confers useful information for psychotherapy is questionable given its low diagnostic reliability, heterogeneity of underlying personality traits, and conflation with the rarer and more severe construct of psychopathy. Furthermore, the inclusion of ASPD in the DSM for several decades has not led to the development of a body of empirical knowledge about effective interventions to reduce antisocial behavior. Instead, the field is replete with ineffective treatments, implausible treatments, harmful treatments, and what has been referred to as "knowledge destruction"; the intentional promotion of conventional wisdom and pseudoscience while dismantling and undermining empirical evidence to the contrary (Cullen & Gendreau, 2001). Psychologists and others in the criminal justice system have made significant progress in providing programs and interventions that reduce recidivism. This work does not directly align with traditional psychotherapy because (1) clients are selected because they have dynamic risk factors that indicate a high overall likelihood of reconviction and (2) treatment effectiveness is often judged in terms of post-treatment reconviction rates. Both of these represent crude proxies for psychological diagnosis and measurement of symptom reduction. However, this approach has proved so far to be a useful place to start. If better translated across into health settings, its further development could result in patients with ASPD, despite the challenges they may pose in the therapy process, being treated more humanely and effectively.

Devon L. L. Polaschek, PhD, DipClinPsyc, MNZM, is a Professor of Psychology with the following affiliations: Te Kura Whatu Oho Mauri | School of Psychology and Te Puna Haumaru | New Zealand Institute of

Security and Crime Science, University of Waikato. She is co-editor of *The Wiley International Handbook of Correctional Psychology* (2019).

References

American Psychiatric Association. (1980). *Diagnostic and Statistical manual of mental disorders (DSM-III)*. 3rd ed. American Psychiatric Association.

American Psychiatric Association.(2022). *Diagnostic and statistical manual of mental disorders, fifth edition, text revision* (DSM-5-TR). American Psychiatric Association.

Black, D. W. (2017). The treatment of antisocial personality disorder. *Current Treatment Options in Psychiatry*, *4*, 295–302. https://doi.org/10.1007/s40501-017-02123-z.

Blackburn, R. (1988). On moral judgements and personality disorders: The myth of the psychopathic personality revisited. *British Journal of Psychiatry*, *153*, 505–512.

Boccaccini, M. T., Turner, D. B., & Murrie, D. C. (2008). Do some evaluators report consistently higher or lower PCL-R scores than others: Findings from a statewide sample of Sexually Violent Predator evaluations. *Psychology, Public Policy, and Law*, *14*, 262–283. https://doi.org/10.1037/a0014523.

Bonta, J., & Andrews, D. A. (2016). *The psychology of criminal conduct*. 6th ed. Routledge.

Bonta, J., Blais, J., & Wilson, H. A. (2014). A theoretically informed meta-analysis of the risk for general and violent recidivism for mentally disordered offenders. *Aggression and Violent Behavior*, *19*, 278–287. https://doi.org/10.1016/j.avb.2014.04.014.

Caldwell, M. F., McCormick, D. J., Wolfe, J., & Umstead, D. (2012). Treatment-related changes in psychopathy features and behavior in adolescent offenders *Criminal Justice and Behavior*, *39*, 144–155. https://doi.org/10.1177/0093854811429542.

Carlisi, C. O., Moffitt, T. E., Knodt, A. R., Harrington, H., Ireland, D., Melzer, T. R., Poulton, R., Ramrakha, S., Caspi, A., Hariri, A. R., & Viding, E. (2020). Associations between life-course-persistent antisocial behaviour and brain structure in a population-representative longitudinal birth cohort. *Lancet Psychiatry*, *7*, 245–253. https://doi.org/10.1016/ S2215-0366(20)30002-X.

Coid, J., Yang, M., Tyrer, P., Roberts, A., & Ullrich, S. (2006). Prevalence and correlates of personality disorder in Great Britain. *British Journal of Psychiatry*, *188*, 423–431. https://doi.org/10.1016/j.ijlp.2009.01.002.

Cullen, F. T., & Gendreau, P. (2001). From nothing works to what works: Changing professional ideology in the 21st century. *The Prison Journal*, *81*(3), 313–338. https://doi.org/10.1177/0032885501081003002.

Cunningham, M. D., & Reidy, T. J. (1998). Antisocial personality disorder and psychopathy: Diagnostic dilemmas in classifying patterns of antisocial behavior in sentencing evaluations. *Behavioral Sciences and the Law*, *16*, 333–351.

DeLisi, M. Drury, A. J., & Elbert, M. J. (2019). The etiology of antisocial personality disorder: The differential roles of adverse childhood experiences and childhood psychopathology. *Comprehensive Psychiatry*, *92*, 1–6. https://doi.org/10.1016/j.comppsych.2019.04.001.

DeMatteo, D., Edens, J. F., Galloway, M., Cox, J., Smith, S. T., Koller, J. P., & Bersoff, B. (2014). Investigating the role of the Psychopathy Checklist–Revised in United States case law. *Psychology, Public Policy and Law*, *20*, 96–1067. https://doi.org/10.1037/a0035452.

DeMatteo, D., Hart, S. D., Heilbrun, K., Boccaccini, M. T., Cunningham, M. D., Douglas, K. S., Dvoskin, J. A., Edens, J. F., Guy, L. S., Murrie, D. C., Otto, R. K., Packer, I. R., & Reidy, T. J. (2020). Statement of concerned experts on the use of the Hare Psychopathy Checklist–Revised in capital sentencing to assess risk for institutional violence. *Psychology, Public Policy, and Law*, *26*(2), 133–144. https://doi.org/10.1037/law0000223.

DeMatteo, D., & Olver, M. E. (2022). Use of the Psychopathy Checklist–Revised in legal contexts: Validity, reliability, admissibility, and evidentiary issues. *Journal of Personality Assessment*, *104*(2), 234–251. https://doi.org/10.1080/00223891.2021.1955693.

Duggan, C., & Kane, E. (2010). Commentary: Developing a National Institute of Clinical Excellence and health guideline for antisocial personality disorder. *Personality and Mental Health*, *4*, 3–8. https://doi.org/10.1002/pmh.109.

Duignan, B. (n.d.). What's the difference between a psychopath and a sociopath? And how do both differ from narcissists? Brittanica. www.britannica.com/story/whats-the-difference-between-a-psychopath-and-a-sociopath-and-how-do-both-differ-from-narcissists.

Edens, J. F., Lilienfeld, S. O., & Kelley, S. E. (2018). DSM-5 Antisocial Personality Disorder: Predictive validity in a prison sample. *Law and Human Behavior*, *39*(2), 123–129. https://doi.org/10.1037/lhb0000105.

Edens, J. F., Marcus, D. K., Lilienfeld, S. O., & Poythress Jr., N. G. (2006). Psychopathic, not psychopathic: Taxometric evidence for the dimensional structure of psychopathy. *Journal of Abnormal Psychology*, *115*, 131–144.

Fazel, S., & Danesh, J. (2002). Serious mental disorder in 23000 prisoners: A systematic review of 62 surveys. *The Lancet*, *359*, 545–550.

Flint-Stevens, G. (1993). Applying the diagnosis antisocial personality disorder to imprisoned offenders: Looking for hay in a haystack. *Journal of Offender Rehabilitation, 19*, 1–2. https://doi.org/10.1300/J076v19n01_01.

Fowles, D. C. (2018). Temperamental and risk factors for psychopathy. In C. J. Patrick (Ed.), *Handbook of psychopathy* (2nd ed., pp. 94–125). Guilford.

Freedman, R., Lewis, D. A., Michels, R., Pine, D. S., Schultz, S. K., Tamminga, C. A., Gabbard, G. O., Gau, S. S., Javitt, D. C., Oquendo, M. A., Shrout, P. E., Vieta, E., & Yager, J. (2013). The initial field trials of DSM-5: New blooms and old thorns. *American Journal of Psychiatry, 170*(1), 1–5. https://doi.org/10.1176/appi.ajp.2012.12091189.

Gao, Y. (2019). Neurological profiles of psychopathy: A neurodevelopmental perspective. In M. DeLisi (Ed.), *Routledge international handbook of psychopathy and crime* (pp. 154–165). Routledge.

Gibbon, S., Khalifa, N. R., Cheung, N. H., Völlm, B. A., & McCarthy, L. (2020). Psychological interventions for antisocial personality disorder. *Cochrane Database of Systematic Reviews* (9), CD007668. https://doi.org/10.1002/14651858.CD007668.pub3.

Goodwin, R. D., & Hamilton, S. P. (2003). Lifetime comorbidity of antisocial personality disoder and anxiety disorders among adults in the community. *Psychiatry Research 117*(2), 159–166.

Gurley, J. R. (2009). A history of changes to the criminal personality in the DSM. *History of Psychology, 12*(4), 285–304. https://doi.org/10.1037/a0018101.

Harding, D. J., Morenoff, J. D., Nguyen, A. P., & Bushway, S. D. (2017). Short- and long-term effects of imprisonment on future felony convictions and prison admissions. *Proceedings of the National Academy of Sciences, 114* (42), 11103–11108. https://doi.org/10.1073/pnas.1701544114.

Hare, R. D. (1980). A research scale for the assessment of psychopathy in criminal populations. *Personality and Individual DIfferences, 1*, 111–119. https://doi.org/10.1016/0191-8869(80)90028-8.

Hare, R. D. (1991). *The Hare Psychopathy Checklist – Revised* Multi-Health Systems.

Hare, R. D. (1996). Psychopathy and antisocial personality disorder: A case of diagnostic confusion. *Psychiatric Times, 8*(1). www.psychiatrictimes.com/antisocial-personality-disorder/psychopathy-and-antisocial-personality-disorder-case-diagnostic-confusion.

Hare, R. D. (1998). The Hare PCL-R: Some issues concerning its use and misuse. *Legal & Criminological Psychology, 3*, 99–119.

Hare, R. D. (2003). *The Hare Psychopathy Checklist – Revised technical manual.* 2nd ed. Multi-Health Systems.

Hare, R. D., & Neumann, C. S. (2010). The role of antisociality in the psychopathy construct: Comment on Skeem and Cooke (2010). *Psychological Assessment, 22*(2), 446–454. https://doi.org/10.1037/a0013635.

Harris, G. T., Rice, M. E., & Cormier, C. (1994). Psychopaths: Is a therapeutic community therapeutic? *Therapeutic Communities: International Journal for Therapeutic and Supportive Organizations, 15*, 283–299.

Hatchett, G. T. (2015). Treatment guidelines for clients with Antisocial Personality Disorder. *Journal of Mental Health Counselling, 37*(1), 15–27.

Hicks, B. M., & Drislane, L. E. (2018). Variants ('subtypes") of psychopathy. In C. J. Patrick (Ed.), *Handbook of psychopathy* (2nd ed., p. 297). Guilford.

Holoyda, B. (2020). The psychedelic renaissance and its forensic implications. *Journal of the American Academy of Science, 48*(1), 1–11. https://doi.org/10 .29158/JAAPL.003917-20.

Howells, K., Day, A., & Thomas-Peter, B. (2004). Changing violent behaviour: Forensic mental health and criminological models compared. *The Journal of Forensic Psychiatry and Psychology, 15*, 391–404.

Kelley, S. E., Edens, J. F., Mowle, E. N., Peonson, B. N., & Rulseh, A. (2019). Dangerous, depraved, and death-worth: A meta-analysis of the correlates of perceived psychopathy in jury simulation studies. *Journal of Clinical Psychology, 75*, 627–643. https://doi.org/10.1002/jclp.22726.

Kiehl, K. A. (2015). *The psychopath whisperer: The science of those without conscience.* Crown.

Latessa, E. J., Johnson, S. L., & Koetzle, D. (2020). *What works (and doesn't) in reducing recidivism.* Routledge.

Lilienfeld, S. O., Smith, S. F., Sauvigné, K. C., Patrick, C. J., Drislane, L. E., Latzman, R. D., & Krueger, R. F. (2016). Is boldness relevant to psychopathic personality? Meta-analytic relations with non-Psychopathy Checklist-based measures of psychopathy. *Psychological Assessment, 28*, 1172–1185. https://doi.org/10.1037/pas0000244.

McGuire, J. (2002). Integrating findings from research reviews. In J. McGuire (Ed.), *Offender rehabilitation and treatment: Effective programmes and policies to reduce re-offending* (pp. 3–38). Wiley.

Moffitt, T. E. (1993). Adolescence-limited and life-course-persistent antisocial behavior: A developmental taxonomy. *Psychological Review, 100*, 674–701.

Motz, R. T., Barnes, J. C., Caspi, A., Arseneault, L., Cullen, F. T., Houts, R., Wertz, J., & Moffitt, T. E. (2020). Does contact with the justice system deter or promote future delinquency? Results from a longitudinal study of British adolescent twins. *Criminology, 58*(2), 307–335. https://doi.org/10 .1111/1745-9125.12236.

Olver, M. E., Stockdale, K. C., Neumann, C. S., Hare, R. D., Mokros, A., Baskin-Sommers, A., Brand, E., Folino, J., Gacono, C., Gray, N. S., Kiehl, K., Knight, R. A., Leon-Mayer, E., Logan, M., Meloy, J. R., Roy, S., Salekin, R. T., Snowden, R. J., Thomson, N., ... Yoon, D. (2020). Reliability and validity of the Psychopathy Checklist–Revised in the assessment of risk for institutional violence: A cautionary note on DeMatteo et al. (2020). *Psychology, Public Policy, and Law*, *26*(4), 490–510. https://doi.org/10.1037/law0000256.

Patrick, C. J., Fowles, D. C., & Krueger, R. F. (2009). Triarchic conceptualization of psychopathy: Developmental origins of disinhibition, boldness, and meanness. *Development and Psychopathology*, *21*, 913–938. https://doi .org/10.1017/S0954579409000492.

Polaschek, D. L. L. (2010). What do mental health services offer to people with antisocial personality disorder? A commentary on the NICE clinical guideline. *Personality and Mental Health*, *4*, 20–29.

Polaschek, D. L. L. (2014). Adult criminals with psychopathy: Common beliefs about treatability and change have little empirical support. *Current Directions in Psychological Science*, *23*, 296–301. https://doi.org/10.1177 /0963721414535211.

Polaschek, D. L. L. (2022). Criminal justice responses to psychopathy. In J. E. Vitale (Ed.), *The complexity of psychopathy* (pp. 571–610). Springer.

Polaschek, D. L. L., & Skeem, J. L. (2018). Treatment of adults and juveniles with psychopathy. In C. J. Patrick (Ed.), *Handbook of psychopathy* (2nd ed., pp. 710–731). Guilford.

Poythress, N. G., Edens, J. F., Skeem, J. L., Lilienfeld, S. O., Douglas, K. S., Frick, P. J., Patrick, C. J., Epstein, M., & Wang, T. (2010). Identifying subtypes among offenders with antisocial personality disorder: A cluster-analytic study. *Journal of Abnormal Psychology*, *119*, 389–400.

Raine, A. (2018). Antisocial personality as a neurodevelopmental disorder. *Annual Review of Clinical Psychology*, *14*, 259–289. https://doi.org/10 .1146/annurev-clinpsy-050817-084819.

Rice, M. E., & Harris, G. T. (1992). Ontario's maximum security hospital at Penetanguishene: Past, present, and future. *International Journal of Law and Psychiatry*, *16*, 195–215.

Rice, M. E., Harris, G. T., & Cormier, C. A. (1992). An evaluation of a maximum security therapeutic community for psychopaths and other mentally disordered offenders. *Law and Human Behavior*, *16*, 399–412.

Robins, L. N., Tipp, J., & Przybeck, T. (1991). Antisocial personality. In L. N. Robins & D. A. Regier (Eds.), *Psychiatric disorders in America* (pp. 258–290). Free Press.

Romer, A., Elliott, M., Knodt, A., Sison, M., Ireland, D., Houts, R., Ramrakha, S., Poulton, R., Keenan, R., Melzer, T., Moffitt, T., Caspi, A., & Hariri, A. (2021). Pervasively thinner neocortex as a transdiagnostic feature of general psychopathology. *American Journal of Psychiatry*, *178* (2), 174–182. https://doi.org/10.1176/appi.ajp.2020.19090934.

Singh, J. P., Desmarais, S. L., Hurducas, C., Arbach-Lucioni, K., Condemarin, C., Dean, K., Doyle, M., Folino, J. O., Godoy-Cervera, V., Grann, M., Mei Yee Ho, R., Large, M. M., Nielsen, L. H., Pham, T. H., Rebocho, M. F., Reeves, K. A., Rettenberger, M., de Ruiter, C., Seewald, K., & Otto, R. K. (2014). International perspectives on the practical application of violence risk assessment: A global survey of 44 countries. *International Journal of Forensic Mental Health*, *13*(3), 193–206. https://doi.org/10.1080/14999013 .2014.922141.

Singleton, N., Melzer, H., & Gatward, R. (1998). *Psychiatric morbidity among prisoners in England and Wales*. The Stationary Office.

Skeem, J. L., & Cooke, D. J. (2010). Is criminal behavior a central component of psychopathy? Conceptual directions for resolving the debate. *Psychological Assessment*, *22*(2), 433–445. https://doi.org/10.1037/ a0008512.

Skeem, J. L., Polaschek, D. L. L., Patrick, C. J., & Lilienfeld, S. O. (2011). Psychopathic personality: Bridging the gap between scientific evidence and public policy. *Psychological Science in the Public Interest*, *12*, 95–162. https://doi.org/10.1177/1529100611426706.

Skeem, J. L., Steadman, H. J., & Manchak, S. M. (2015). Applicability of the Risk–Need–Responsivity Model to persons with mental illness involved in the criminal justice system. *Psychiatric Services*, *66*(9), 916–922. https://doi .org/10.1176/appi.ps.201400448.

Taylor, S. (2013). The real meaning of "good" and "evil": How are saintly people different from "evil" ones? What does 'good' really mean? *Out the Darkness*. www.psychologytoday.com/intl/blog/out-the-darkness/201308/ the-real-meaning-good-and-evil.

Van den Bosch, L. M.C, Rijckmans, M. J. N., Decoene, S., & Chapman, A. L. (2018). Treatment of antisocial personality disorder: Development of a practice focused framework. *International Journal of Law and Psychiatry*, *58*, 72–78. https://doi.org/10.1016/j.ijlp.2018.03.002.

Waldman, I. D., Rhee, S. H., LoParo, D., & Park, Y. (2018). Genetic and environmental influences on psychopathy and antisocial behavior. In C. J. Patrick (Ed.), *Handbook of psychopathy* (pp. 335–353). Guilford.

Walsh, A., & Wu, H. (2008). Differentiating antisocial personality disorder, psychopathy, and sociopathy: Evolutionary, genetic, neurological, and sociological considerations. *Criminal Justice Studies*, *21*(2), 135–152. https://doi.org/10.1080/14786010802159814.

Walters, G. D., Gray, N. S., Jackson, R. L., Sewell, K. W., Rogers, R., Taylor, J., & Snowden, R. J. (2008). A taxometric analysis of the Psychopathy Checklist: Screening Version (PCL:SV): Further evidence of dimensionality. *Psychological Assessment*, *19*, 330–339.

Wermink, H., Blokland, A., Nieuwbeerta, P., Nagin, D., & Tollenaar, N. (2010). Comparing the effects of community service and short-term imprisonment on recidivism. *Journal of Experimental Criminology*, *6*, 325–349. https://doi .org/10.1007/s11292-010-9097-1.

Werner, K. B., Few, L. R., & Bucholz, K. K. (2015). Epidemiology, comorbidity, and behavioral genetics of Antisocial Personality Disorder and psychopathy. *Psychiatric Annals*, *45*(4), 195–199. https://doi.org/10.3928 /00485713-20150401-08.

Wormith, J. S., & Zidenberg, A. M. (2018). The historical roots, current status, and future applications of the Risk–Need–Responsivity Model (RNR). In E. L. Jeglic & C. Calkins (Eds.), *New frontiers in offender treatment* (pp. 11–41). Springer Nature.

Yakeley, J. (2012). Treating the untreatable: The evolution of a psychoanalytically informed service for antisocial personality disorder. In A. Lemma (Ed.), *Contemporary developments in adult and young adult therapy* (pp. 179–204). Routledge.

Yang, M., Wong, S. C. P., & Coid, J. W. (2010). The efficacy of violence prediction: A meta-analytic comparison of nine risk assessment tools. *Psychological Bulletin*, *136*, 740–767.

Yoon, D., Eher, R., & Mokros, A. (2022). Incremental validity of the Psychopathy Checklist–Revised above and beyond the diagnosis of antisocial personality disorder regarding recidivism in sexual offenders. *Journal of Criminal Justice*, *80*, 101780. https://doi.org/https://doi.org/10.1016/j.jcrimjus.2020.101780.

15

Personality

Joel Paris

The diagnosis of mental disorders is far from an exact science. The classification systems we use are imprecise and problematic (Frances, 2013). Nevertheless, clinicians and patients place great faith in diagnoses, believing that they are as valid as those made for medical illness. But they are not. In mental health practice, we need to tolerate this level of uncertainty, and to avoid thinking that our evaluations are necessarily grounded in empirical data.

As the science for a topic gets weaker, the door widens for pseudoscience. In diagnostic evaluations, this involves treating an inexact diagnosis as if it were definite. This is a problem that affects the evaluation of almost all mental disorders. Personality disorder (PD) is a particularly tricky construct, which leaves it even more open to pseudoscience. (Note: this chapter will use the convention of abbreviating PD when discussing general personality disorder and will write out any specific personality disorder that is mentioned.)

PD has a detailed definition in the *Diagnostic and Statistical Manual of Mental Disorders* (DSM-5-TR; American Psychiatric Association, 2022). It can be best summarized as a domain of mental disorder characterized by long-term dysfunction in self, mood, and interpersonal relationships (Paris, 2015). The DSM-5-TR includes ten primary PDs – examples mentioned in this chapter include avoidant personality disorder, narcissistic personality disorder, obsessive-compulsive personality disorder, borderline personality disorder, and antisocial personality disorder (the last of which is discussed in detail in Chapter 14 of this book).

Borderline personality disorder is especially common both in the community and in the clinic. Because almost all of the research on PD and its treatment concerns this diagnosis, borderline personality disorder will receive the most attention in this chapter. Borderline personality disorder has a community prevalence of 1–2% in the United States (Trull et al., 2010). The disorder is much more common in mental health clinics, where it can be found in up to 9% of patients (Zimmerman et al., 2005).

There are more published research articles about borderline personality disorder than any other category of PD. It is also the disorder that makes the most trouble in clinical settings (Chartonas et al., 2017). Moreover, this diagnosis carries a strong stigma (Aviram et al., 2006) that often contributes to questionable clinical decisions.

15.1 Pseudoscience and Questionable Ideas

15.1.1 Diagnostic Controversies

Evaluating PDs requires clinical judgment and experience. Patients with PDs have a reputation of being both difficult to treat and to engage in therapy, resulting in many clinicians disliking their patients with PDs (Chartonas et al., 2017). They may prefer to diagnose them on the basis of symptoms such as anxiety and depression, and to leave personality on the back burner. Last but not least, borderline personality disorder is characterized by chronic suicidality, making it frightening for many, if not most, clinicians.

Patients with PDs do not always have the dramatic symptoms seen in other mental disorders. Instead, they have a personality that gets them into serious trouble in life. The main exception concerns patients with borderline personality disorder, who present with high levels of mood instability, impulsivity, and suicidality (Paris, 2020a). This level of symptomatology may lead clinicians to focus on these symptomatic features of all PDs, failing to recognize the context of personality in which symptoms develop.

One of the problems with recognizing PDs is that core features may not be seen by patients as a problem, because the core features are egosyntonic, or viewed as part of the self. When patients present with psychoses or severe depression, almost everyone sees them as something separate from the person. They are viewed as ill, but people who do not get along with other people due to PD may be seen differently – more as difficult than as disordered.

This problem is particularly noticeable in narcissistic personality disorder, in which patients often feel entitled to feel grandiosity and to act on these fantasies (Campbell & Miller, 2011). In obsessive-compulsive personality disorder, patients tend to see others as not meeting their high standards (Diedrich & Voderholzer, 2015). Patients with antisocial personality disorder are more likely to make others suffer rather than feel distress themselves, which is why they rarely seek help from health professionals (Black, 2013). Avoidant personality disorder, on the other hand, is a diagnosis in which patients do suffer inwardly, largely due to the pain of social isolation (Lampe & Malhi, 2018). Patients with schizotypal personality disorder seem to lie on a schizophrenic spectrum, but they too rarely ask for help (Torgersen et al., 2002).

Another reason for the failure to diagnose PD is the problematic nature of our classification system. The categorical definitions of ten PDs in the DSM-5-TR go back 40 years, and many of them have little research support. The most studied disorders are borderline personality disorder and antisocial personality disorder. Yet Zimmerman and colleagues (2005) found that the most common PD in clinical settings is diagnosed as unspecified (i.e., a clinical picture that meets overall criteria for a PD but does not fit into any category).

One attempt to resolve these difficulties is the use of dimensional diagnoses. This method has been promoted by trait psychologists and has several advantages, such as the avoidance of artefactual comorbidity between PDs (Krueger & Markon, 2014). Some researchers (e.g., Kotov et al., 2017) have suggested that *all* diagnoses in psychiatry should be dimensional rather than categorical. Dimensionality recognizes that traits are continuous with disorders, avoiding arbitrary boundaries around diagnosis. However, clinicians have been slow to adopt a system that is more familiar to researchers. While full dimensionality or a hybrid system is being promoted by groups of committed scholars, neither is yet in wide use in practice.

The alternative model of personality disorders (AMPD; Krueger & Markon, 2014) is included in Section III of the DSM-5-TR and is comprised of a list of potential diagnoses and models requiring further research. This is a hybrid model that builds up five categories from a set of dimensional measures of functioning. While the AMPD has a good grounding in research, it is not yet clear to what extent this system will be adopted by clinicians.

The *International Classification of Diseases* (ICD-11; World Health Organization, 2018) has adopted a more radically dimensional system for the classification of PDs. All former categories except for borderline personality disorder have been replaced by a scoring system focusing on traits and intensity. Again, it is too soon to know how widely this system will be used in practice.

15.1.2 Myths that Influence Treatment

15.1.2.1 Myth: Personality Disorder Diagnoses Should Be Avoided to Minimize Stigma

Sometimes, clinicians avoid diagnosing PDs due to stigma. Across the lifespan, many patients with borderline personality disorder threaten suicide or attempt it, and somewhere between 5% and 10% eventually die by their own hand (Paris, 2020a). Chronic suicidality is worrying, and not all clinicians are prepared to deal with this anxiety. In addition, patients with borderline personality disorder are often considered to be uncooperative and difficult to treat. Hospital emergency rooms tend to be many patients' entry point to the mental health system. Physicians and psychiatrists who cover the emergency room know this population well, and they often resent those who threaten to kill themselves. But when patients are difficult to manage, professionals can be tempted to give them a different diagnosis – one that leads to a more familiar form of treatment with which the clinician feels comfortable.

15.1.2.2 *Myth: Borderline Personality Disorder Is Untreatable*

Patients with borderline personality disorder have a wide range of symptoms, including mood swings and interpersonal distress. These mood swings often involve a range of impulsivity that includes suicide attempts, self-harm, substance use, chaotic intimate relationships, as well as micro-psychotic phenomena such as depersonalization, paranoid trends, or hallucinations under stress (Paris, 2020a). Patients with borderline personality disorder are chronically distressed by emotional dysregulation that is often mistaken for classical presentations of anxiety and depression, even though this population does not respond to typical anxiety or depression treatment (Newton-Howes et al., 2006). Patients with borderline personality disorder use impulsive behaviors to cope with these emotions, but their mood swings and lack of anger control make their relationships equally unstable.

Research has found that the diagnosis of borderline personality disorder may be entirely missed because when clinicians assess mental disorders, they focus on symptoms that can be targeted by treatment methods with which they are familiar (Zimmerman & Mattia, 1999; Zimmerman et al., 2005). Diagnosis is often driven by the need to identify a treatable condition. An incorrect perception of incurability tends to make clinicians reluctant to make a diagnosis. Diagnoses that describe patients who are believed to be untreatable, at least by usual methods, tend to be unpopular. Yet when effective therapy is available, conditions may be overdiagnosed. This happens in depression, bipolar disorder, attention-deficit/hyperactivity disorder, and posttraumatic stress disorder (Paris, 2020b). Fortunately, in recent years, the success of interventions like dialectical behavior therapy (DBT; Linehan, 1993) may have reduced the reluctance to diagnose borderline personality disorder. Regardless, this important condition continues to be missed, underdiagnosed, or misdiagnosed.

15.1.2.3 Myth: Treatments That Work for Other Disorders Also Work for Borderline Personality Disorder

If a patient suffers from depression and anxiety, physicians tend to prescribe antidepressants, and most psychologists tend to offer standard cognitive-behavioral therapy, both of which often help patients with depression and anxiety. But these interventions typically fail to consider the PD that underlies symptomatic features. Offering standard treatment that works for patients who do not have a PD tends to be ineffective for this patient population (Paris, 2020a).

15.1.2.4 Myth: Adolescents Cannot Meet the Diagnostic Criteria for Borderline Personality Disorder

Many clinicians believe that a borderline personality disorder diagnosis should not be made in patients younger than 18. Actually, the DSM-5 clearly states that young people may be diagnosed if symptoms persist for at least a year. However, mental health professionals may still be reluctant to identify a potentially chronic condition in the midst of adolescent development.

Research shows that most cases of borderline personality disorder actually begin in adolescence, that the clinical features of the disorder are almost identical, and that effective treatment methods are much same (Chanen & McCutcheon, 2013). Adolescents who have a PD that is not diagnosed may not be able to benefit from the specific therapies that have been designed for emotion dysregulation and impulsivity.

15.1.3 Other Conditions Diagnosed in Place of Borderline Personality Disorder

There are several common ways borderline personality disorder is misdiagnosed as other conditions that have a different etiology and a different method of treatment. In each of these scenarios, patients will not be directed to the evidence-based methods that have been shown to be effective for PDs.

15.1.3.1 Major Depression

Patients with borderline personality disorder often have prominent mood symptoms, but mood is not, as in classical depression, consistently low. Instead, it is unstable and mercurial, marked by problematic responses to environmental challenges (Zanarini, 2005). Therefore, it is not surprising that they do not respond well to treatment with antidepressants (Binks et al., 2012) and may benefit more from specialized therapy than from standard forms of cognitive-behavioral therapy (Binks et al., 2012).

The problem is that clinicians can readily diagnose patients with major depressive disorder, a category with a relatively lower bar (i.e., 2 weeks of symptoms, of which only five of nine are required). While some avoid diagnosing a PD, but look for a more treatable depression, many more mistakenly think that even if there is a PD, they can treat a "depressive component" with medication. Moreover, psychiatrists and family physicians have been taught that depression can be managed through the prescription of multiple drugs. Patients with mood disorders who do not respond to these agents are often referred to as treatment-resistant. Instead of reconsidering the diagnosis and asking whether a PD is present, physicians tend to follow treatment algorithms that involve prescribing additional drugs (i.e., antipsychotics, mood stabilizers, anxiolytics). Clinicians who practice in this way appear to know how to add, but not how to subtract. The end of this road is polypharmacy, and some patients end up taking six or more drugs for years on end. This type of practice reflects the triumph of hope over evidence.

Ultimately, it is not unusual for patients with borderline personality disorder to be on six or more drugs for extended periods without a formal PD diagnosis. This all too common scenario is an example of pseudoscience in action, even if carried out with good intentions. Polypharmacy is rarely scientific, and it often reflects desperation on the part of the prescriber. Yet another factor is the concept of treatment-resistant depression, which is associated with a recommendation by clinical treatment guidelines for aggressive pharmacological intervention (Voineskos et al., 2020). All too often, patients are subjected to polypharmacy and fail to be referred to specialized forms of psychotherapy. Luckily, misdiagnosis of a PD as a major depressive episode may be changing, as more clinicians become aware that borderline personality disorder has a reasonably good prognosis, and that recovery does not, as previously believed, require years of therapy.

15.1.3.2 Bipolar Disorder

Patients with borderline personality disorder have prominent mood swings, as do patients with bipolar disorder. For some researchers, all mood swings are a feature of bipolarity, which is seen as lying behind a broad spectrum of mental disorders (Akiskal, 2002). However, mood changes in borderline personality disorder do not meet criteria for hypo-mania – they are rapid, lasting hours rather than days or weeks, and are environmentally sensitive (Paris et al., 2007). Patients with borderline personality disorder do not experience manic or hypomanic episodes that are continuously present for at least four days. Moreover, patients with borderline personality disorder do not respond to the drugs used for bipolarity. Neither lithium nor the anticonvulsant drugs known as mood stabilizers qualify as evidence-based treatments for borderline person-ality disorder (Binks et al., 2012; Crawford et al., 2018).

Unfortunately, clinicians who see borderline personality disorder as a form of bipolarity will treat their patients with the same drugs used for classical bipolar illness. Many patients are prescribed medications for months to years without benefit. A combination of placebo effects, misplaced trust in prescribers, and lack of access to psychotherapies all reinforce the tendency to offer these pseudoscientific regimes.

15.1.3.3 Posttraumatic Stress Disorder (PTSD)

PTSD is a popular diagnosis. It has been used to explain the development of a variety of mental disorders in patients exposed to trauma, particu-larly in patients who have experienced childhood sexual abuse (Horwitz, 2018; McNally, 2016). This framework provides another way to avoid making a personality disorder diagnosis.

Trauma is real, and a history of severe adversity adds drama to clinical practice. But it is a mistake to routinely attribute causality to traumatic histories by themselves. It is true that at least a third of borderline personality disorder patients report some form of childhood sexual abuse, and that this history of abuse worsens the course and prognosis of the disorder (Soloff et al., 2005). But trauma is not the entire picture.

The etiology of borderline personality disorder derives from complex interactions between biological, psychological, and social risk factors (Paris, 2020a). Thus, temperamental vulnerability (emotion dysregula-tion) interacts with failures of validation and social support, amplifying instability in mood and relationships. PD is a complex phenomenon that can only be understood in a multidimensional model based on the inter-play between genes and the environment.

Those who see trauma as the main cause of borderline personality disorder may prefer to describe their patients as suffering from PTSD and are often described as having complex PTSD (Brewin et al., 2017). Complex PTSD is a recently accepted category in the ICD-11 classification of mental disorders, but not the DSM-5-TR. In this diagnosis, a wide range of symptoms are understood as a response to childhood trauma. If you look at the diagnostic criteria for complex PTSD, however, they are largely a description of borderline personality disorder.

Like the pharmacological reformulations of borderline personality disorder as a mood disorder, diagnosing complex PTSD leads to a different kind of treatment. This will usually be some form of trauma-focused cognitive-behavioral therapy, which was originally designed for classic cases of PTSD (Deblinger et al., 2006). But patients with borderline personality disorder and traumatic histories will be directed away from evidence-based psychotherapies for PDs, such as dialectical behavior therapy, and may be given therapy that does not have as strong a base in research. These therapies, unlike dialectical behavior therapy, do not focus on the core features of borderline personality disorder related to personality traits, emotion dysregulation, and impulsivity.

15.1.3.4 Dissociative Disorders

Making a diagnosis of dissociative identity disorder is particularly likely in patients who have similar symptoms and who can be more easily convinced to "recover" memories of trauma and produce dissociated identities known as alters (Piper & Merskey, 2004). Dissociative disorders may be artifacts of bad therapy driven by pseudoscientific theories, and most cases seen by clinicians in the last few decades were influenced by highly suggestive methods of psychotherapy (Lilienfeld et al., 1999). The entire field of dissociative disorders is a particularly problematic (see Paris, 2012 for a more thorough critique in addition to Chapter 7 on Dissociation of this volume).

This is not to say that patients with notable dissociative features do not have a mental disorder. More likely, they have borderline personality disorder with unusually prominent dissociative symptoms. If these patients fall into the hands of misguided therapists who want to shape pathology by invoking repressed and recovered memories, their prognosis will be guarded.

15.1.3.5 Attention-Deficit/Hyperactivity Disorder (ADHD)

ADHD has been well-researched in children, although it is likely over-diagnosed in adults (Paris et al., 2015). Even in children, it is difficult to separate hyperactivity and impulsivity from conduct disorder, or to separate deficits in attention from anxiety or depression. Moreover, the prevalence of ADHD varies greatly around the world (Smith, 2017). In the last few decades, as the diagnosis of ADHD in adults has dramatically increased, there has been an explosive increase in the prescription of stimulant drugs in medical and mental health practices (Olfson et al., 2013).

Some of the features of ADHD overlap with borderline personality disorder, including impulsivity and emotion dysregulation. Some cases of adult ADHD seem to show apparent comorbidity that can be used to justify prescribing stimulants. The problem is that if stimulant medication is given to patients with borderline personality disorder, the PD's core features are not addressed.

15.1.4 Ineffective Treatments

Even when borderline personality disorder is recognized and treated as such, pseudoscience can still obscure the picture. This is because disorders that are both serious and chronic tend to attract quick fixes.

When borderline personality disorder was first described over 80 years ago, it was noted that patients did not do well in psychoanalysis (Stern, 1938). One could argue that since little evidence has supported psychoanalysis as an effective therapy with plausible mechanism of change, this treatment method continues to be characterized as questionable at best, if not wholly pseudoscientific (Paris, 2019). Psychoanalysis, which can be both lengthy and regressive, may do more harm than good in this highly vulnerable population.

One of the most persistently damaging ideas in the field of PDs is an underlying assumption is that if patients have had problems for a long time, they will need to be in therapy for a long time. It follows that patients with chronic symptoms require open-ended therapy. Actually, there is no research supporting such a conclusion.

This point of view has been most strongly held by psychodynamically oriented therapists, but it also has influenced other frameworks. For example, even though dialectical behavior therapy has been shown to be an effective therapy for borderline personality disorder in a 12-month framework, Linehan (1993) also suggested that full treatment with her method could take several years. However, several years of therapy can be prohibitively expensive. Most patients and families cannot even afford a 12-month treatment, and patients with borderline personality disorder typically have no access to any form of evidence-based psychotherapy. Moreover, even in clinics that are affordable, longer treatment means longer waiting lists. This is hardly the best situation for patients who already have trouble waiting.

Several brief therapies have been found to be efficacious for border-line personality disorder, and many patients improve within only 3 months (Laporte et al., 2018). Even the most dysfunctional cases may not benefit from extending treatment beyond one year. The burden of proof should be on those who promote longer and more costly courses of therapy to provide evidence supporting their recommendations.

15.2 Research-Supported Approaches

All therapists who treat patients with PDs should be guided by research showing that that heritable personality traits lead to emotion dysregulation (Livesley & Kang, 2008). In other words, the patients have trouble regulating intense emotions due to a combination of genes and the environment (Linehan, 1993). If such individuals are raised in an emotionally supportive environment, high reactivity may not be a problem, and may even offer advantages (Belsky & Pluess, 2009). Brought up in an unsupportive environment, however, children with PDs may not learn how to regulate strong feelings.

This etiological pathway supports treatment methods like dialectical behavior therapy (Linehan, 1993) that teach patients the emotion regulation skills they lack. Methods that hyperfocus on traumatic events in the past ignore skills training in areas like impulsivity control and establishment of stable relationships. Briefer and more targeted methods of therapy avoid the high cost of dialectical behavior therapy and other specialized methods such as mentalization-based treatment or transference-focused psychotherapy, all of which are costly because they last at least a year or more (see review in Paris, 2020a).

Using research-supported approaches, most patients with a PD have a good long-term prognosis (Paris, 2015). Knowledge of these research findings is now weakening pseudoscientific ideas that bipolar disorder is incurable or requires life-long therapy. This level of research has been stimulated by clinical demand. Whether similarly effective approaches can be developed for other PDs remains a subject for future investigation.

15.3 Conclusion

The treatment of PDs has suffered from misdiagnosis and mistreatment for decades. Because patients with PDs have broad diagnostic comorbidities, it is easy to see them as having other disorders that require very different forms of treatment. Consequently, difficult cases are frequently misunderstood and patients lack access to treatments from which they are most likely to benefit. The most common and problematic examples include the overuse of medication, polypharmacy, and therapies that focus entirely on past trauma.

By and large, pseudoscience in this population is not being offered to patients so much by alternative practitioners, but by trained professionals who misunderstand the problems presented by those with PDs. Some patients may also have the misfortune of being treated by therapists who promote pseudoscientific methods for all of their clients. This practice ranges from the marginally scientific (as is the case with some trauma-based therapies) to the clearly unscientific (like treatment methods designed for dissociative disorders; Paris, 2012). Pseudoscience enters into the picture whenever psychopathology is complex and difficult to treat, and PDs are no exception to the rule.

Joel Paris, MD, is an Emeritus Professor of Psychiatry at McGill University in Canada. He is author of the book *Treatment of Borderline Personality Disorder: A Guide to Evidence-Based Practice, Second Edition* (2020).

References

Akiskal, H. S. (2002). Classification, diagnosis and boundaries of bipolar disorders. *Bipolar Disorder*, 5, 1–95.

Aviram, R. B., Brodsky, B. S., & Stanley, B. (2006). Borderline personality disorder, stigma, and treatment implications. *Harvard Review of Psychiatry*, *14*, 249–256.

American Psychiatric Association.(2022). *Diagnostic and statistical manual of mental disorders, fifth edition, text revision* (DSM-5-TR). American Psychiatric Association.

Belsky, J., & Pluess, M. (2009). The nature (and nurture?) of plasticity in early human development. *Perspectives in Psychological Science*, *4*, 345–351.

Binks, C. A., Fenton, M., McCarthy, L., Lee, T., Adams, C. E., & Duggan, C. (2012). Pharmacological interventions for people with borderline personality disorder. *Cochrane Database of Systematic Reviews*, (1), CD005653.

Black, D. W. (2013). *Bad boys, bad men: Confronting antisocial personality disorder*. 2nd ed. Oxford University Press.

Brewin, C. R., Cloitre, M., Hylandc, P., Shevlind, M., Maerker, A., Bryant, R. A., Humayun, A., Jones, L. M., Kagee, A., Rousseau, C., Somasundaram, D., Suzuki, Y., Wessely, S., van Ommeren, M., & Reed, G. M. (2017). A review of current evidence regarding the ICD-11 proposals for diagnosing PTSD and complex PTSD. *Clinical Psychology Review*, *58*, 1–15.

Campbell, W. K., & Miller, J. D. (2011). *Handbook of narcissism and narcissistic personality disorder*. Wiley.

Chanen, A. M., & McCutcheon, L. (2013). Prevention and early intervention for borderline personality disorder: Current status and recent evidence. *British Journal of Psychiatry, 202*, S24–29.

Chartonas, D., Kyratsous, M., Dracass, S., Lee, T., & Bhui, K. (2017). Personality disorder: Still the patients that psychiatrists dislike? *BJPsych Bulletin, 41*, 12–17.

Crawford, M., Sanatinia, R., Barrett, B. M., & Cunningham, G. (2018). The clinical effectiveness and cost-effectiveness of lamotrigine in borderline personality disorder: A randomized placebo-controlled trial. *American Journal of Psychiatry, 175*, 576–580.

Deblinger, E., Mannarino, A. P., Cohen, J. A., & Steer, R. A. (2006). A follow-up study of a multisite, randomized, controlled trial for children with sexual abuse-related PTSD symptoms. *Journal of the American Academy of Child & Adolescent Psychiatry, 45*, 1474–1484.

Diedrich, A., & Voderholzer, U. (2015). Obsessive-compulsive personality disorder: A current review. *Current Psychiatry Reports, 17*(2), 2. https://doi .org/10.1007/s11920-014-0547-8.

Frances, A. (2013). The past, present and future of psychiatric diagnosis. *World Psychiatry, 12*(2), 111–112.

Horwitz, A. V. (2018). *PTSD*. Johns Hopkins Press.

Kotov, R., Krueger, R. F., Watson, D., Achenbach, T. M., Althoff, R. R., Bagby, R. M., & Zimmerman, M. (2017). The Hierarchical Taxonomy of Psychopathology (HiTOP): A dimensional alternative to traditional nosologies. *Journal of Abnormal Psychology, 126*, 454–477.

Krueger, R. F., & Markon, K. E. (2014). The role of the DSM-5 personality trait model in moving toward a quantitative and empirically based approach to classifying personality and psychopathology. *Annual Review of Clinical Psychology, 10*, 477–501.

Lampe, L., &Malhi, G. S. (2018). Avoidant personality disorder: Current insights. *Psychology Research and Behavior Management, 11*, 55–66.

Laporte, L., Paris, J., Zelkowitz, P., & Cardin, J. F. (2018). Clinical outcomes of a Stepped Care program for the treatment of borderline personality disorder. *Personality and Mental Health, 12*, 252–264.

Lilienfeld, S. O., Lynn, S. J., Kirsch, I., Chaves, J. F., Sarbin, T. R., Ganaway, G. K., & Powell, R. A. (1999). Dissociative identity disorder and the sociocognitive model: Recalling the lessons of the past. *Psychological Bulletin, 125*, 507–523.

Linehan, M. (1993). *Cognitive Behavior Therapy for Borderline Personality Disorder*. Guilford.

Livesley, W. J., & Jang, K. L. (2008). The behavioral genetics of personality disorder. *Annual Review of Clinical Psychology, 4,* 247–274.

McNally, R. J. (2016). The expanding empire of psychopathology: The case of PTSD. *Psychological Inquiry, 27*(1), 46–49.

Newton-Howes, G., Tyrer, P., & Johnson, T. (2006). Personality disorder and the outcome of depression: Meta-analysis of published studies. *British Journal of Psychiatry, 188,* 13–20.

Olfson, M., Blanco, C., Wang, S., & Greenhill, L. L. (2013). Trends in office-based treatment of adults with stimulants in the United States. *Journal of Clinical Psychiatry, 74,* 43–50.

Paris, J. (2012). The rise and fall of dissociative disorders. *Journal of Nervous and Mental Diseases, 200,* 1076–1079.

Paris, J. (2015). *A concise guide to personality disorders.* American Psychological Association.

Paris, J. (2019). *An evidence-based critique of contemporary psychoanalysis.* Routledge.

Paris, J. (2020a). *Treatment of borderline personality disorder: A guide to evidence-based practice,* 2nd ed., revised and updated. Guilford.

Paris, J. (2020b). *Overdiagnosis in psychiatry,* 2nd ed. Oxford University Press.

Paris, J., Bhat, V., & Thombs, B. (2015). Is adult ADHD being over-diagnosed? *Canadian Journal of Psychiatry, 60,* 324–328.

Paris, J., Gunderson, J., & Weinberg, I. (2007). The interface between borderline personality disorder and bipolar spectrum disorders. *Comprehensive Psychiatry, 48*(2), 145–154.

Piper, A., & Merskey, H. (2004). The persistence of folly: A critical examination of dissociative identity disorder. Part I. The excesses of an improbable concept. *Canadian Journal of Psychiatry, 49,* 592–600.

Soloff, P. H., Lis, J. A., Kelly, T., Cornelius, J., & Ulrich, R. (2005). Risk factors for suicidal behavior in borderline personality disorder: A review and update. *Medical Psychiatry, 31,* 333–367.

Smith, M. (2017). Hyperactive around the world? The history of ADHD in global perspective. *Social History of Medicine, 30*(4), 767–787.

Stern, A. (1938). Psychoanalytic investigation of and therapy in the borderline group of neuroses. *Psychoanalytic Quarterly, 7,* 467–489.

Torgersen, S., Edwardsen, P., Øien, S., Onstad, S., Skre, I., Lygren, S., & Kringlen, E. (2002). Schizotypal personality disorder inside and outside the schizophrenic spectrum. *Schizophrenia Research, 54,* 33–40.

Trull, T. J., Jahng, S., & Tomko, R. L. (2010). Revised NESARC personality disorder diagnosis: Gender, prevalence, and comorbidity with substance dependence disorders. *Journal of Personality Disorders, 24,* 412–426.

Voineskos, D., Daskalakis, Z. J., & Blumberger, D. M. (2020). Management of treatment-resistant depression: Challenges and strategies. *Neuropsychiatric Disease and Treatment*, *16*, 221–234.

World Health Organization. (2018). *International classification of diseases*, 11th ed. WHO.

Zanarini, M. C. (2005). *Textbook of borderline personality disorder*. Taylor & Francis.

Zimmerman, M., & Mattia, J. (1999). Differences between clinical and research practices in diagnosing borderline personality disorder. *American Journal of Psychiatry*, *156*, 1570–1574.

Zimmerman, M., Rothschild, L., & Chelminski, I. (2005). The prevalence of DSM-IV personality disorders in psychiatric outpatients. *American Journal of Psychiatry*, *162*, 1911–1918.

16

Psychosis and Schizophrenia

Brandon A. Gaudiano, Katherine Visser, and Elizabeth Thompson

When you hear the word psychosis, what comes to mind? Many people think of the term's use in mainstream culture to describe individuals as crazy, insane, violent, jealous, or a host of other undesirable traits. In actuality, psychosis refers to a category of mental illness that is marked by a disconnection from reality causing confusion, distress, and difficulties functioning in everyday life. Pseudoscientific explanations may flourish because psychotic disorders are often chronic, difficult to treat, heterogeneous in presentation among people, and hard for unaffected individuals to understand.

Depictions of what was most likely psychosis, often referred to as madness, or lunacy, have existed throughout much of recorded history and extend back thousands of years. Many ancient and contemporary cultures attribute psychosis to supernatural origins, and given the shroud of mystery and intrigue surrounding psychotic experiences, these phenomena have attracted pseudoscientific ideas like moths to a flame. Throughout history, people with psychosis have been subjected to having holes drilled in their skulls to release evil spirits (trepanning), magical rituals, herbal treatments, prayers to appease divine punishment, and even exorcism in attempts to expel evil spirits. Some of these practices continue to this day (Foerschner, 2010).

Pseudoscience is not just a relic of the past. Despite great strides in mental health research over the past century, dubious explanations for psychosis persist in modern times. In 2004, Jarl Flensmark published a paper in the journal *Medical Hypotheses* noting that cases of schizophrenia emerged 1,000 years ago, shortly after the invention of footwear with heels. He then went on to conclude that these types of shoes caused schizophrenia and alternatively, flat footwear promoted brain health. In the following sections, we offer more examples of faulty reasoning and unsubstantiated claims and review various myths and misunderstandings surrounding the etiology and treatment of psychosis. Before we delve further into the discussion of specific myths, however, we will first take a closer look at what psychosis actually is.

Psychosis, broadly speaking, is characterized by disruptions in thoughts and perceptions associated with hearing, seeing, or believing in things that are not based in reality. The term psychosis can refer to isolated experiences, brief periods of symptoms, or a diagnosable psychotic disorder. Due to the variability seen in symptom expression and course, psychotic disorders are thought of as residing along a spectrum of illnesses, with a range of symptom presentations. All psychotic spectrum disorders are defined by the presence of *positive symptoms*, labelled positive because they indicate the presence of atypical, excess experiences that did not occur prior to illness (positive does not refer to a qualitative valence but instead to the presence – as opposed to the absence – of symptoms). Positive symptoms include hallucinations (sensory experiences in the absence of stimuli, such as hearing voices or seeing things that are not real), delusions (fixed and false beliefs), and disorganized thoughts or behavior (thoughts, speech, or behavior that is confusing or bizarre, marked by a lack of planning or control). If any of these symptoms are present and accompanied by distress and functional interference, an individual may have one of several psychotic spectrum disorders (American Psychiatric Association [APA], 2022). In addition to positive symptoms, many individuals with psychosis also have so-called *negative symptoms* (which refer to behavioral deficits), such as a lack of motivation, emotional flattening, and social withdrawal, as well as cognitive symptoms such as difficulty with attention, concentration, and memory. Taken together, it is easy to see how psychosis can cause a great deal of emotional distress and interfere with one's ability to function, feel happy, and be fulfilled in everyday life, especially when the public misunderstands and stigmatizes mental health difficulties related to psychosis.

Schizophrenia is one specific, commonly referenced type of psychotic disorder that is defined by symptom persistence for 6 months or longer, with marked interference in school, work, or social interactions (APA, 2022). Other psychotic spectrum disorders include those with a shorter course of symptoms (schizophreniform disorder or brief psychotic disorder), disorders marked primarily by delusions (delusional disorder), those that include major mood episodes (depression or mania) along with psychotic episodes (e.g., schizoaffective disorder or mood disorders with psychotic symptoms), psychosis caused by a substance or medical condition, catatonia (immobility or abnormal movements that cause significant interference in functioning), or other psychotic symptoms that cause difficulty for the individual experiencing them (e.g., attenuated psychosis, marked by symptoms subthreshold for full diagnosis). Given the range of currently recognized diagnostic categories pertaining to psychosis, it is not surprising that these conditions have been the subject of much controversy and confusion over the years.

16.1 Pseudoscience and Questionable Ideas

16.1.1 Diagnostic Confusion

Much of the misunderstanding surrounding psychosis stems from common misuses of the term schizophrenia. The word schizophrenia literally means *split* (schizo) *mind* (phrene) and is commonly credited to psychiatrist Eugen Bleuler who, in the early 1900s, studied and helped define symptoms of psychosis (Ashok et al., 2012). With the term schizophrenia, Bleuler was referring to a "split" between the disease process and the person's normal personality. Unfortunately, the media and public have often misinterpreted schizophrenia as being defined by having various personalities. However, dissociative identity disorder, or DID (formerly called multiple personality disorder) is a separate mental disorder from psychosis, and is characterized by exhibiting distinct identities that are perceived to control the person's behavior at times. This confusion pertaining to schizophrenia versus DID is perpetuated in modern media and mainstream representations of schizophrenia, such as in the 2000 movie starring Jim Carrey and Renée Zellweger, *Me, Myself, and Irene*.

Also concerning is the media and public's misassociation of schizophrenia with violence, lack of remorse or empathy, and criminal behavior. These features are often present in a different mental illness called antisocial personality disorder (often erroneously called psychopathy or sociopathy). As discussed above, none of these characteristics are included in the definition of psychosis. While there is evidence that anger and violence may be present in some individuals with psychosis, aggression stemming from psychosis is most likely attributed to the person's confusion about reality, paranoia, and responses to internal stimuli (experiencing threatening voices or visions). Effective treatment of these symptoms can address associated agitation and unsafe behaviors. Furthermore, evidence suggests that the link between violent crimes and psychosis is largely accounted for by drug or alcohol misuse (Fazel et al., 2009), which is common among individuals with and without psychosis. It is also important to note that individuals with schizophrenia are far more likely to have violence perpetrated against them than they are to perpetrate violence, yet media bias often focuses on the links between schizophrenia and violence perpetration, rather than victimization (Wehring & Carpenter, 2011).

16.1.2 Questionable Assessment Practices

Given the diagnostic confusion surrounding psychosis, it is not surprising that questionable assessment practices also abound. The first hurdle to accessing appropriate treatment for psychosis is obtaining a thorough and clinically informative assessment of symptoms. Traditionally, this is done by a trained clinician who asks direct questions about symptoms and experiences to both clients and support persons such as family members, while also making behavioral observations. This method of clinical interviewing is the cornerstone of psychological assessment and the most reliable method of delineating symptoms against diagnostic criteria laid out in standardized psychiatric classification systems such as the *Diagnostic and Statistical Manual of Mental Disorders* (DSM-5-TR; APA, 2022) and the *International Classification of Diseases, 11th Revision* (ICD-11; World Health Organization, 2018).

One method designed to tap into underlying characteristics of illness includes the use of projective tests, such as the Rorschach ink blot test or the Thematic Apperception Test (TAT). Projective tests are designed to assess a patient's interpretation of ambiguous stimuli, such as ink blots or pictures. Clinicians then interpret results using various scoring systems to determine how the patients' responses may indicate personality, emotional, or diagnostic characteristics. Projective tests are often subjectively interpreted and have been criticized for lacking reliability and validity (Hines, 2023; Lilienfeld et al., 2000). These tests, and the Rorschach in particular, may offer some utility in determining an individual's level of thought disorder. However, these methods do not outperform traditional clinical interviewing, and scores linked to thought disorder do not necessarily indicate a formal diagnosis (Lilienfeld et al., 2000).

Given the inconsistency and uncertainty inherent in projective assessments like the Rorschach, researchers have sought to identify more direct observational methods of confirming diagnosis. For many years, the search for a genetic marker for psychosis has become something of a holy grail of psychiatric diagnosis. However, the search has revealed complex genetic layers and environmental interactions which, for the most part, have yet to yield fruitful diagnostic tools (as described in more detail below). Similarly, there are no brain scans or imaging techniques that can be used to reliably diagnose psychosis. Unfortunately, despite various promising avenues of research, a reliable diagnostic shortcut does not yet exist. Good old-fashioned, clinician-administered diagnostic interviews and symptom scales are our best measures of psychosis at this time.

16.1.3 Myths that Influence Treatment

Throughout history there have been many implausible beliefs about the cause or etiology of psychosis. While much progress has been made, many myths still exist that influence treatment.

Myth: There is a gene that will unlock the secrets of psychosis.
   Truth: There is no single gene responsible for psychosis, and gene therapy for psychosis is unlikely.

It is well-established that schizophrenia has a genetic component and runs in families. For example, an identical twin of someone with schizophrenia has an approximately 33–50% probability of developing the illness (Hilker et al., 2018; Tsuang, 2000), and the probability is about 6–17% for someone with a parent or sibling with schizophrenia. Thus, first-degree relatives are at elevated risk for developing schizophrenia compared to the general population, whose risk is about 1% (Tsuang, 2000). However, research does not support any single gene or specific collection of genes as primarily responsible for schizophrenia. Instead, a large number of gene linkage studies have revealed many possible gene candidates that individually have small effects and complex interactions with each other, but in aggregate may result in a higher likelihood of developing the disorder (Karayiorgou & Gogos, 2006; Trifu et al., 2020). Most tellingly, the amount of heritability in schizophrenia currently explained by identified genes is only about 2% (Trifu et al., 2020). Thus, much of the genetic architecture of psychosis remains unexplained. Accordingly, genetic testing is not currently a viable avenue for the diagnosis of psychotic disorders, nor can blood tests tell us much about an individual's true level of risk. Given that the search for genetic markers of psychosis has only revealed more complexity, at this time gene therapy as a treatment for psychosis is unlikely. Despite disappointment in identifying an explanatory genetic underpinning, this line of research has served to combat pessimism related to schizophrenia being an unmodifiable genetic condition (Fleming & Martin, 2011). Recognition of the interplay between biological and environmental factors in its etiology has motivated more hopeful attitudes toward resilience and recovery, as well as spurred the development of more viable methods of prevention and intervention focused on modifiable factors such as behavior, environmental stressors, and interpersonal relationships.

Myth: It's all the mother's fault!

Truth: The etiology of psychosis stems from a complex combination of genetic and environmental factors (which can include the home environment among many others). Blaming one source alone can result in missed opportunities for intervention, and blaming mothers specifically is sexist and wrong.

The "schizophrenogenic mother" is an outdated concept originating from a 1948 hypothesis that mothers who show elements of being both rejecting and overprotective will cause psychosis (Fromm-Reichmann, 1948). The "schizophrenogenic mother" concept has been dismissed based on research showing that mothers who used higher rates of rejection and overprotection were not more likely to have children with psychotic spectrum diagnoses (Parker, 1982). Even in the time during which this notion was conceived, the idea clearly placed too much emphasis on mothers over fathers.

Although the concept of the "schizophrenogenic mother" has been debunked, family environment is known to play a role in the course of psychosis. Research has indicated that high levels of expressed emotion (which consists of greater volume of critical comments, emotional over-involvement, or hostility by family members) are linked to poorer prognoses and a host of undesirable outcomes in psychotic disorders (e.g., more hospital admissions, increased frequency of symptom relapse, poorer coping, and greater perceived caregiver burden; Cechnicki et al., 2013; Kuipers et al., 2010). Accordingly, changing family communication patterns can be very helpful in improving outcomes for individuals with early psychosis, helping to improve prognosis overall (Claxton et al., 2017). Importantly, family interventions are likely to be maximally helpful as part of an individualized intervention package rather than a single, one-size-fits-all intervention (Thompson et al., 2015).

Myth: Smoking marijuana causes schizophrenia.

Truth: This myth has some elements of truth. Cannabis can produce psychotic experiences and may trigger psychotic illness, but probably in those already vulnerable to developing psychosis due to other or additive risk factors.

The contribution of substance use to the development of psychosis is a valid concern (Colizzi & Bhattacharyya, 2020). In particular, marijuana or cannabis use is consistently highlighted as possibly increasing risk for developing psychosis (Bechtold et al., 2016; Colizzi & Bhattacharyya, 2020; Radhakrishnan et al., 2014). As rates of cannabis legalization increase globally, this issue draws significant public health attention. Indeed, research indicates that increased cannabis use predicts psychosis, especially within those with a family history of psychotic spectrum disorders (Bersani et al., 2002; Radhakrishnan et al., 2014). However, there is also evidence suggesting that risk depends on the concentration of tetrahydrocannabinol (THC) present in the particular cannabis strain, with greater concentrations resulting in greater risk (Di Forti et al., 2015). Furthermore, evidence suggests that cannabidiol (CBD), another compound present in cannabis, may have beneficial properties for those diagnosed with psychosis; in particular, research has noted an ameliorative effect on positive symptoms (Bhattacharyya et al., 2018; McGuire et al., 2018). Overall, research is clear that THC use may result in increased likelihood of developing psychosis in those at risk, but it is unclear if cannabis use is a frequent cause of psychotic spectrum disorders in the general public. Moreover, marijuana does not trigger psychotic illness for the large majority of users. The complete picture regarding cannabis is complicated and requires further investigation.

Myth: Schizophrenia has no cure, and people with schizophrenia will never live productive lives.

Truth: Recovery is absolutely possible, and many people go on to work, have families, and live according to their goals.

Unfortunately, the perception persists that psychosis is an incurable illness that destroys the ability to function in society. Until recently, traditional medical treatment narrowly focused on symptom remission alone, generally without considering other dimensions of recovery. However, research shows that up to 20% of those with schizophrenia recover completely (i.e., experienced either full symptom remission or at most, only very mild symptoms, with improved social functioning over 2 years) and many more significantly improve and can manage their condition successfully in the community (Jääskeläinen et al., 2013). Research and practice have now begun to consider a wider view of recovery, reconceptualizing it as both an outcome and a process focusing on a variety of person-centered principles (Vita & Barlati, 2018). One influential recovery model was generated by the Substance   Abuse   and   Mental   Health   Services   Administration

(SAMHSA, 2010) and focuses on a holistic and person-centered process of recovery from serious mental illness. It is composed of ten different aspects and predicated on four core dimensions: home, health, purpose, and community. This recovery model provides a lens through which to view and sculpt treatment packages, leading to the development of skills, resources, and hope for living a full and satisfying life despite symptoms.

16.1.4 Implausible and/or Ineffective Treatments

Just as there are multiple myths influencing treatment development and attitudes toward treatment, myths also exist concerning what types of treatments are effective. Given the pervasiveness, acuity, and distress linked to schizophrenia, it is no surprise that people have sought out a multiplicity of diverse interventions. Some of them are effective and safe, some are ineffective and safe, some are outright harmful, and some are outright dubious. These treatments are detailed below, beginning with the implausible.

16.1.4.1 Homeopathy

Homeopathy is the debunked practice of progressively diluting an ingredient that, in larger quantities, is claimed to produce the very symptoms it purports to treat. For example, solutions of the plants belladonna, *Datura stramonium* (thornapple or jimsonweed), and *Hyoscyamus* (henbane or stinking nightshade) were documented as supposed treatments for psychotic disorders as recently as 2017 (Grise et al., 2017; Merizalde, 2018). Homeopathic practitioners believe that the smaller the amount of the harmful ingredient dissolved in solution, the more potent and curative it becomes. Thus, homeopathy is said to rely on the "law of similars," which states that a substance known in detectable quantities to produce symptoms can be used, in increasingly smaller quantities (known as the "law of infinitesimals"), to cure the very same symptoms. Accordingly, greater dilution is thought to increase strength and effectiveness (Merizalde, 2018).

Homeopathy was introduced in the late eighteenth and early nineteenth centuries by physician Samuel Hahnemann to treat a wide variety of conditions (Merizalde, 2018). However, homeopathy is unsupported by consistent or rigorous scientific evidence, and the idea that a solution of decreasing strength increases in efficacy lacks connection with established facts in physics, chemistry, and biology. In fact, modern homeopathic remedies extract (literally) every single molecule of the original active agent during the extensive serial dilution process, effectively producing completely inert tinctures. In essence, homeopathic remedies are little more than placebos. In rigorous drug trials, patients in the nontreatment arm receive sugar pills or other inactive substances to compare outcomes to the medication being tested. Even though they lack an active ingredient, placebos may nevertheless be associated with subsequent improvement due to nonspecific factors including natural remission of illness, a patient's expectations for improvement, attention and support by providers, and other influences. While some reports from uncontrolled case studies have suggested benefits from homeopathy for individuals with psychosis (Grise et al., 2017), the so-called placebo effect is a more likely explanation when studied under randomized controlled conditions (Brien et al., 2011).

16.1.4.2 Psychoanalysis

In the late 1800s, the Austrian neurologist Sigmund Freud created a form of talk therapy called psychoanalysis. Psychoanalysis posits that unconscious mental processes repressed from childhood cause psychological problems but can be brought into conscious awareness using dream interpretation and free association (Ferenczi & Rank, 1986). Freud originally warned against using this new approach to treat schizophrenia because he did not think it would be appropriate (Mueser & Berenbaum, 1990). Unfortunately, Freud's admonition did not stop his successors from promoting psychoanalysis for this very purpose. Psychoanalysis for schizophrenia and the modern variant of this approach, called psychodynamic therapy, became the dominant treatment in many psychiatric settings up through the 1980s (Mueser & Berenbaum, 1990).

Despite its widespread use, research conducted on psychoanalysis and psychodynamic therapy concluded that these interventions were either ineffective or potentially harmful for people with schizophrenia (for a comprehensive review, see Mueser & Berenbaum, 1990). For example, naturalistic studies of patients undergoing intensive psychodynamic therapy showed poorer functioning and higher rates of suicide at follow-up, and randomized controlled trials failed to show beneficial effects either when used alone or in combination with antipsychotic medication. A recent rigorously conducted Cochrane systematic review of randomized controlled trials concluded that there is no evidence to support psychodynamic therapy for schizophrenia (Malmberg et al., 2001). Nevertheless, this approach continues to be used by many clinicians who cite anecdotal evidence that it is effective for their patients (Lombardi et al., 2019).

16.1.4.3 Vitamin Therapy

Complementary and alternative medicine has become popular for treating a host of medical and psychiatric conditions, with vitamins and nutritional supplements increasingly being promoted for schizophrenia (Brown & Roffman, 2014). For example, the popular website WebMD.com has a recent article promoting the following regimen for schizophrenia: B vitamins, omega-3 fatty acids, CBD, amino acids, melatonin, antioxidants, and gluten-free or ketogenic diets (Svobada, 2020). Within this context, it is helpful to remember the history of vitamin therapy for schizophrenia, because it provides a cautionary tale in light of the increasingly strong claims being made about its benefits for this population today.

Linus Pauling was a preeminent chemist who is the only person ever to be awarded two Nobel prizes (in chemistry and, later, peace; Weiss, 2017). However, today he is probably best known for his tireless efforts to promote the use of vitamin C. Pauling started using vitamin C himself following a recommendation from a colleague, later claiming that it cured him of chronic colds (Offit, 2013). He then went on to promote "mega-dosing" the vitamin (i.e., taking up to 3,000 mg per day representing 50 times the recommended allowance), and his 1970 book, *Vitamin C and the Common Cold*, became an international best-seller. Pauling also asserted that vitamin C could cure a host of other maladies, including cancer. However, subsequent research invalidated Pauling's claims about Vitamin C's health benefits (Barrett, 1995).

In the 1960s, Pauling also developed an interest in using vitamin therapy to treat mental illness. He coined the term "orthomolecular psychiatry," claiming that some mental illnesses were caused by nutrient deficiencies in the brain undetectable by blood tests, but which could produce psychiatric illnesses including schizophrenia (Weiss, 2017). Based on his "orthomolecular" model, Pauling recommended megadosing vitamin B3, claiming it could be successfully used to treat schizophrenia when other traditional medical approaches failed. Pauling's claims were roundly criticized in a 1973 American Psychiatric Association Task Force report, concluding that the studies offered by vitamin therapy proponents lacked adequate methods and controls, and that independently conducted and controlled trials failed to replicate the supposed benefits of vitamin therapy for schizophrenia (APA, 1973).

Recent clinical trials suggest that certain B vitamins (e.g., B6, B8, and B12) may improve overall psychiatric symptoms in patients with schizophrenia when added to antipsychotic medication; however, the evidence is generally of low quality and requires further replication (Firth et al., 2017). Nevertheless, Pauling's vitamin deficiency hypothesis has never been supported as a causal factor in the development of schizophrenia. While some vitamins and nutritional supplements may provide certain health benefits to subgroups of patients with schizophrenia with poor health due to lifestyle factors, there remains a lack of evidence that vitamins improve psychotic symptoms specifically or can cure psychosis (Magalhães et al., 2016).

16.1.4.4 Other Implausible Treatments

Examples of other implausible treatments include the use of natural rock crystals like lepidolite, ruby, sugilite, emerald, and tiger's eye for their purported healing properties as well as reiki therapy, which relies on the manipulation and unblocking of purportedly invisible energy fields found in the body (Morero et al., 2021). No reliable, controlled research exists to support these treatments for psychosis. These strategies remain implausible because they lack a credible scientific explanation for their effects.

16.1.5 Potentially Harmful Treatments

Benjamin Rush, the eighteenth-century physician, often credited founder of American psychiatry, and signer of the Declaration of Independence, believed that mental illness was caused by problems with blood vessels in the brain (Levin, 2019). Rush employed a host of potentially ineffective and harmful treatments for psychiatric patients living in asylums including bloodletting, hot and cold-water baths, mercury doses, and immobilizing chairs. Similarly, harmful medical procedures were commonly used well into the modern era, often justified on the grounds that schizophrenia required extreme interventions.

16.1.5.1 Lobotomy

Lobotomy was first introduced by Antonio Egas Moniz, a Portuguese neurologist who coined the term *psychosurgery*, in the 1930s (Tan & Yip, 2014). Moniz theorized that schizophrenia was caused by abnormal brain connections and used physical and chemical methods to destroy or sever the connections between the prefrontal cortex (responsible for executive and other higher-order cognitive functions) and the other parts of the brain. A commonly used instrument was the leucotome, a thin, needle-like device with a retractable wire that cut through brain tissue via a hole drilled in the skull (Tan & Yip, 2014). Moniz was later awarded the Nobel Prize for his discovery, a decision that remains controversial to this day. American physicians Walter Freeman and James Watts expanded upon Moniz's procedure, which required general anesthesia, by inserting a sharp instrument resembling an ice pick through the top of the eye socket, thus destroying brain tissue while the patient was still conscious (Gross, 2011).

Using lobotomies, Moniz initially claimed that 35% of cases were healed, 35% were improved, and 30% were unchanged, all with minimal side effects (Gross, 2011). However, later scientific reviews of psycho-surgical procedures found little evidence that lobotomies reduced psychotic symptoms, and any clinical benefits observed came at serious costs to patients, including irreversible brain damage and severe functional impairment (Soares et al., 2013). Critics began to question whether destroying parts of the brain should be considered a legitimate form of treatment. Indeed, the theoretical neurological assumptions underlying the lobotomy were weak. Moniz and other proponents minimized the procedure's harms and inaccurately extolled its benefits, perhaps motivated by professional gain (Valenstein, 1986). Lobotomies fell out of favor after the discovery of more effective pharmacological treatments in the 1950s (Tan & Yip, 2014).

16.1.5.2 Insulin Coma and Convulsive Therapies

Also starting in the 1930s, so-called shock therapies were developed to induce comas and seizures using various techniques, such as electrical stimulation or injections of insulin or camphor (Tan & Yip, 2014). These shocks to the system were thought to jolt the person out of a psychotic episode. German physician Manfred Sakel first used insulin injections to treat patients with schizophrenia by inducing hypoglycemic shock comas daily over a period of several weeks or months (Wright-Mendoza, 2018). After one or two hours in a coma-like state, the process would be reversed with an injection of glucose and the patient would regain consciousness. At the time, insulin coma therapy was considered a breakthrough treatment for schizophrenia and many noted physicians sang its praises. However, the treatment produced serious complications, including obesity, brain damage, and even death (Jones, 2000).

In the 1950s, a paper was published in the prestigious journal the *Lancet* entitled "The insulin myth." The author, a young physician named Harold Bourne (1953), concluded that there was no scientific rationale for the use of insulin to treat schizophrenia, that early clinical studies used unreliable methods, and that any benefits observed were probably due to the nonspecific effects of extra attention and support provided by medical staff delivering the intensive intervention over many days and weeks. Once again, the advent of modern psychopharmacological treatments starting in the 1950s served as the death knell for insulin coma therapy and it is no longer used today.

In 1934, Hungarian psychiatrist Ladislas Meduna chemically induced seizures in patients with schizophrenia using injections of camphor. It had been previously observed that patients with malaria who had seizures showed improvements in their symptoms, so seizures were induced for psychosis in the hopes of providing similar symptom relief (Fink, 2000). Later, the method was refined by placing electrodes on the temples to pass electricity through the brain, a procedure known as electroconvulsive therapy (or ECT). During the early years of treatment, seizures were induced without anesthesia, resulting in violent body shaking and subsequent bone fractures. In 1975, the coercive and abusive practices of early ECT were graphically depicted in the movie, *One Flew Over the Cuckoo's Nest*, which resulted in much public outcry over the procedure.

It should be noted that modern forms of ECT are relatively safe and efficacious. ECT is indicated in the treatment of severe mood episodes, especially related to affective psychosis, if the patient has not first responded to medication or therapy (Kaster et al., 2021). Today, the procedure is done under general anesthesia, the electrical stimulation to the brain is more limited, and muscle relaxants are given to prevent physical injuries during convulsions (Fink, 2000). However, critics continue to question ECT's costs versus benefits, and significant side effects remain, such as temporary memory loss and headaches (Read & Bentall, 2010). In addition, relapse rates are high (50% within a year), so other follow-up treatments are needed to promote long-term recovery (Jelovac et al., 2013).

16.1.5.3 Exorcism

In addition to early medical treatments, spiritually based approaches have been practiced to treat psychosis. Not surprisingly, the delusions, hallucinations, and other disorganized behavior exhibited by people

with psychosis have been interpreted by religious traditions throughout history as indicating possession by evil spirits or the devil.
Exorcism is a religious ritual designed to expel such invaders from
the body through prayers and other rites, and it is practiced by various
religions including, but not limited to, Buddhism, Christianity,
Hinduism, Islam, and Judaism (Thomason, 2008). Research indicates
that religious delusions are quite common in psychosis, occurring in
20–60% of patients (Cook, 2015). Pfeifer (1994) surveyed 343 outpatients in a Swiss psychiatric clinic and found that 30% of patients
sought out exorcisms, with the highest rates occurring in patients with
schizophrenia (up to 70%). Reports suggest that the demand for
exorcisms has been on the rise in recent years (Mariani, 2018). The
psychiatrist Richard Gallagher (2016) even claims that he has personally witnessed paranormal phenomena and has consulted with clergy
on several hundred cases over 25 years to help them identify demonic
possessions requiring exorcism.

Exorcisms often require the purportedly possessed person to be
restrained to prevent them from harming themselves or others during
the ritual (Hall, 2016). Abuse and torture of victims of exorcism have
resulted in suffocation, various injuries, and even death (Libaw, 2006). In
one infamous case, Anneliese Michel, a 23-year-old German woman who
experienced epilepsy and psychosis, was subjected to 67 exorcisms and
other forms of maltreatment, ultimately resulting in her death from
malnutrition (Getler, 1978). Michel's parents and two Catholic priests
were later convicted of negligent homicide.

The Catholic Church asserts that exorcisms are infrequently performed and careful evaluations are conducted by trained professionals
first to determine if the person has a psychiatric or medical condition that
would explain their behavior (United States Conference of Catholic
Bishops, n.d.). Then, they claim that exorcisms are only officially sanc-
tioned in the rare cases in which other natural causes have been carefully
ruled out. However, there is no clear standard of care or independent
oversight of those who practice exorcism to provide confidence in the
adequacy of any such evaluation process, and no scientific evidence exists
that exorcism is helpful even when it is not directly harmful to the subject
(Tajima-Pozo et al., 2011). Furthermore, misconceptions about the nature of mental illness being caused by evil spirits or the devil result in
other opportunity costs, such as delaying or preventing individuals from
seeking appropriate medical care that could otherwise alleviate their
symptoms (Pietkiewicz et al., 2021).

16.2 Research-Supported Approaches

This chapter has reviewed many treatments claiming to be effective for people with psychosis that are not supported by science and may even be harmful. However, evidence-based therapies do exist and can improve symptoms, reduce relapse, and increase quality of life and functioning in those with schizophrenia. Antipsychotic medications are considered the current frontline treatment for acute psychosis. Research-supported psychological therapies used adjunctively to medication can significantly improve outcomes for patients with psychosis beyond pharmacotherapy alone. For example, cognitive-behavioral therapy for psychosis is a modern psychotherapeutic approach that helps patients examine and challenge their psychotic experiences and develop strategies to actively cope with them in an effort to improve functioning. The United Kingdom's National Collaborating Centre for Mental Health (2014) clinical guideline on the treatment of psychosis and schizophrenia recommends that cognitive-behavioral therapy be provided to patients in all phases of illness, from the early stages of psychosis through acute episodes in addition to maintenance stages.

Recently, Lincoln and Pedersen (2019) conducted a comprehensive review of the available evidence for various psychotherapeutic interventions for schizophrenia. They similarly concluded that strong evidence supports cognitive-behavioral therapy's ability to improve psychotic symptoms in the short and long term. Additionally, family psychoeducation reduces relapses and rehospitalizations. They also found emerging evidence for a number of other allied therapies, including acceptance and commitment therapy (ACT), mindfulness therapies, meta-cognitive therapy, social skills training, and systemic family therapy. Given the clinical variety of efficacious therapeutic approaches, it is essential that clinicians, patients, and their family members become better informed about these options so that they don't fall prey to unscrupulous claims about nonsupported approaches commonly promoted online and in the popular media.

16.3 Conclusion

As we have seen, schizophrenia and other psychotic disorders are chronic illnesses that have vexed both providers and patients throughout human history. It is not surprising that public perception of schizophrenia is often incorrect or misleading. Fortunately, modern, evidence-based interventions, including pharmacological and psychological therapies, can reduce symptoms and improve individuals' chances for recovery. Nevertheless, relapse rates remain high and people may still experience significant symptoms and continued impairment, even when receiving the best available treatments. Sadly, this has left a vacuum that is all too often filled by promoters of questionable or pseudoscientific treatments claiming to cure schizophrenia.

The Latin phrase *post hoc, ergo propter hoc* translates to "after this, therefore because of this." This common error in thinking underlies pseudoscientific notions about the etiology and treatment of psychosis, as many people fail to take heed of the well-known adage that correlation is not the same as causation. Unfortunately, patients with schizophrenia and their loved ones may try just about anything to allay feelings of hopelessness with the allure of simple cures. Therefore, it remains essential for educators, health professionals, and consumers to redouble their efforts to dispel myths about psychosis, while ensuring that the treatments being offered to vulnerable patients are safe, effective, and backed by sound research. Failing to do so will continue to result in direct and indirect harms to society, ultimately keeping individuals with psychosis from receiving the help that they need to foster long-term recovery from this pernicious illness.

Brandon A. Gaudiano, PhD, is a Professor in the Department of Psychiatry and Human Behavior at the Warren Alpert Medical School of Brown University and in the Department of Behavioral and Social Sciences at the Brown School of Public Health. He is also Director of the Transitional Outpatient Program at Butler Hospital, and a Research Psychologist at the Providence VA Medical Center. He is editor of the book *Incorporating Acceptance and Mindfulness into the Treatment of Psychosis: Current Trends and Future Directions* (2015).

Katherine Visser, PhD, obtained her doctorate in clinical psychology and currently is a Staff Psychologist with the Lifespan Physician's Group in Providence, RI.

Elizabeth Thompson, PhD, is a clinical psychologist and an Assistant Professor of Psychiatry and Human Behavior at the Warren Alpert Medical School of Brown University. She also is a Research Scientist at Rhode Island Hospital.

References

American Psychiatric Association. (1973). *Task Force Report 7: Megavitamin and orthomolecular therapy in psychiatry*. American Psychiatric Association.
American Psychiatric Association. (2022). *Diagnostic and statistical manual of mental disorders, fifth edition, text revision* (DSM-5-TR). American Psychiatric Association.

Ashok, A. H., Baugh, J., & Yeragani, V. K. (2012). Paul Eugen Bleuler and the origin of the term schizophrenia (SCHIZOPRENIEGRUPPE). *Indian Journal of Psychiatry*, *54*, 95–96.

Barrett, S. (1995). The dark side of Linus Pauling's legacy. *Skeptical Inquirer*, *19*, 18–20.

Bechtold, J., Hipwell, A., Lewis, D. A., Loeber, R., & Pardini, D. (2016). Concurrent and sustained cumulative effects of adolescent marijuana use on subclinical psychotic symptoms. *American Journal of Psychiatry*, *173* (8), 781–789.

Bersani, G., Orlandi, V., Kotzalidis, G. D., & Pancheri, P. (2002). Cannabis and schizophrenia: Impact on onset, course, psychopathology and outcomes. *European Archives of Psychiatry and Clinical Neuroscience*, *252*(2), 86–92.

Bhattacharyya, S., Wilson, R., Appiah-Kusi, E., O'Neill, A., Brammer, M., Perez, J., Murray, R., Allen, P., Bossong, M. G., & McGuire, P. (2018). Effect of cannabidiol on medial temporal, midbrain, and striatal dysfunction in people at clinical high risk of psychosis: A randomized clinical trial. *JAMA Psychiatry*, *75*(11), 1107–1117.

Bourne, H. (1953). The insulin myth. *The Lancet*, *262*, 964–968.

Brien, S., Lachance, L., Prescott, P., McDermott, C., & Lewith, G. (2011). Homeopathy has clinical benefits in rheumatoid arthritis patients that are attributable to the consultation process but not the homeopathic remedy: A randomized controlled clinical trial. *Rheumatology*, *50*, 1070–1082.

Brown, H. E., & Roffman, J. L. (2014). Vitamin supplementation in the treatment of schizophrenia. *CNS Drugs*, *28*, 611–622.

Cechnicki, A., Bielańska, A., Hanuszkiewicz, I., & Daren, A. (2013). The predictive validity of expressed emotions (EE) in schizophrenia. A 20-year prospective study. *Journal of Psychiatric Research*, *47*(2), 208–214.

Claxton, M., Onwumere, J., & Fornells-Ambrojo, M. (2017). Do family interventions improve outcomes in early psychosis? A systematic review and meta-analysis. *Frontiers in Psychology*, *8*, 371.

Colizzi, M., & Bhattacharyya, S. (2020). Is there sufficient evidence that cannabis use is a risk factor for psychosis? In A. Thompson & M. Broome (Eds.), *Risk factors for psychosis* (pp. 305–331). Academic Press.

Cook, C. C. (2015). Religious psychopathology: The prevalence of religious content of delusions and hallucinations in mental disorder. *International Journal of Social Psychiatry*, *61*, 404–425.

Di Forti, M., Marconi, A., Carra, E., Fraietta, S., Trotta, A., Bonomo, M., Bianconi, F., Gardner-Sood, P., O'Connor, J., Russo, M., Stilo, S. A., Marques, T. R., Mondelli, V., Dazzan, P., Pariente, C., David, A. S., Gaughran, F., Atakan, Z., Iyegbe, C., ... Murray, R. M. (2015). Proportion of patients in south London with first-episode psychosis attributable to use of high potency cannabis: A case-control study. *The Lancet Psychiatry, 2*(3), 233–238.

Fazel, S., Gulati, G., Linsell, L., Geddes, J. R., & Grann, M. (2009). Schizophrenia and violence: Systematic review and meta-analysis. *PLoS Medicine*, 6, e1000120.

Ferenczi, S., & Rank, O. (1986). The development of psychoanalysis. *Classics in Psychoanalysis Monograph Series*, Mo *4*, 68.

Fink, M. (2000). Electroshock revisited: Electroconvulsive therapy, once vilified, is slowly receiving greater interest and use in the treatment of mental illness. *American Scientist, 88*, 162–167.

Firth, J., Stubbs, B., Sarris, J., Rosenbaum, S., Teasdale, S., Berk, M., & Yung, A. R. (2017). The effects of vitamin and mineral supplementation on symptoms of schizophrenia: A systematic review and meta-analysis. *Psychological Medicine, 47*, 1515–1527.

Fleming, M. P., & Martin, C. R. (2011). Genes and schizophrenia: A pseudoscientific disenfranchisement of the individual. *Journal of Psychiatric and Mental Health Nursing*, 18, 469–478.

Flensmark, J. (2004). Is there an association between the use of heeled footwear and schizophrenia? *Medical Hypotheses, 63*, 740–747.

Foerschner, A. M. (2010). The history of mental illness: From "skull drills" to "happy pills." *Inquiries Journal, 2*(9), 1–4.

Fromm-Reichmann, F. (1948). Notes on the development of treatment of schizophrenics by psychoanalytic psychotherapy. *Psychiatry, 11*, 263–273.

Gallagher, R. (2016). As a psychiatrist, I diagnose mental illness. Also, I help spot demonic possession. *The Washington Post*. https://wrpvincent.com/wp-content/uploads/2016/07/As-a-psychiatrist-I-diagnose-mental-illness.-Also-I-help-spot-demonic-possession.pdf.

Getler, M. (1978). Cries of a woman possessed. *The Washington Post*. www.washingtonpost.com/archive/politics/1978/04/21/cries-of-a-woman-possessed/94bf2fd3-8e64-482d-869d-1f929851ca8f/.

Grise, D. E., Peyman, T., & Langland, J. (2017). Remission of schizoaffective disorder using homeopathic medicine: 2 case reports. *Alternative Therapies in Health & Medicine*, 24, 50–56.

Gross, D., & Schäfer, G. (2011). Egas Moniz (1874–1955) and the "invention" of modern psychosurgery: A historical and ethical reanalysis under special consideration of Portuguese original sources. *Neurosurgical Focus, 30*, E8.

Hall, H. (2016). Exorcism, religious freedom and consent: The devil in the detail. *Journal of Criminal Law, 80*, 241–253.

Hilker, R., Helenius, D., Fagerlund, B., Skytthe, A., Christensen, K., Werge, T. M., Nordentoft, M., & Glenthøj, B. (2018). Heritability of schizophrenia and schizophrenia spectrum based on the nationwide Danish twin register. *Biological Psychiatry, 83*, 492–498.

Hines, T. (2023). Projective tests and personality. In S. Hupp & R. Wiseman (Eds.), *Investigating pop psychology: Pseudoscience, fringe science, and controversies*. Routledge.

Jääskeläinen, E., Juola, P., Hirvonen, N., McGrath, J. J., Saha, S., Isohanni, M., Veijola, J., & Miettunen, J. (2013). A systematic review and meta-analysis of recovery in schizophrenia. *Schizophrenia Bulletin, 39*, 1296–1306.

Jelovac, A., Kolshus, E., & McLoughlin, D. M. (2013). Relapse following successful electroconvulsive therapy for major depression: A meta-analysis. *Neuropsychopharmacology, 38*, 2467–2474.

Jones, K. (2000). Insulin coma therapy in schizophrenia. *Journal of the Royal Society of Medicine, 93*, 147–149.

Karayiorgou, M. & Gogos, J.A. (2006). Schizophrenia genetics: Uncovering positional candidate genes. *European Journal of Human Genetics, 14*, 512–519.

Kaster, T. S., Vigod, S. N., Gomes, T., Sutradhar, R., Wijeysundera, D. N., & Blumberger, D. M. (2021). Risk of serious medical events in patients with depression treated with electroconvulsive therapy: A propensity score-matched, retrospective cohort study. *The Lancet Psychiatry, 8*, 686–695.

Kuipers, E., Onwumere, J., & Bebbington, P. (2010). Cognitive model of caregiving in psychosis. *British Journal of Psychiatry, 196*, 259–265.

Levin, A. (2019). The life of Benjamin Rush reflects troubled age in U.S. medical history. *Psychiatric News*. https://psychnews.psychiatryonline.org/doi/10.1176/appi.pn.2019.2a23.

Libaw, O. (2006). Exorcism thriving in U.S., say experts. *ABC News*. https://abcnews.go.com/US/story?id=92541.

Lilienfeld, S. O., Wood, J. M., & Garb, H. N. (2000). The scientific status of projective techniques. *Psychological Science in the Public Interest, 1*, 27–66.

Lincoln, T. M., & Pedersen, A. (2019). An overview of the evidence for psychological interventions for psychosis: Results from meta-analyses. *Clinical Psychology in Europe, 1*, 1–23.

Lombardi, R., Rinaldi, L., & Thanopulos, S. (Eds.) (2019). *Psychoanalysis of the psychoses: Current developments in theory and practice*. Routledge.

McGuire, P., Robson, P., Cubala, W. J., Vasile, D., Morrison, P. D., Barron, R., Taylor, A., & Wright, S. (2018). Cannabidiol (CBD) as an adjunctive therapy in schizophrenia: A multicenter randomized controlled trial. *American Journal of Psychiatry, 175*(3), 225–231.

Magalhães, P. V., Dean, O., Andreazza, A. C., Berk, M., & Kapczinski, F. (2016). Antioxidant treatments for schizophrenia. *Cochrane Database of Systematic Reviews*, (2), CD008919.

Malmberg, L., Fenton, M., & Rathbone, J. (2001). Individual psychodynamic psychotherapy and psychoanalysis for schizophrenia and severe mental illness. *Cochrane Database of Systematic Reviews*, (3), CD001360.

Mariani, M. (2018). American exorcism. *The Atlantic*. www.theatlantic.com /magazine/archive/2018/12/catholic-exorcisms-on-the-rise/573943/.

Merizalde, B. A. (2018). Homeopathy and psychiatry. In D. A. Moni & A. B. Newberg (Eds.), *Integrative psychiatry and brain health* (2nd ed.). Oxford University Press.

Morero, J. A. P., de Souza Pereira, S., Esteves, R. B., & Cardoso, L. (2021). Effects of reiki on mental health care: A systematic review. *Holistic Nursing Practice, 35,* 191–198.

Mueser, K. T., & Berenbaum, H. (1990). Psychodynamic treatment of schizophrenia: Is there a future? *Psychological Medicine, 20,* 253–262.

National Collaborating Centre for Mental Health (UK). (2014). *Psychosis and schizophrenia in adults: Treatment and management.* National Institute for Health and Care Excellence (UK).

Offit, P. (2013). The vitamin myth: Why we think we need supplements. *The Atlantic, 7,* 19.

Parker, G. (1982). Re-searching the schizophrenogenic mother. *The Journal of Nervous and Mental Disease, 170,* 452–462.

Pfeifer, S. (1994). Belief in demons and exorcism in psychiatric patients in Switzerland. *British Journal of Medical Psychology, 67,* 247–258.

Pietkiewicz, I. J., Kłosińska, U., & Tomalski, R. (2021). Delusions of possession and religious coping in schizophrenia: A qualitative study of four cases. *Frontiers in Psychology, 12,* 842.

Radhakrishnan, R., Wilkinson, S. T., & D'Souza, D. C. (2014). Gone to pot – A review of the association between cannabis and psychosis. *Frontiers in Psychiatry, 5,* 54.

Read, J., & Bentall, R. (2010). The effectiveness of electroconvulsive therapy: A literature review. *Epidemiology and Psychiatric Sciences, 19,* 333–347.

Soares, M. S., Paiva, W. S., Guertzenstein, E. Z., Amorim, R. L., Bernardo, L. S., Pereira, J. F., Fonoff, E. T., & Teixeira, M. J. (2013). Psychosurgery for schizophrenia: history and perspectives. *Neuropsychiatric Disease and Treatment, 9,* 509–515.

Substance Abuse and Mental Health Services Administration. (2012). SAMHSA's working definition of recovery. SAMHSA. https://store .samhsa.gov/sites/default/files/d7/priv/pep12-recdef.pdf.

Svoboda, E. (2020). Complementary treatments for schizophrenia. *WebMD.* www .webmd.com/schizophrenia/schizophrenia-complementary-treatments.

Tajima-Pozo, K., Zambrano-Enriquez, D., de Anta, L., Moron, M. D., Carrasco, J. L., Lopez-Ibor, J. J., & Diaz-Marsá, M. (2011). Practicing exorcism in schizophrenia. *BMJ Case Reports,* 2011, bcr1020092350.

Tan, S. Y., & Yip, A. (2014). António Egas Moniz (1874–1955): Lobotomy pioneer and Nobel laureate. *Singapore Medical Journal, 55,* 175–176.

Thomason, T. C. (2008). Possession, exorcism, and psychotherapy. *Professional Issues in Counseling*, *8*, 3–22.

Thompson, E., Millman, Z. B., Okuzawa, N., Mittal, V., DeVylder, J., Skadberg, T., Buchanan, R. W., Reeves, G. M., & Schiffman, J. (2015). Evidence-based early interventions for individuals at clinical high risk for psychosis: A review of treatment components. *Journal of Nervous and Mental Disease*, *203*, 342–351.

Trifu, S.C., Kohn, B., Vlasie, A., & Patrichi, B. (2020). Genetics of schizophrenia. *Experimental and Therapeutic Medicine*, *20*, 3462–3468.

Tsuang, M. (2000). Schizophrenia: Ggenes and environment. *Biological Psychiatry*, *47*, 210–220.

United States Conference of Catholic Bishops. (n.d.). Exorcism. www.usccb.org/prayer-and-worship/sacraments-and-sacramentals/sacramentals-blessings/exorcism.

Valenstein, E. S. (1986). *Great and desperate cures: The rise and decline of psychosurgery and other radical treatments for mental illness*. Basic Books.

Vita, A., & Barlati, S. (2018). Recovery from schizophrenia: Is it possible? *Current Opinion inPsychiatry*, *31*, 246–255.

Wehring, H. J., & Carpenter, W. T. (2011). Violence and schizophrenia. *Schizophrenia Bulletin*, *37*, 877–878.

Weiss, K. J. (2017). Linus Pauling, Ph.D. (1901–1994): From chemical bond to civilization. *American Journal of Psychiatry*, *174*, 518–519.

World Health Organization. (2018). *International classification of diseases for mortality and morbidity statistics* (11th revision). https://icd.who.int/browse11/l-m/en.

Wright-Mendoza, J. (2018). The (unproven, deadly) common cure for schizophrenia. *JSTOR Daily*. https://daily.jstor.org/the-unproven-deadly-common-cure-for-schizophrenia/.

17

Autism Spectrum and Intellectual Disability

Jason C. Travers

Autism spectrum disorder (ASD) is a developmental disorder that affects social development, communication, and behavior (American Psychiatric Association [APA], 2022). ASD is typically diagnosed using clinical criteria in the *Diagnostic and Statistical Manual of Mental Disorders* (APA, 2022) that also includes an indication of the severity of impairment. Specifically, a child must have persistent deficits in social–emotional reciprocity and nonverbal communication. They also must demonstrate deficits with developing, maintaining, and understanding relationships. The severity of these impairments can range from relatively mild (e.g., average IQ but stilted conversations, flat affect, limited social initiations) to severe (e.g., very low IQ with absent speech and high rates of repetitive behavior and self-stimulation). Accordingly, some individuals who have mild impairments have average to above average intelligence and use speech and language to communicate but experience social difficulties that negatively impact quality of life throughout adulthood. Conversely, other individuals with ASD may have moderate or severe intellectual impairments, do not use speech, have very limited understanding of language, and need support for daily living. Thus, an individual may have ASD with or without an intellectual disability.

Intellectual disability is indicated when impairments in intellectual functioning such as reasoning, problem solving, planning, academic skills, and abstract thinking occur during childhood and persist throughout the life span (APA, 2022). Such impairments are most often identified via cognitive testing but also can be evident in assessment of adaptive skills (e.g., functional daily-living skills assessments like the Vineland Adaptive Behavior Scale; Sparrow et al., 2016). For example, an individual with an intellectual disability may not perform various skills consistent with others of the same age and sociocultural experiences including but not limited to communication, self-care, and social interactions (APA, 2022). The distinctive adaptive skill profiles of individuals with intellectual disabilities indicate that cognitive tests, which have been criticized, are not necessary for making a clinical diagnosis.

While ASD appears to have a genetic etiology (Taylor et al., 2020), intellectual disabilities may be the result of genetic makeup, another disabling condition (e.g., Down syndrome, fetal alcohol syndrome, fragile X syndrome), and/or environmental factors (e.g., lead poisoning, phenylalanine toxicity, malnutrition). Although some individuals with ASD also have an intellectual disability, others have only one disorder or the other.

17.1 Pseudoscience and Questionable Ideas

ASD and intellectual disabilities have historically been attributed to various superstitious and spurious causes that, in turn, were treated with pseudoscientific and questionable interventions. One popular albeit pseudoscientific belief was that parents (and mothers in particular) caused psychological damage to their children by way of neglect or insufficient emotional attachment. So-called "refrigerator mothers" were largely considered the cause of ASD due to renowned yet infamous psychologist Bruno Bettelheim. Bettelheim (1967) claimed ASD was a psychogenetic disorder caused by poor parenting with symptoms that were similar to the psychological damage experienced by survivors of the Holocaust. He analogized parents of children with ASD to Nazis and implicated them as weak, uncaring, and emotionally absent from their child. Bettelheim published numerous accounts of successful psychodynamic treatment, but his career was later found to be rife with research fraud, plagiarism, and blatant fabrications (Pollak, 1998). Bettelheim's claims became increasingly disfavored when evidence revealed ASD to be a developmental disorder with a genetic etiology (Folstein & Rutter, 1977). Unfortunately, that did not stop new pseudoscientific treatments from emerging.

The notion that vaccines cause ASD is perhaps one of the most well-known, discredited claims filling the void when a psychogenic etiology was debunked. Initially promoted by Andrew Wakefield, it was later found to be the result of fraudulent research (Offit, 2008). Offit, a world-renowned vaccine expert, explained that Wakefield stood to gain financially from sales of his patented alternative to the leading vaccine for measles, mumps, and rubella (MMR). Unfortunately, the claim that the existing MMR vaccine caused autism gained attention before the fraud was realized, and concerns about increased ASD prevalence increased. These conditions likely contributed a cottage industry of quacks and charlatans selling various biomedical treatments aimed at mitigating supposed harm from ingredients like thimerosal, a preservative commonly used in MMR vaccines.

Dubious treatments emerged alongside increased awareness of ASD, while screening and diagnostic practices simultaneously improved. As the ability to identify ASD increased, so too did fears about an autism epidemic in popular media. During a time when confidence in e-commerce ballooned, fears of rising ASD incidence likely contributed to a belief in dubious causes of the disorder coupled with unsupported and dangerous treatments (Travers et al., 2016). For example, the notion that vaccines, and thimerosal specifically, cause autism led to the popular albeit discredited use of chelation therapy, a treatment for heavy metal toxicity such as mercury poisoning (Crisponi et al., 2015). Proponents claimed chelation therapy led to marked improvements in social, behavioral, and intellectual functioning, effectively "curing" ASD. However, no studies have ever found such effects. Chelation is considered a dangerous and potentially deadly treatment (Baxter & Krenzelok, 2008).

Other purported treatments (e.g., auditory integration training, secretin hormone treatment) also were popularized based on unsubstantiated anecdotes of improved psychological and intellectual function. Purveyors of pseudoscientific treatments capitalized on the compassion and empathy among those in helping professions, including psychotherapists, psychologists, educators, and others (Metz et al., 2016). Marketing tactics also likely exploited fears by capitalizing on the contradiction of significant intellectual impairment coupled with savant skills in some people with ASD (Travers et al., 2016). These and other factors served as fertile ground for diagnostic controversies, questionable assessment practices, myths, and misconceptions about the etiology of ASD. In turn, implausible and ineffective treatments emerged, waned, and in some cases returned in new forms while discouraging or misleading professionals away from evidence-based interventions.

17.1.1 Myths That Influence Treatment

17.1.1.1 *Myths about Diagnosis*

One common diagnostic controversy emerging over the past few decades relates to sensory processing disorder. It is commonly believed that individuals exhibiting self-stimulatory behavior and atypical responses to sensory stimuli have a sensory processing disorder. Ayres (1972) initially suggested that neurological dysfunction complicates the brain's interpretation of sensory information, leading to difficulty filtering relevant sensation and subsequent adverse responses (e.g., aggression to escape a loud room; body rocking to access sensory experience).

One diagnostic criterion for ASD is hyper- or hyporeactive responses to sensory stimuli, including adverse responses to specific sounds or textures, apparent indifference to temperature or pain, excessive touching or smelling of objects, and visual fascination with lights or movement (e.g., body rocking and hand flapping; APA, 2022). Sensory processing disorder may seem reasonable given this criterion and the behavioral characteristics of individuals with ASD. That is, the notion that ASD is caused or explained by impairments or differences in brain processing seems plausible. However, this perspective is largely descriptive (rather than prescriptive), has many hallmarks of pseudoscience, and has ushered in various treatments that are unsupported by rigorous experimental evidence.

Sensory integration treatment emerged following Ayres' (1972) seminal paper, in which she reported that children with learning disabilities (e.g., dyslexia) who received the treatment showed significant decreases in sensory integration dysfunction when compared to matched controls. The treatment procedures were not described with replicable precision, but instead offered a general explanation that individualized programs were developed based on sensory profiles of participants. Ayres interpreted the findings as evidence for the "normalization of sensory integrative processes, especially at the brain-stem level" (p. 27) following treatment, but those claims were not supported by any measures or observations of brain functioning in the study. This and similar claims associated with sensory processing disorder and sensory integration treatment (typically administered by occupational therapists) are common and arguably represent how pseudoscientific nonsense is easily disguised with neurobabble to convince unscrupulous researchers, professionals, and consumers alike.

Psychotherapists might perceive sensory processing disorder a legitimate diagnosis and sensory integration treatment as potentially useful when viewing these through a treatment lens focused on systematic desensitization to build tolerance of unpleasant stimuli (e.g., Koegel et al., 2004). They also may accept these ideas as grounds for applying exposure-based treatments commonly used for the ritualistic and repetitive behaviors associated with obsessive-compulsive disorder (e.g., Zandt et al., 2007). Such treatments may be appropriate for some individuals with ASD, but they are not predicated on or substantiated by evidence that sensory processing disorder is a legitimate neurological condition. Indeed, the American Academy of Pediatrics published a policy statement explaining that sensory processing disorder is not a recognized diagnosis and its treatments remain controversial (Zimmer & Desch, 2012). There remains no rigorous experimental evidence that sensory integration treatment improves repetitive, stereotypical, or self-stimulatory behavior in people with ASD. To the contrary, a systematic review found experimental evidence that sensory integration treatment may exacerbate problems rather than resolve them (Lang et al., 2012). Psychotherapists and other professionals who evaluate or treat individuals with ASD and/or intellectual disability should be wary of treatment recommendations based on reports that attribute behavioral excesses and deficits to a sensory processing disorder, as well as recommendations for sensory integration treatment aimed at reducing behavioral excesses and deficits.

17.1.1.2 Myths about Etiology

There are many misconceptions about the etiology of ASD. Two were mentioned above – the psychogenic cause (i.e., "refrigerator mothers") and vaccine-induced toxicity. Mercer and colleagues (2006) found parents often believed these myths, and in addition, they blamed diets with gluten and casein (a milk protein) as a cause of ASD. Additionally, early researchers suggested that difficulties encountered by people with ASD reflected poor adherence to a pattern of typical child development, leading to a few discredited, albeit somewhat popular, developmental models of treatment. These myths are worth exploring in more detail so professionals might readily identify and avoid them.

17.1.1.3 Myths about Biomedical Cures

ASD and intellectual disabilities are developmental in nature, and although early intervention can significantly improve the long-term outcomes for individuals, they are not believed to be curable. That is, evidence-based treatments and interventions can lessen the negative effects that ASD symptoms have on a person's quality of life, but the person will experience disability throughout their lifetime. Some comorbid conditions (e.g., food allergies, digestive disorders, skin conditions) may merely be incidental and unrelated to an individual's developmental disability.

While pharmacological treatments may be useful for addressing a variety of behavioral and medical conditions (e.g., anxiety, seizures), many complementary and alternative medicine approaches have emerged. Proponents of alternative treatments assert that inflammation in the body causes or exacerbates symptoms associated with ASD. Such inflammation is claimed to be caused by food allergies, particularly gluten and casein, although studies have repeatedly failed to find any such relationship (e.g., Elder et al., 2006; González-Domenech et al., 2020; Mulloy et al., 2010). Other alternative treatments lack evidentiary support but remain popular, including the use of vitamins and supplements, "detoxifying" salt baths, and consumption of activated charcoal to improve communication and behavior. Various probiotic, antibiotic, and antiyeast pharmaceutical regimens are claimed without credible evidence to reduce purported bacterial infections exacerbating severe behavior.

17.1.1.4 *Myths about Repairing Relationships*

Developmental theories of ASD and intellectual disability were arguably most popular during the 1970s and 1980s when treatment options were relatively rare and crude. Developmental treatments are predicated on the idea that associated symptoms (e.g., atypical speech, limited communication, behavioral excesses and deficits, reduced social skills and social competence) result from poor relationship development during childhood. The interventions that emerged based on this perspective emphasize repairing relationships by increasing attachment, affect, and social bonds (Heflin & Simpson, 1998). Travers and colleagues (2016) identified three popular albeit unsupported developmental treatments including gentle teaching, the Son-Rise™ program, and Floortime. These and similar methods harken back to the debunked psychogenetic theory of ASD and are associated with questionable practices and unsupported claims. For example, the Son-Rise™ program involves adults imitating socially inappropriate behavior (e.g., repeating phrases, imitating body rocking, and hand-flapping) as a means of fostering the relationship. Son-Rise™ proponents have claimed their method cures ASD, although no experimental evidence shows beneficial effects let alone miraculous cures. Floortime is another relatively popular intervention that uses techniques associated with applied behavior analysis (an evidence-based treatment approach), such as recognizing the person's interest and supporting appropriate communication with prompting, reinforcement, and redirection. However, Floortime's procedures and outcomes are usually explained in general terms and often lack sufficient specificity associated with experimental research and independent replication.

17.1.1.5 Myths about Motor Abilities

An increasingly popular myth is that many people with ASD actually have normal or above average intellectual ability, but experience motor impairments that affect speech and behavior. This idea has origins in the facilitated communication craze that swept the United States and other countries in the 1990s. Facilitated communication and similar methods are described in more detail below, but first it is important to delineate the association and attached pseudoscientific ideas that underpin this popular myth. Proponents argue that individuals with ASD have sensory and motor difficulties that affect control of their body, but they can overcome such challenges to communicate complex and abstract ideas when provided with emotional and physical support (Leary & Donnellan, 2013). This idea lacks credible evidence yet is promoted in popular books like *The Reason I Jump* (Higashida, 2007), which was recently made into a full-length feature documentary film. Other popular books include *Carly's Voice* (Fleischmann & Fleischmann, 2012), *How Can I Talk if My Lips Don't Move* (Mukhopadhyay, 2008), and *Underestimated: An Autism Miracle* (Handley, 2021). Many people with ASD do have average or above average intelligence. However, there is no reliable evidence to support the claim that individuals with intellectual impairments truly have average or advanced intellectual ability accompanied by motor impairments that affect speech.

17.1.2 Implausible, Ineffective, and Potentially Harmful Treatments

All ineffective treatments are associated with some degree of harm. For example, Travers (2017) explains that lost time, effort, material resources, and money harm helping professionals. Clients also are harmed by loss of opportunity, failure to benefit, and delayed therapeutic improvements that may be urgent. Additionally, clients who are treated with an ineffective intervention have likely lost financial resources (i.e., paying for treatment that provides no benefit). Pseudoscience and credulous behavior warrant careful consideration when making treatment decisions, thus justifying an ethical obligation to adhere to evidence-based treatments that are likely to benefit individuals with ASD and intellectual disability. Unfortunately, the field is rife with implausible, ineffective, and harmful treatments.

17.1.2.1 Facilitated Communication and Its Variants

Many people with ASD or intellectual disability benefit from augmentative communication devices. Yet, arguably the most prominent pseudoscientific method is facilitated communication. Unlike effective communication interventions, facilitated communication involves a so-called facilitator who holds the hand, wrist, or elbow of a person with ASD or intellectual disability to point to letters and spell words representative of their thoughts (Biklen, 1993). In some cases, facilitated communication entails holding a communication device like a keyboard or placard with printed letters underneath the hand of the client. These variants are sometimes called spelling to communicate, rapid prompting method, letterboarding, or informative pointing (Todd, 2016).

Many individuals in the helping professions likely have learned about facilitated communication in the context of a history lesson about the dangers of sweeping pseudoscientific fads that emerge without empirical evidence. Some readers may recall a documentary called *Prisoners of Silence* by Palfreman (1993) that originally aired on the PBS show *Frontline*. The film explained the craze associated with facilitated communication and featured prominent researchers who investigated experimental methods revealing the bogus nature of facilitated communication.

Irrespective of the label or style of deception, an abundant corpus of evidence from very well-controlled experimental studies revealed that people with ASD or intellectual disability were not the ones generating the messages during facilitated communication. In fact, the facilitators generated the messages, often without realizing it due to a phenomenon known as the ideomotor effect (Lilienfeld et al., 2014; Mostert, 2001; 2010; Schlosser et al., 2014). The ideomotor effect is the phenomenon that accounts for debunked claims associated with Ouija board, dowsing, and automatic writing (Todd, 2016). Unfortunately, facilitated communication and its variants have been associated with multiple false allegations of sexual and physical abuse, often against professionals and parents, unwittingly generated by facilitators (Konstantareas, 1998; Travers et al., 2014). Accordingly, professionals would be wise to abstain from treating individuals who use facilitated communication lest they become the focus of facilitated false allegations.

17.1.2.2 Other Treatments

Additional treatments have enjoyed popular use despite dubious rationales. Hyperbaric oxygen chamber treatment is predicated on the notion that ASD is associated with oxidative stress and neuroinflammation. The treatment involves placing a child in a chamber where atmospheric pressure is reduced. Multiple studies have investigated this assertion and found no beneficial effects (Granpeesheh et al., 2010; Jepson et al., 2011). Other dubious methods that claim to reorganize neural networks in the brain also have been promoted with some success. Fast ForWord is a computer-based system aimed at treating language and literacy delays with rapid auditory processing activities and games alleged to improve neural functioning. Although popular, the method has been repeatedly studied with meta-analyses finding no beneficial effects (e.g., Strong et al., 2011). Auditory integration training is a similar intervention based on similar assertions and involves listening to music that has been filtered and otherwise modified. Claims of its ability to cure ASD and intellectual disability have been thoroughly debunked (Sinha et al., 2011).

17.1.3 Undermining Evidence-Based Treatments

All individuals with ASD and intellectual disabilities have strengths, interests, and preferences that professionals should learn about and leverage for better outcomes. Individuals with ASD can have significant impacts on society, impacting their families and communities in positive ways. Some proponents of the neurodiversity movement, however, argue that ASD and other mental health conditions are simply part of normal human variation. Consequently, they are opposed to treatment aimed at functional improvement in favor of acceptance and accommodation. Yet many (if not most) people with ASD also experience barriers to quality of life and high degrees of suffering that mere acceptance will not alleviate. It seems reasonable, then, to find a balance between respecting neurodivergence with a desire to reduce the suffering that many individuals with ASD encounter (e.g., Kapp et al., 2013; Tincani et al., 2009). Sadly, vocal opposition to evidence-based treatments has become a prominent theme of the neurodiversity movement, particularly on social media and in some academic circles (e.g., disability studies; Broderick & Roscigno, 2021). In particular, some neurodiversity proponents aim to undermine evidence-based treatments rooted in applied behavior analysis.

Applied behavior analysis is considered the standard of care for people with ASD and intellectual disability, but various critiques and misconceptions are common. The earliest applied behavior analysis research included punishment to reduce dangerous and disruptive behavior without understanding why it occurred. (This was known as behavior modification, and is different from today's commonly used applied behavior analysis approaches.) Due to significant practical and ethical advances since the 1960s and 1970s, punishment is now generally unused with a few exceptions (such as loss of privileges aimed at decreasing unwanted behavior) and only after reinforcement-based interventions have failed (Behavior Analyst Certification Board, 2017).

Common misunderstandings about applied behavior analysis include the false belief that systematic instruction (i.e., breaking down complex tasks into discrete steps for teaching) is synonymous with dog training (Milton, 2018). Critics also disavow the use of rewards to support various types of skill acquisition as coercion, falsely believing applied behavior analysis forces eye contact and rigid behavioral compliance (e.g., Sandoval-Norton & Shkedy, 2019). These and other common myths and misconceptions appear motivated by an extreme antitreatment ideology that wrongly perceives behavioral interventions as focusing on an internal pathology of individuals (Trump et al., 2018). In fact, applied behavior analysis emphasizes flawed environments and past experiences as the primary changeable source of a person's impaired functioning and therefore focuses treatment on environmental arrangement (Cooper et al., 2020). Furthermore, applied behavior analysis is not a curriculum or prescription that identifies what behavioral changes ought to be made, but rather a technology for helping people achieve desired behavior change.

17.2 Research-Supported Approaches

Applied behavior analysis is a distinct field of study that aims to understand the relationship between a person's experience, current environment, and behavior in order to support behavior change and overall wellbeing. Most of the evidence-based treatments for people with ASD and intellectual disability are based on applied behavior analysis. These include antecedent-based interventions, discrete trial teaching, prompting, time delay, reinforcement, response interruption and redirection, task analysis, modeling, conversational scripting, visual supports, and functional communication training (Hume et al., 2021; Wong et al., 2015).

Functional communication training uses contextual behavior assessment results to elucidate the needs being met by specific behaviors (Cooper et al., 2020). This treatment is commonly used for individuals with limited speech and language, but it also has been effective for individuals with challenging behaviors such as aggression, property destruction, and self-injury. Functional communication training begins by identifying and assessing behavioral difficulties in context (e.g., examining documented incidents, reviewing records, observing the individual). If, for example, assessment results indicate an individual hits others in order to access a preferred item, then functional communication training involves teaching that person to use an easier, more effective, and socially acceptable way to tell someone they want the item (i.e., a replacement behavior). A person might be taught to say a word or phrase, push a button on a communication device, give a printed symbol or word, or use a gesture or manual sign that conveys their desire to access the preferred item. With repeated experience, the person learns that access to the preferred item is easily and consistently achieved via the replacement behavior and that the challenging behavior (hitting others) is ineffective, more effortful, and therefore no longer occurs.

17.3 Conclusion

People with ASD and/or intellectual disability experience a range of social, communicative, and behavioral challenges that require evidence-based treatments primarily rooted in applied behavior analysis. As the reported prevalence of ASD has increased in past decades, quacks and charlatans have manufactured bogus causes and used emotional manipulation to promote unsupported, discredited, and wholly pseudoscientific treatments. Some such treatments appear benign while others are quite harmful. Professionals who recognize that ASD and intellectual disabilities are not mysterious disorders, but developmental disabilities that cause lifelong impairments, may be less inclined to use, recommend, or inadvertently promote pseudoscientific treatments. Adhering to an evidence-based approach will not only serve clients and their families, but they may enhance professional success while limiting the spread of harmful treatments.

Jason C. Travers, PhD, BCBA-D, is an Associate Professor of Teaching and Learning at Temple University. He is author of the book *Sexuality Education* (2018).

References

American Psychiatric Association. (2022). *Diagnostic and statistical manual of mental disorders, fifth edition, text revision* (DSM-5-TR). American Psychiatric Association.

Ayres, A. J. (1972). Improving academic scores through sensory integration. *Journal of Learning Disabilities*, 5(6), 338–343.

Baxter, A. J., & Krenzelok, E. P. (2008). Pediatric fatality secondary to EDTA chelation. *Clinical Toxicology*, *46*, 1083–1084.

Behavior Analyst Certification Board. (2017). Professional and ethical compliance code for behavior analysts. www.bacb.com/wp-content/uploads/2020/05/BACB-Compliance-Code-english_190318.pdf.

Bettelheim, B. (1967). *The empty fortress: Infantile autism and the birth of the self.* The Free Press.

Biklen, D. (1993). *Communication unbound: How facilitated communication is challenging traditional views of autism and ability/disability.* Teachers College Press.

Broderick, A. A., & Roscigno, R. (2021). Autism, inc.: The autism industrial complex. *Journal of Disability Studies in Education*, *2*(1), 77–101.

Cooper, J. O., Heron, T. E., & Heward, W. L. (2020). *Applied behavior analysis* (3rd ed.). Pearson.

Crisponi, G., Nurchi, V. M., Lachowicz, J. I., Crespo-Alonso, M., Zoroddu, M. A., & Peana, M. (2015). Kill or cure: Misuse of chelation therapy for human diseases. *Coordination Chemistry Reviews*, *284*, 278–285.

Donnellan, A. M., Hill, D. A., & Leary, M. R. (2013). Rethinking autism: Implications of sensory and movement differences for understanding and support. *Frontiers in Integrative Neuroscience*, *6*, 124.

Elder, J. H., Shankar, M., Shuster, J., Theriaque, D., Burns, S., & Sherrill, L. (2006). The gluten-free, casein-free diet in autism: Results of a preliminary double blind clinical trial. *Journal of Autism and Developmental Disorders*, *36*(3), 413–420.

Fleischmann, A. & Fleischmann, C. (2012). *Carly's voice*. Simon & Schuster.

Folstein, S., & Rutter, M. (1977). Infantile autism: A genetic study of 21 twin pairs. *Journal of Child Psychology and Psychiatry*, *18*(4), 297–321.

González-Domenech, P. J., Atienza, F. D., Pablos, C. G., Soto, M. L. F., Martínez-Ortega, J. M., & Gutiérrez-Rojas, L. (2020). Influence of a combined gluten-free and casein-free diet on behavior disorders in children and adolescents diagnosed with autism spectrum disorder: A 12-month follow-up clinical trial. *Journal of Autism and Developmental Disorders*, *50*(3), 935–948.

Granpeesheh, D., Tarbox, J., Dixon, D. R., Wilke, A. E., Allen, M. S., & Bradstreet, J. J. (2010). Randomized trial of hyperbaric oxygen therapy for children with autism. *Research in Autism Spectrum Disorders*, *4*, 268–275.

Handley, J. B. (2021). *Underestimated: An autism miracle*. Skyhorse Publishing.

Heflin, L. J., & Simpson, R. L. (1998). Interventions for children and youth with autism: Prudent choices in a world of exaggerated claims and empty promises. Part I: Intervention and treatment option review. *Focus on Autism and Other Developmental Disabilities*, *13*, 194–211.

Higashida, N. (2013). *The reason I jump: The inner voice of a thirteen-year-old boy with autism.* Random House.

Hume, K., Steinbrenner, J. R., Odom, S. L., Morin, K. L., Nowell, S. W., Tomaszewski, B., Szendrey, S., McIntyre, N. S., Yücesoy-Özkan, S., & Savage, M. N. (2021). Evidence-based practices for children, youth, and young adults with autism: Third generation review. *Journal of Autism and Developmental Disorders, 51,* 4013–4032.

Jepson, B., Granpeesheh, D., Tarbox, J., Olive, M. L., Stott, C., Braud, S., Yoo, J. H., Wakefield, A., & Allen, M. S. (2011). Controlled evaluation of the effects of hyperbaric oxygen therapy on the behavior of 16 children with autism spectrum disorders. *Journal of Autism and Developmental Disorders, 41,* 575–588.

Kapp, S. K., Gillespie-Lynch, K., Sherman, L. E., & Hutman, T. (2013). Deficit, difference, or both? Autism and neurodiversity. *Developmental Psychology, 49*(1), 59–71.

Koegel, R. L., Openden, D., & Koegel, L. K. (2004). A systematic desensitization paradigm to treat hypersensitivity to auditory stimuli in children with autism in family contexts. *Research and Practice for Persons with Severe Disabilities, 29*(2), 122–134.

Konstantareas, M. M. (1998). Allegations of sexual abuse by nonverbal autistic people via facilitated communication: Testing of validity. *Child Abuse & Neglect, 22,* 1027–1041.

Lang, R., O'Reilly, M., Healy, O., Rispoli, M., Lydon, H., Streusand, W., Davis, T., Kang, S., Sigafoos, J., Lancioni, G., Didden, R., & Giesbers, S. (2012). Sensory integration therapy for autism spectrum disorders: A systematic review. *Research in Autism Spectrum Disorders, 6,* 1004–1018.

Lilienfeld, S. O., Marshall, J., Todd, J. T., & Shane, H. C. (2014). The persistence of fad interventions in the face of negative scientific evidence: Facilitated communication for autism as a case example. *Evidence-Based Communication Assessment and Intervention, 8*(2), 62–101.

Mercer, L., Creighton, S., Holden, J. J. A., & Lewis, M. E. S. (2006). Parental perspectives on the causes of an autism spectrum disorder in their children. *Journal of Genetic Counseling, 15*(1), 41–50.

Metz, B., Mulick, J. A., & Butter, E. M. (2016). Autism: A late 20th century fad magnet. In R. M. Foxx, & J. A. Mulick (Eds.), *Controversial therapies for developmental disabilities* (2nd ed., pp. 237–263). Routledge.

Milton, D. (2018). A critique of the use of applied behavioural analysis (ABA): On behalf of the Neurodiversity Manifestor Steerint Group. Unpublished manuscript. https://kar.kent.ac.uk/69268/1/Applied%20behaviour%20ana lysis.pdf.

Mostert, M. P. (2001). Facilitated communication since 1995: A review of published studies. *Journal of Autism and Developmental Disorders, 31,* 287–313.

Mostert, M. P. (2010). Facilitated communication and its legitimacy – Twenty-first century developments. *Exceptionality, 18*, 31–41.

Mukhopadhyay, T. (2008). *How can I talk if my lips don't move: Inside my autistic mind.* Arcade.

Mulloy, A., Lang, R., O'Reilly, M., Sigafoos, J., Lancioni, G., & Rispoli, M. (2010). Gluten-free and casein-free diets in the treatment of autism spectrum disorders: A systematic review. *Research in Autism Spectrum Disorders, 4*(3), 328–339.

Offit, P. (2008). *Autism's false prophets.* Columbia University Press.

Palfreman, J. (1993). *Frontline: Prisoners of silence.* WGBH Public Television.

Pollak, R. (1998). *The creation of Doctor B: A biography of Bruno Bettelheim.* Simon and Schuster.

Sandoval-Norton, A. H., & Shkedy, G. (2019). How much compliance is too much compliance: Is long-term ABA therapy abuse? *Cogent Psychology, 6*, 1641258.

Schlosser, R. W., Balandin, S., Hemsley, B., Iacono, T., Probst, P., & von Tetzchner, S. (2014). Facilitated communication and authorship: A systematic review. *Augmentative and Alternative Communication, 30*(4), 359–368.

Sinha, Y., Silove, N., Hayen, A., & Williams, K. (2011). Auditory integration training and other sound therapies for autism spectrum disorders (ASD). *Cochrane Database of Systematic Reviews*, (12), CD003681.

Sparrow S. S., Cicchetti D. V. & Saulnier C. A. (2016) *Vineland Adaptive Behavior Scales* (3rd ed.). Pearson.

Strong, G. K., Torgerson, C. J., Torgerson, D., & Hulme, C. (2011). A systematic meta-analytic review of evidence for the effectiveness of the 'Fast ForWord' language intervention program. *Journal of Child Psychology and Psychiatry, 52*(3), 224–235.

Taylor, M. J., Rosenqvist, M. A., Larsson, H., Gillberg, C., D'Onofrio, B. M., Lichtenstein, P., & Lundström, S. (2020). Etiology of autism spectrum disorders and autistic traits over time. *JAMA psychiatry, 77*(9), 936–943.

Tincani, M., Travers, J. C., & Boutot, A. B. (2009). Race, culture, and autism spectrum disorders: Understanding the role of diversity in successful educational interventions. *Research and Practice in Severe Disabilities, 34*, 81–90.

Todd, J. T. (2016). Old horses in new stables: Rapid prompting, facilitated communication, science, ethics, and the history of magic. In R. M. Foxx & J. A. Mulick (Eds.), *Controversial therapies for autism and intellectual disabilities: Fad, fashion, and science in professional practice* (2nd ed., pp. 372–409). Routledge.

Travers, J. C. (2017). Evaluating claims to avoid pseudoscientific and unproven practices in special education. *Intervention in School and Clinic, 52*, 195–203. https://doi.org/10.1177/1053451216659466.

Travers, J. C., Ayers, K., Simpson, R. L., & Crutchfield, S. (2016). Fad, pseudoscientific, and controversial interventions. In R. Lang, T. B. Hancock, & N. N. Singh (Eds.), *Early intervention for young children with autism spectrum disorder* (pp. 257–293). Springer.

Travers, J. C., Tincani, M., & Lang, R. (2014). Facilitated communication denies people with disabilities their voice. *Research and Practice in Severe Disabilities*, *39*, 195–202.

Trump, C. E., Pennington, R. C., Travers, J. C., Ringdahl, J. E., Whiteside, E. E., & Ayres, K. M. (2018). Applied behavior analysis in special education: Misconceptions and guidelines for use. *Teaching Exceptional Children*, *50* (6), 381–393.

Wong, C., Odom, S. L., Hume, K. A., Cox, A. W., Fettig, A., Kucharczyk, S., Brock, M. E., Plavnick, J. B., Fleury, V. P., & Schultz, T. R. (2015). Evidence-based practices for children, youth, and young adults with autism spectrum disorder: A comprehensive review. *Journal of Autism and Developmental Disorders*, *45*(7), 1951–1966.

Zandt, F., Prior, M., & Kyrios, M. (2007). Repetitive behaviour in children with high functioning autism and obsessive compulsive disorder. *Journal of Autism and Developmental Disorders*, *37*(2), 251–259.

Zimmer, M., & Desch, L. (2012). Sensory integration therapies for children with developmental and behavioral disorders. *Pediatrics*, *129*(6), 1186–1189.

18

Inattention and Hyperactivity

J. Russell Ramsay

Attention-deficit/hyperactivity disorder (ADHD) emerged as a diagnostic entity in the second edition of the *Diagnostic and Statistical Manual of Mental Disorders* (American Psychiatric Association [APA], 1968) via an economical 22-word description of what was then branded as hyperkinetic reaction of childhood (or adolescence). This cursory sketch emphasized problems related to overt motoric overactivity with a single mention of short attention span, symptoms which reportedly would remit before adulthood.

The ADHD diagnosis currently resides under the umbrella of neurodevelopmental disorders in the DSM-5-TR (APA, 2022), with a relatively consistent 18-item symptom list. Across some editions of the DSM, some alterations have been made to aspects of the diagnostic criteria relevant to the persistence of ADHD into adulthood. These changes are among several topics reviewed in this chapter. ADHD is associated with risk for significant life impairments but, at the same time, there are effective, research-based treatments. However, there are questionable ideas and treatments whose reputations outdistance the data to be discussed.

18.1 Pseudoscience and Questionable Ideas

Many of the issues addressed in the sections that follow are not necessarily "pseudoscientific," per se. Several compelling ideas continue to be debated, while interventions with mixed outcomes require more honing and research in order to firmly establish their effectiveness. That said, some ideas are just plain wrong. This review will begin with issues related to the diagnosis of adult ADHD. Subsequent questions about symptoms in adulthood, later in life onset, and claims that ADHD is not a mental disorder worthy of a diagnosis will be addressed. Later sections target questionable nonmedical treatments that frequently appear in lists of options for adult ADHD. Namely, these treatments are neurofeedback training, other neurocognitive training, dietary supplementation, and "medical marijuana."

18.1.1 Diagnostic Changes and Controversies

Compared to the previous edition, the DSM-5 (APA, 2013) modified the diagnostic criteria for ADHD to include an extended age-of-onset for emergence of symptoms (up from 7 years old to 12 years old); yet, Barkley and colleagues (2008) make a compelling empirical argument for a threshold of 16 years of age. The DSM-5 also changed the symptom endorsement criterion for adults by lowering the minimum number of symptoms to at least five out of nine (compared to the six-symptom threshold for children) to account for the fact adults often "age out" of some extant criteria.

The persistence rates of ADHD from childhood to adulthood range from around 50% to upwards of 80% (Barkley, 2015). The lower-end rates result from the use of strict criteria (including age-of-onset), whereas the upper-end rates often reflect persistence of residual symptoms and ongoing functional impairments, if not the full syndrome (Biederman et al., 2010; 2011; Volkow & Swanson, 2013). In fact, adults with ADHD who met all diagnostic criteria in childhood except for the strict age-of-onset (7 years old at the time of the study) were clinically indistinguishable from those meeting full criteria (Faraone et al., 2006). These persistence rates do not account for late-diagnosed adults who are first identified with ADHD later in life, although this clinical group has led to questions about whether ADHD can emerge *de novo* in adulthood.

18.1.1.1 Adult-Onset ADHD

Adult-onset ADHD refers to cases in which adults fulfill current diagnostic criteria for ADHD without ever before showing symptoms. Adult-onset ADHD has been the target of media fodder for several years, and researchers have also investigated this phenomenon (Agnew-Blais et al., 2016; Caye et al., 2016; Moffitt et al., 2015). Using retrospective assessments of childhood symptoms along with assessments of current symptoms and impairments in adulthood (and ruling out other causes), studies identified groups of adults with ADHD who did not have emergence of symptoms in childhood. In two examples (Agnew-Blais et al., 2016; Caye et al., 2016), the adult samples were comprised of 18- and 19-year-olds, a hazy line between adolescence and adulthood (Faraone & Biederman,

2016). However, Moffitt and colleagues' (2015) study was comprised of developmentally mature adults, which raised the possibility of a new, distinct ADHD presentation.

Critiques pointed out that, as with past studies revealing low persistence rates of childhood ADHD into adulthood, the above-mentioned research relied upon parent ratings for childhood symptoms and young adult self-ratings for current symptoms (Faraone & Biederman, 2016). Although both assessments are commonly used in diagnostic evaluations for the respective age groups, switching measures may have introduced error, as young adults tend to underreport symptoms (Barkley et al., 2008). Recall of symptoms is often imperfect, and both parent and adult memories may estimate childhood age of onset as being 5–7 years older than in reality (Barkley, 2016b). Hence, the low persistence rates seen in adult-onset studies may have resulted from such measure switching.

Adult-onset studies are also limited when the absence of the full ADHD syndrome in childhood was used as the definition of a negative history of ADHD (Faraone & Biederman, 2016). Diagnostic guidelines for adult ADHD do not require a previous diagnosis or even retrospectively established childhood diagnosis, but rather that "many symptoms" emerged and persisted in childhood. Symptoms may worsen over time and when using strict, categorical definitions, a single symptom may promote or preclude a diagnosis (Barkley, 2016b). Thus, late-onset cases may reflect adults who had many earlier symptoms and struggles but were not diagnosed until in adulthood.

There also may be other explanations for emergent, ADHD-like difficulties, which are considered in any clinical assessment. Sibley and colleagues (2018) performed repeated evaluations of children with ADHD, following them into young adulthood. The results indicated that adult-onset ADHD cases almost always represented ADHD-like symptoms from non-ADHD factors. The issue of accurate evaluation is important because an ADHD diagnosis may be the gateway to seeking help for one's longstanding struggles. Skepticism about treatments, though, often stems from doubts about the seriousness of ADHD.

18.1.1.2 Discrediting the Significance of ADHD

Some professionals deny the significance or existence of ADHD (see Novella, 2017a; 2017b). However, ADHD is one of the more impairing disorders encountered in outpatient behavioral health practices. Academic and occupational functioning are two life domains requiring intact self-regulatory functioning, and adults with ADHD routinely report problems in these areas (Faraone et al., 2021; Kooij et al., 2019). Most other spheres of adult life also require intact self-regulation, including roles that have effects on others. Risks for social and relationship problems, psychiatric and substance use disorders, legal problems, poor health outcomes (including decreased life expectancy), and lower self-esteem are all greater for adults with ADHD than the general population (Barkley, 2015; Barkley & Fischer, 2019; Faraone et al., 2021; Kooij et al., 2019; Nigg, 2013).

Despite these dire prospects, there are many medical and psychosocial research-supported treatments for adult ADHD. At the same time, treatments with equivocal or weak empirical support are often viewed as equally viable. That said, some treatments that may be promising or reasonable adaptations of established treatments that are not yet empirically established fill a clinical need and offer relatively safe bets for patients. Clinicians should strive for transparency in their treatment protocols, allowing patients to make informed decisions by weighing the risks and benefits of different options.

18.1.2 Ineffective Technological Treatments

18.1.2.1 Neurofeedback

Neurofeedback training is essentially biofeedback training for the brain (Ramsay, 2010). Biofeedback is a research-supported approach that involves gathering analog readings of automatic physiological processes like heart rate or galvanic skin response. These processes usually operate outside of one's awareness unless attention is directed toward them. Relevant data from measured physiological processes are translated into a form that can be used by individuals to regulate these signals in a desired direction. For example, a tone reflecting one's pulse can be used to regulate breathing and slow one's heart rate for stress management (Masters et al., 1987).

Neurofeedback, on the other hand, uses electroencephalography to read the brain's electrical activity via sensors placed on the scalp. The resulting analog brain-wave data are translated, often in a gamified format, and used to help adults with ADHD shape their attentional skills to achieve symptomatic improvement.

There have been ambiguous findings of the symptomatic and functional benefits of neurofeedback training for ADHD across age groups. For example, meta-analyses of neurofeedback training for children and adolescents have resulted in a consensus that it is not a recommended treatment, despite small gains in some studies (Kooij et al., 2019). A systematic review of neurofeedback for adult ADHD found discordant findings across studies, including positive results that were no different than those achieved by sham (placebo) controls (Fullen et al., 2020).

18.1.2.2 Neurocognitive Training

The related domain of neurocognitive training encompasses computerized training protocols for attention and executive function skills, and specifically working memory training. These approaches work on an assumption that cognitive skills and other brain-based capacities may be strengthened through practice.

In fact, there were encouraging preliminary findings from well-designed, laboratory-based studies of computerized working memory training for children with ADHD (see Ramsay, 2010 and Simons et al., 2016). Based on these results, a commercially available working memory training program was released that could be conducted remotely and monitored via a remote training coach (see Ramsay, 2010 for a review). Subsequent independent studies and meta-analyses of working memory training and other neurocognitive training technologies, however, did not find sufficient evidence of either the durability of gains from training or improvements in academic functioning (Simons et al., 2016).

An illustrative example of the limits of neurocognitive training is a randomized study of adults with ADHD who were assigned to either a computerized program that provided escalating challenges to match trainees' progress, or a placebo version of the same program kept at the basic level (Stern et al., 2016). Both groups reported significant improvements in ratings of ADHD symptoms, job performance, and measures of executive functions, measures of neurocognitive performance or quality of life revealed no significant improvements. Although positive results were associated with the training, the placebo condition achieved similar gains.

As with neurofeedback, inconsistent results occur in neurocognitive training studies of adults with ADHD (Simons et al., 2016). The expectancy effect, or the belief that improvements will occur simply because a treatment is in place, appears to be a primary mechanism for the positive results achieved (Lee & Suhr, 2019; Schönenberg et al., 2021). More research and development are likely needed to tether computerized practices to real-world outcomes, perhaps with Virtual or Augmented Realities or other emerging technologies. Hopefully, computerized training and psychoeducation will be designed to augment existing psychosocial approaches for adult ADHD.

18.1.3 Questionable Dietary and Nutrition Approaches

18.1.3.1 Supplementation

Diet and nutrition have been claimed to play a role in ADHD (Schnoll et al., 2003). Vitamins, minerals, and other supplements thought to target symptoms of ADHD have been considered, although these approaches have not appeared in systematic reviews of nonpharmacologic treatments for adult ADHD (De Crescenzo et al., 2017; Nimmo-Smith et al., 2020). Well-designed studies have yielded small but significant improvements from omega-3 fatty acid supplementation, although they were not associated with clinical or functional improvements (Sonuga-Barke et al., 2013). Similarly, studies of an assortment of vitamin–mineral and micronutrient supplementation approaches for adults have reported modest symptomatic improvements but not necessarily functional improvements apart from some benefits to overall wellbeing (Rucklidge et al., 2014; Rucklidge & Kaplan, 2014).

Past studies of the use of zinc or iron supplementation to ameliorate deficiencies achieved mild symptomatic improvements on ADHD symptom ratings until levels were normalized, but did not necessarily reflect treatments for ADHD (see Ramsay, 2010). The circumscribed symptoms that have been targeted by supplementation and other dietary interventions did not reflect the wide-ranging, self-dysregulation and functional difficulties characteristic of clinic-referred ADHD cases. Any achieved results for ADHD symptoms relative to the strict demands of supplementation/dietary protocols, apart from the obvious health benefits of correcting deficiencies, fell at the low end of a cost/benefit analysis of time and effort compared with other available treatments for ADHD.

18.1.3.2 Medical Marijuana

Cannabis-based products, including medical marijuana, have been purported to treat adult ADHD symptoms, but their evidence is unconvincing. To date, the United States Food and Drug Administration (FDA) has not approved any cannabis-derived products for the treatment of ADHD. However, one cannabis-derived product and three cannabis-related products (Epidiolex [cannabidiol]), and three synthetic cannabis-related drug products: (Marinol [dronabinol], Syndros [dronabinol], Cesamet [nabilone]) have been approved for the treatment of seizures and anorexia due to acquired immunodeficiency syndrome (AIDS).

Online information on marijuana use for ADHD has exploded. A study of Internet content over the span of a decade (2004–2014) revealed prevalent testimonials for its benefits (Mitchell et al., 2016). The review found that 30% of online posts indicated cannabis was helpful for ADHD (25% cited it as helpful and 5% as both helpful and harmful); 8% found it harmful and 2% reported no effects on ADHD, with the remainder of coded posts accounted for by individuals without reported ADHD dealing with other symptoms. In forum posts, the suggested benefits of cannabis for ADHD did not generalize to non-ADHD symptoms or daily life coping. Moreover, 59% of the forums reviewed included posts commending the benefits of cannabis for ADHD, with "cannabis" employed as an umbrella category for any sort of cannabis product. In some cases, they were tied to specific symptoms like inattention while others described indiscriminate benefits. The view that cannabis has medicinal effects for ADHD has been steadily rated higher than its negative effects since 2006, more and more justified by the increasing endorsement of the benefits of medical marijuana for other conditions and its standing as a "natural" medicine (Mitchell et al., 2016). Such piggy-backing of medical marijuana's benefits for other conditions amounts to "effectiveness by association" that gradually shapeshifts into accepted fact.

Questions related to the effectiveness and safety of cannabis-based products for ADHD deserves quality research. A closer inspection of positive media accounts shows that these reports are often based on conference papers (Dumas-Mallet & Gonon, 2020). Such papers have not undergone rigorous peer review required for publication. In general, only about half of papers on any topic presented at conferences are eventually published.

Along with cannabidiol (CBD), tetrahydrocannabinol (THC) is the most common cannabinoid in use (Canadian ADHD Resource Alliance [CADDRA], 2020). THC is the chemical responsible for the euphoria associated with marijuana. Regarding medical or recreational marijuana use, there is no peer-reviewed, published evidence that THC provides any benefits for adult ADHD and its use is patently discouraged for people with ADHD at any age (CADDRA, 2020). There are several known adverse effects of THC on brain development (Volkow et al., 2014), and these are more pronounced in teens with ADHD (Tamm et al., 2013). CBD is a common ingredient in therapeutic preparations, as it does not have THC's psychoactive profile (CADDRA, 2020). Although CBD research for psychiatric conditions is still in an early stage, there is tentative support for its use with some disorders (Sarris et al., 2020). These preliminary results come with cautions.

Recent comprehensive reviews of studies did not find any support for the benefits of CBD for adult ADHD (Black et al., 2019; Sarris et al., 2020). One controlled study of a CBD preparation for adult ADHD reported nominal improvements in performance on a computerized continuous performance task as well as symptom ratings, but these finding were nonsignificant after controlling for multiple testing (Cooper et al., 2017). Research will likely continue, but there is currently no empirical support for the use of cannabis-based products or medical marijuana for the symptoms of ADHD.

18.2 Research-Supported Approaches

A helpful framework for discerning the usefulness of various treatments for specific features of ADHD involves categorization as broad-band or narrow-band approaches (Faraone & Antshel, 2014). Pharmacotherapy, for example, is a broad-band treatment as medications for ADHD target multiple symptoms including inattention, hyperactivity, and impulsivity. Associated symptom reduction sets the stage for cascading benefits in a broad array of life domains. There are several approved stimulant and nonstimulant medication options for ADHD that, when taken as prescribed, are safe and effective (Faraone et al., 2021). A recent meta-analysis revealed amphetamine-based preparations as the more effective option for adults and methylphenidate-based preparations for children with ADHD (Cortese et al., 2018).

However, symptom improvement does not inexorably lead to adequate functional gains or better coping skills for many clinic-referred adults with ADHD (Barkley, 2015). Consequently, narrow-band treatments promote improved performance in specific domains of functioning without directly targeting core symptoms. Said differently, narrow-band treatments target focused life problems associated with ADHD. For example, cognitive-behavioral therapy is an research-supported narrow-band treatment adapted for adult ADHD (Fullen et al., 2020; Ramsay, 2021). Apart from its core symptom criteria, ADHD is a neurodevelopmental syndrome of impaired self-regulation, meaning that it involves executive dysfunction (Barkley, 2016a). Executive dysfunction, which overlaps with the core symptoms of ADHD, creates a downstream, documented lifetime risk for impairments (Barkley, 2015; Friedman & Robbins, 2022). It is these impairments – difficulties planning, organizing, and enacting behaviors across time toward personally valued goals – for which people seek help. In other words, ADHD is not a knowledge problem but a performance problem manifesting as difficulties carrying out the essential coping strategies (Ramsay & Rostain, 2016).

Cognitive-behavioral therapy for adult ADHD promotes the implementation of coping skills and other compensatory strategies for working around the characteristic self-regulation difficulties that define the disorder. It has the added benefit of being efficacious for treating co-occurring mood, anxiety, and substance use problems (Fordham et al., 2021). Although measures of ADHD symptoms are included in most outcome studies, the main target and measure of effectiveness of cognitive-behavioral therapy for adult ADHD is functioning and wellbeing (Ramsay, 2017; 2021), often concurrent with pharmacotherapy.

Despite the existing evidence base, there is more work to be done to refine psychotherapeutic approaches for adult ADHD. To date, research has not yet been conducted to identify the precise mechanisms of change in cognitive-behavioral therapy for adult ADHD. Existing manuals provide detailed interventions tailored to the needs of adults with ADHD and are well-suited to identify a foundation of coping skills for its psychosocial management.

One example, Adult ADHD Coaching, is a psychosocial support service with strategies that overlap with cognitive-behavioral therapy, generally promoting coping skill development and use (Wright, 2014). To date, ADHD Coaching is not a licensed behavioral health profession or a healthcare service covered by insurance. Nevertheless, it is based on solid and growing evidence, including randomized controlled trials supporting its efficacy, particularly for college students with ADHD (see Ahmann et al., 2018 for a review).

Mindfulness is another research-supported approach for adult ADHD (Fullen et al., 2020; Zylowska & Mitchell, 2021). Mindfulness-based approaches are ubiquitous in the psychological treatment literature and have strong empirical support for treating anxiety and depression (Blanck et al., 2018). Similar to other psychosocial approaches for ADHD, mindfulness was adapted for use with adults with ADHD due to their proneness to distraction, restlessness, and poor follow through. Mindfulness is known to improve executive functioning, including emotion regulation, and other facets of adult ADHD (Zylowska & Mitchell, 2021). Mindfulness can be used to augment psychosocial treatment protocols or as a stand-alone treatment. The unfolding research on mindfulness for adult ADHD has yielded patient-oriented resources (Zylowska, 2012) and a clinician-oriented manual (Zylowska & Mitchell, 2021).

Narrow-band supports that address specific functional ADHD domains continue to emerge. For example, ADHD-affected couples' treatments are drawn from existing evidence-supported approaches and are based on promising early outcome studies (Hirvikoski et al., 2015; Pera & Robin, 2016). Such approaches may not yet be firmly established, but ongoing, active research reveals them to be credible options filling a treatment need for many adults with ADHD.

18.3 Conclusion

Adult ADHD is one of the more impairing conditions encountered in outpatient behavioral healthcare. There is virtually no domain of life that is immune from possible negative consequences related to its core symptoms and executive dysfunctions. Yet many research-supported approaches, both medical and psychosocial, offer both symptom relief and functional improvements. Conversely, there are several popular approaches whose promised benefits do not match their purported outcomes. While all patients have a right to self-determination, choosing unsupported interventions may result in lost time and money, while delaying the more promising benefits offered by established, evidence-based treatments.

J. Russell Ramsay, PhD, ABPP, is a Professor of Psychology at the University of Pennsylvania Perelman School of Medicine. He is author of the book *Rethinking Adult ADHD: Helping Clients Turn Intentions Into Actions* (Ramsay, 2020).

References

Agnew-Blais, J. C., Polanczyk, G. V., Danese, A., Wertz, J., Moffitt, T., & Arseneault, L. (2016) Evaluation of the persistence, remission, and emergence of attention-deficit/hyperactivity disorder in young adulthood. *JAMA Psychiatry*, *73*(7), 713–720. https://doi.org/10.1001/jamapsychiatry.2016.0465.

Ahmann, E., Tuttle, L. J., Saviet, M., & Wright, S. D. (2018). A descriptive review of ADHD coaching results: Implications for college students. *Journal of Postsecondary Education and Disability*, *31*(1), 17–39. www.ahead.org/professional-resources/publications/jped/archived-jped/jped-volume-31.

American Psychiatric Association. (1968). *Diagnostic and statistical manual of mental disorders* (2nd ed.). American Psychiatric Association.

American Psychiatric Association. (2013). *Diagnostic and statistical manual of mental disorders* (5th ed.). https://doi.org/10.1176/appi.books.9780890425596.

American Psychiatric Association. (2022). *Diagnostic and statistical manual of mental disorders, fifth edition, text revision* (DSM-5-TR). American Psychiatric Association.

Barkley, R. A. (Ed.) (2015). *Attention-deficit hyperactivity disorder: A handbook for diagnosis and treatment* (4th ed.). Guilford.

Barkley, R. A. (2016a). Attention-deficit/hyperactivity disorder and self-regulation: Taking an evolutionary perspective on executive functioning. In K. D. Vohs & R. F. Baumeister (Eds.), *Handbook of self-regulation: Research, theory, and applications* (3rd ed., pp. 497–513). Guilford.

Barkley, R. A. (2016b). Is there an adult onset type of ADHD? Issues in establishing persistence and remission of ADHD from childhood to adulthood. *The ADHD Report*, 28(8), 6–13.

Barkley, R. A., & Fischer, M. (2019). Hyperactive childhood syndrome and estimate life expectancy at young adult follow-up: The role of adult ADHD and other potential predictors. *Journal of Attention Disorders, 23* (9), 907–923. https://doi.org/10.1177/1087054718816164.

Barkley, R. A., Murphy, K. R., & Fischer, M. (2008). *ADHD in adults: What the science says.* Guilford.

Biederman, J., Petty, C. R., Clarke, A., Lomedico, A., & Faraone, S. V. (2011). Predictors of Persistent ADHD: An 11-year follow-up study. *Journal of Psychiatric Research*, 45(2), 150–155. https://doi.org/10.1016/j.jpsychires.2010.06.009.

Biederman, J., Petty, C. R., Evans, M., Small, J., & Faraone, S. V. (2010). How persistent is ADHD? A controlled 10-year follow-up study of boys with ADHD. *Psychiatry Research, 177*(3), 299–304. https://doi.org/10.1016/j.psychres.2009.12.010.

Black, N., Stockings, E., Campbell, G., Tran, L. T., Zagic, D., Hall, W. D., Farrell, M., & Degenhardt, L. (2019). Cannabinoids for the treatment of mental disorders and symptoms of mental disorders: A systematic review and meta-analysis. *Lancet Psychiatry*, 6(12), 995–1010. https://doi.org/10.1016/S2215-0366(19)30401-8.

Blanck, P., Perleth, S., Heidenreich, T., Kröger, P., Ditzen, B., Bents, H., & Mander, J. (2018). Effects of mindfulness exercises as stand-alone interventions on symptoms of anxiety and depression: Systematic review and meta-analysis. *Behaviour Therapy and Research, 102*, 25–35. https://doi.org/10.1016/j.brat.2017.12.002.

Canadian ADHD Resource Alliance. (2020). Cannabis and ADHD: A CADDRA policy statement. www.caddra.ca/cannabis-and-adhd-a-caddra-policy-statement/.

Caye, A., Rocha, T. B., Anselmi, L., Murray, J., Menezes, A. M. B., Barros, F. C., Gonçalves, H., Wehrmeister, F., Jensen, C. M., Steinhausen, H. C., Swanson, J. M., Kieling, C., & Rohde, L. A. (2016). Attention-Deficit/Hyperactivity Disorder trajectories from childhood to young adulthood: Evidence from a birth cohort supporting a late-onset syndrome. *JAMA Psychiatry*, 73(7), 705–712. https://doi.org/10.1001/jamapsychiatry.2016.0383.

Cooper R. E., Williams, E., Seegobin, S., Tye, C., Kuntsi, J., & Asherson, P. (2017). Cannabinoids in attention-deficit/hyperactivity disorder: A randomized controlled trial. *European Neuropsychopharmacology*, *27*(8), 795–808.

Cortese, S., Adamo, N., Del Giovane, C., Mohr-Jensen, C., Hayes, A. J., Carucci, S., Atkinson, L. Z., Tessari, L., Banaschewski, T., Coghill, D., Hollis, C., Simanoff, E., Zuddas, A., Barbui, C., Purgato, M., Steinhausen, H. C., Shakraneh, F., Xia, J., & Cipriani, A. (2018). Comparative efficacy and tolerability of medications for attention-deficit hyperactivity disorder in children, adolescents, and adults: A systematic review and network meta-analysis. *Lancet Psychiatry*, *5*(9), P727–738. https://doi.org/10.1016/S2215-0366(18)30269-4.

De Crescenzo, F., Cortese, S., Adamo, N., & Janiri, L. (2017). Pharmacological and non-pharmacological treatment of adults with ADHD: A meta-review. *Evidence Based Mental Health*, *20*(1), 1–11. https://doi .10.1136/eb-2016-102415.

Dumas-Mallet, E., & Gonon, F. (2020). Messaging in biological psychiatry: Misrepresentations, their causes, and potential consequences. *Harvard Review of Psychiatry*, *28*(6), 395–403. https://doi.org/10.1097/HRP .0000000000000276.

Faraone, S. V. & Antshel, K. M. (2014). ADHD: nonpharmacologic interventions. *Child & Adolescent Psychiatric Clinics of North America*, *23*(4), P965–972. https://doi.org/10.1016/j.chc.2014.06.003.

Faraone, S. V., Banaschewski, T., Coghill, D., Zheng, Y., Biederman, J., Bellgrove, M. A., Newcorn, J. H., Gignac, M., Al Saud, N. M., Manor, I., Rohde, L. A., Yang, L., Cortese, S., Almagor, D., Stein, M. A., Albatti, T. H., Aljoudi, H. F., Alqahtani, M. M. J., Asherson, P., … Wang, Y. (2021). The World Federation of ADHD international consensus statement: 208 evidence-based conclusions about the disorder. *Neuroscience and Biobehavioral Reviews*, *128*, 789–818. https://doi.org/10 .1016/j.neubiorev.2021.01.022.

Faraone, S. V., & Biederman, J. (2016). Can attention-deficit/hyperactivity disorder onset occur in adulthood? *JAMA Psychiatry*, *73*(7), 655–656. https:// doi.org/10.1001/jamapsychiatry.2016.0400.

Faraone, S. V., Biederman, J., Spencer, T., Mick, E., Murray, K., Petty, C., Adamson, J. J., & Monuteaux, M. C. (2006). Diagnosing adult attention deficit hyperactivity disorder: Are late onset and subthreshold diagnoses valid? *American Journal of Psychiatry*, *163*(10), 1720–1729. https://doi.org /10.1176/ajp.2006.163.10.1720.

Fordham, B., Sugavanam, T., Edwards, K., Stallard, P., Howard, R., das Nair, R., Copsey, B., Lee, H., Howick, J., Hemming, K. , & Lamb, S. E. (2021). The evidence for cognitive behavioral therapy in any condition, population or context: a meta-review of systematic reviews and panoramic meta-analysis. *Psychological Medicine*, *51*, 21–29. https://doi.org/10.1017/S0033291720005292.

Friedman, N. P., & Robbins, T. W. (2022). The role of prefrontal cortex in cognitive control and executive function. *Neuropsychopharmacology*, *47* (1), 72–89.

Fullen, T., Jones, S. L., Emerson, L. M., & Adamou, M. (2020). Psychological treatments in adult ADHD: A systematic review. *Journal of Psychopathology and Behavioral Assessment*, *42*, 500–518. https://doi.org /10.1007/s10862-020-09794-8.

Hirvikoski, T., Waaler, E., Lindstrom, T., Bolte, S., & Jokinen, J. (2015). Cognitive behavior therapy-based psychoeducational groups for adults with ADHD and their significant others (PEGASUS): An open clinical feasibility trial. *ADHD Attention-Deficit Hyperactivity Disorder*, *7*, 88–99. https://doi.org/10.1007/s12402-014-0141-2.

Kooij, J. J. S., Bijlenga, D., Salerno, L., Jaeschke, R., Bitter, I., Balázs, J., Thome, J., Dom, G., Kasper, S., Nunes Filipe, C., Stes, S., Mohr, P., Leppämäki, S., Casas, M., Bobes, J., McCarthy, J. M., Richarte, V., Kjems, A., Philipsen, A., . . . Asherson, P. (2019). Updated European consensus statement on diagnosis and treatment of adult ADHD. *European Psychiatry*, *56* (1), 14–34. https://doi.org/10.1016/j.eurpsy.2018.11.001.

Lee, G. J., & Suhr, J. A. (2019). Expectancy effects on self-reported attention-deficit/hyperactivity disorder symptoms in simulated neurofeedback: A pilot study. *Archives of Neuropsychology*, *34*(2), 200–205. https:// doi.org/10.1093/arclin/acy026.

Masters, J. C., Burish, T. G., Hollon, S. D., & Rimm, D. C. (1987). *Behavior therapy: Techniques and empirical findings* (3rd ed.). Harcourt, Brace, Jovanovich College Publishers.

Mitchell, J. T., Sweitzer, M. M., Tunno, A. M., Kollins, S. H., & McClernon, F. J. (2016) "I use weed for my ADHD": A qualitative analysis of online forum discussions on cannabis use and ADHD. *PLoS ONE*, *11*(5), e0156614. https://doi.org/10.1371/journal.pone.0156614.

Moffitt, T. E., Houts, R., Asherson, P., Belsky, D. W., Corcoran, D. L., Hammerle, M., Harrington, H. L., Hogan, S., Meier, M. H., Polanczyk, G. V., Poulton, R., Ramrakha, S., Sugden, K., Williams, B., Rohde, L. A., & Caspi, A. (2015). Is adult ADHD a childhood-onset neurodevelopmental disorder? Evidence from a four-decade longitudinal cohort study. *American Journal of Psychiatry*, *172*(10), 967–977. https://doi .org/10.1176/appi.ajp.2015.14101266.

Nigg, J. T. (2013). Attention-deficit/hyperactivity disorder and adverse health outcomes. *Clinical Psychology Review*, *33*(2), 215–228. https://doi.org/10 .1016/j.cpr.2012.11.005.

Nimmo-Smith, V., Merwood, A., Hank, D., Brandling, J., Greenwood, R., Skinner, L., Law, S., Patel, V., & Rai, D. (2020). Non-pharmacological interventions for adult ADHD: A systematic review. *Psychological Medicine, 50*, 529–541. https://doi.org/10.1017/S0033291720000069.

Novella, S. (2017a). The ADHD controversy. https://sciencebasedmedicine.org/the-adhd-controversy/.

Novella, S. (2017b). Another ADHD denier. https://sciencebasedmedicine.org/another-adhd-denier/.

Pera, G., & Robin, A. L. (Eds.) (2016). *Adult ADHD-focused couple therapy: Clinical intervention.* Routledge.

Ramsay, J. R. (2010). *Nonmedication treatments for adult ADHD: Evaluating impact on daily functioning and well-being.* American Psychological Association.

Ramsay, J. R. (2017). Assessment and monitoring of treatment response in adult ADHD patients: Current perspectives. *Neuropsychiatric Disease and Treatment, 13*, 221–232. https://doi.org/10.2147/NDT.S104706.

Ramsay, J. R. (2021). Adult attention-deficit/hyperactivity disorder. In A. Wenzel (Ed.), *Handbook of Cognitive Behavioral Therapy, Volume 2, Applications* (pp. 389–421). American Psychological Association. https://doi.org/10.1037/0000219-012.

Ramsay, J. R., & Rostain, A. L. (2016). Adult ADHD as an implementation problem: Clinical significance, underlying mechanisms, and psychosocial treatment. *Practice Innovations, 1*(1), 36–52. https://doi.org/10.1037/pri0000016.

Rucklidge, J. J., Frampton, C. M., Gorman, B., & Boggis, A. (2014). Vitamin–mineral treatment of attention-deficit hyperactivity disorder in adults: Double-blind randomized placebo-controlled trial. *British Journal of Psychiatry, 204*, 306–315. https://doi.org/10.1192/bjp.bp.113.132126.

Rucklidge, J. J., & Kaplan, B. J. (2014). Broad-spectrum micronutrient treatment for attention-deficit/hyperactivity disorder: Rationale and evidence to date. *CNS Drugs, 28*(9), 775–785. https://doi.org/10.1007/s40263-014-0190-2.

Sarris, J., Sinclair, J., Karamacoska, D., Davidson, M., & Firth, J. (2020). Medicinal cannabis for psychiatric disorders: A clinically-focused systematic review. *BMC Psychiatry, 20*, article 24. https://bmcpsychiatry.biomedcentral.com/articles/10.1186/s12888-019-2409-8.

Schnoll, R., Burshteyn, D., & Cea-Aravena, J. (2003). Nutrition in the treatment of attention-deficit hyperactivity disorder: A neglected but important aspect. *Applied Psychophysiology and Biofeedback, 28*(1), 63–75.

Schönenberg, M., Weingärtner, A. L., Weimer, K., & Scheeff, J. (2021). Believing is achieving – On the role of treatment expectation in neurofeedback applications. *Progress in Neuropsychopharmacology & Biological Psychiatry, 105*, article 110129. https://doi.org/10.1016/j.pnpbp.2020.110129.

Sibley, M. H., Rohde, L. A., Swanson, J. M., Hechtman, L.T., Molina, B. S. G., Mitchell, J. T., Arnold, L. E., Caye, A., Kennedy, T. M., Roy, A., Stehli, A., for the members of the Multimodal Treatment Study of Children with ADHD (MTA) (2018). Late-onset ADHD reconsidered with comprehensive repeated assessments between ages 10 and 25. *American Journal of Psychiatry*, *175*(2), 140–149. https://doi.org/10.1176/appi.ajp.2017.17030298.

Simons, D. J., Boot, W. R., Charness, N., Gathercole, S. E., Chabirs, C. F., Hambrick, D. Z., & Stine-Morrow, E. A. L. (2016). Do "brain training" programs work? *Psychological Science in the Public Interest*, *17*(3), 103–186. https://doi.org/10.1177/1529100616661983.

Sonuga-Barke, E. J. S., Brandeis, D., Cortese, S., Daley, D., Ferrin, M., Hotmann, M., Stevenson, J., Danckaerts, M., van der Oord, S., Döpfner, M., Dittmann, R. W., Simonoff, E., Zuddas, A., Banaschewski, T., Buitelaar, J., Coghill, D., Hollis, C., Konofal, E., Lecendreux, M., … Sergeant, J. (2013). Nonpharmacological interventions for ADHD: Systematic review and meta-analyses of randomized controlled trials of dietary and psychological treatments. *American Journal of Psychiatry*, *170* (3), 275–289. https://doi.org/10.1176/appi.ajp.2012.12070991.

Stern, A., Malik, E., Pollak, Y., Bonne, O., & Maeir, A. (2016). The efficacy of computerized cognitive training in adults with ADHD: A randomized controlled trial. *Journal of Attention Disorders*, *20*(12), 991–1003. https://doi.org/10.1177/1087054714529815.

Tamm, L., Epstein, J. N., Lisdahl, K. M., Tapert, S., Hinshaw, S. P., Arnold, L. E., Velanova, K., Abikoff, H., Swanson, J. M., & MTA Neuroimaging Group. (2013). Impact of ADHD and cannabis use on executive functioning in young adults. *Drug and Alcohol Dependence*, *133*(1), 607–614. https://doi.org/10.1016/j.drugalcdep.2013.08.001.

Volkow, N. D., Baler, R. D., Compton, W. M., & Weiss, S. R. B. (2014). Adverse effects of marijuana use. *New England Journal of Medicine*, *370*, 2219–2227. https://doi.org/10.1056/NEJMra1402309.

Volkow, N. D., & Swanson, J. M. (2013). Adult attention deficit-hyperactivity disorder. *New England Journal of Medicine*, *369*, 1935–1944. https://doi.org/10.1056/NEJMcp1212625.

Wright, S. (2014). *ADHD coaching matters: The definitive guide*. ACO Books.

Zylowska, L. (2012). *The mindfulness prescription for adult ADHD*. Trumpeter.

Zylowska, L., & Mitchell, J. T. (2021). *Mindfulness for adult ADHD: A clinician's guide*. Guilford.

19

Tics

Kirsten Bootes, Brianna Wellen, Emily Braley, and Michael B. Himle

Tic disorders are a class of childhood-onset neurodevelopmental disorders that affect approximately 1% of the population (Robertson, 2008) and are defined by the presence of involuntary, recurrent, nonrhythmic movements and/or vocalizations (i.e., motor and vocal tics; American Psychiatric Association, 2022). Tics typically first appear in early childhood, take a fluctuating course with general worsening over time, and reach peak severity around 10–12 years of age (Bloch & Leckman, 2009). Although studies have shown that most individuals with tic disorders will show symptom improvement in adulthood (Bloch & Leckman, 2009), some tics persist in most cases (Coffey et al., 2004) and often cause impairment in physical, social, educational, and occupational functioning (Conelea et al., 2013).

The *Diagnostic and Statistical Manual of Mental Disorders* (DSM-5-TR) lists four hierarchically arranged diagnostic categories of tic disorders that are differentiated by the types of tics present (i.e., motor, vocal, or both) and the persistence of symptoms since initial onset (i.e., more or less than one year; APA, 2022). Tourette's disorder involves the presence of presence of at least one vocal and multiple motor tics that have been present, although not necessarily concurrently, for at least one year; persistent (chronic) motor or vocal tic disorder involves the presence of motor or vocal tics, but not both, for at least one year; and provisional tic disorder involves motor and/or vocal tics that have been present for less than one year. Each of these diagnoses requires onset prior to age 18 and that the tics are not the direct physiological result of substance exposure or another medical condition. Finally, other specified tic disorder involves the presence of motor and/or vocal tics that do not meet full criteria for the other tic disorder diagnoses, such as when onset begins after age 18 years or when there is evidence to suggest that the tics are secondary to another medical condition or substance use. This latter designation is the only diagnostic category that requires that the tics cause clinically significant distress or impairment in functioning (APA, 2022).

19.1 Pseudoscience and Questionable Ideas

19.1.1 Conceptualization and Diagnosis: Controversies, Myths, and Misunderstandings

19.1.1.1 Dichotomy between Psychological and Neurological Explanations

The first formal description of tic disorders can be traced to an 1885 case series published by French neurologist Georges Gilles de la Tourette wherein he described nine adult patients who displayed a heterogeneous collection of involuntary movements and vocalizations that he hypothesized to be neurological in origin but that were inconsistent with the symptoms of known neurological disorders at the time (Lajonchere et al., 1996). Among these seminal patients, he also documented several phenomenological features that are now known to characterize tic disorders, including the tendency for symptoms to fluctuate, responsiveness to context and apparent controllability, and high rates of what were then called "hysterical" symptoms (i.e., psychiatric comorbidity; Lajonchere et al., 1996). These later features were of particular interest to psychodynamically oriented physicians who conceptualized tics as expressions of unconscious psychological conflict, repressed impulses, a high need for attention, and/or weak character resulting from early life experiences (Ferenczi, 1921; Kushner, 1999). The psychodynamic model failed to produce effective treatments and was eventually dismissed as a plausible conceptual model of tic disorders. Emerging research elucidated the biological underpinnings of tic disorders, and clinical studies demonstrated the efficacy of neuroleptics for suppressing tics (Shapiro & Shapiro, 1968). As a result, the conceptual pendulum swung to a somewhat restrictive biological view of tic disorders that dominated research and clinical practice guidelines for several subsequent decades. Although this shift resulted in a better understanding of the biological correlates of tics and the development of new medication options, available medical treatments remained somewhat limited due to intolerable side effects and modest symptom reduction (Erenberg, 1988).

The biological model of tics continued to dominate the research and clinical landscape throughout the late twentieth century until studies demonstrating the efficacy of behavioral interventions began to emerge in the late 1970s. Most notable among these was collection of behavioral techniques called habit reversal training (Azrin & Nunn, 1973). However, despite numerous published studies demonstrating the efficacy of habit reversal training, it struggled to gain acceptance as a legitimate treatment option within the broader medical field for several decades. Lack of uptake likely stemmed in part from behaviorism's reputation for ignoring the importance of biological determinants of behavior and lingering fears that incorporating psychological conceptualizations would result in a return to a psychodynamic view of tic disorders (Chang et al., 2007). In addition, studies examining the efficacy of habit reversal training largely utilized single-case research designs and direct observation rather than randomized controlled trials and psychometrically validated instruments, which remain the gold standard within the medical research field (Himle et al., 2006).

Over the past 10 years, the psychological versus neurological dichotomy has given way to an integrated biopsychosocial model of tic disorders, and resistance to behavioral interventions has largely subsided. One primary reason for this shift has been empirical studies that advanced our understanding of the influence of environmental factors on tics, including two large randomized controlled trials demonstrating the efficacy and safety of a behavioral treatment package referred to as Comprehensive Behavioral Intervention for Tics (CBIT) for reducing tics in both children and adults (Piacentini et al., 2010; Wilhelm et al., 2012).

19.1.1.2 Controversies Surrounding the Classification of Tic Disorders in the DSM

In the first publication of the DSM, tics were described as symptoms of neurosis and classified as "neurotic traits," which reflected the predominant psychodynamic view at the time (APA, 1952, p. 42). In later iterations of the DSM, tic disorders were moved to the section of disorders usually first diagnosed in infancy, childhood, and adolescence (DSM-IV; APA, 1994), and subsequently the section on neurodevelopmental disorders (DSM-5; APA, 2013), the latter of which better captures and appreciates their neurobiological etiology and typical clinical course. There has been some debate regarding whether tic disorders should be placed within the obsessive-compulsive spectrum disorders section of the DSM given the high rates of comorbidity between tic and obsessive-compulsive disorders (OCD) and similarities in some symptom features (e.g., compulsions and complex tics). However, expert consensus did not support the inclusion of tic disorders in this category due to several clear distinctions between the two diagnoses, including differences in defining symptoms, age of onset and developmental course, response to differing pharmacological and behavioral interventions, and differences in how the disorders are perceived among the public and medical professionals (e.g., psychological versus neurological etiology; Walkup et al., 2010).

19.1.1.3 Unitary Condition or Broad Psychiatric Syndrome?

Although motor and vocal tics are the only symptoms required for a tic disorder diagnosis, most individuals also experience comorbid psychiatric symptoms, including obsessive and compulsive behaviors, inattention and hyperactivity, and disinhibition (i.e., impulsivity, reactive aggression, etc.). It is relatively well established that these associated problems often cause significant functional impairment beyond that caused by tics (Storch et al., 2007). Furthermore, longitudinal studies examining the prognosis of individuals with "pure tic disorder" (those without comorbidity) and those with tic disorder+ (those with comorbid OCD and/or attention-deficit/hyperactivity disorder [ADHD]) have shown that more than half of patients show a changing clinical phenotype over the course of the disorder. For example, one study prospectively followed 100 individuals with a tic disorder over the course of 10 years and found that, among those with "pure tic disorder," 42% of met criteria for tic disorder+OCD ten years later, and 100% of those with tic disorder +ADHD changed clinical phenotypes (at 10-year follow-up, 62% had pure tic disorder, 35% had tic disorder+OCD, and 2% had tic disorder +ADHD+OCD; Rizzo et al., 2012). These and similar findings have led some to argue that tic disorders should not be considered a unitary condition but rather a broader psychiatric syndrome that extends beyond tics and that represents increasing degrees of abnormality within the basal ganglia and associated brain structures (Kurlan, 1994); however, the extent to which tic disorders and common comorbid conditions share an underlying pathophysiology remains unclear (O'Rourke et al., 2009).

19.1.1.4 The Significance of Motor versus Vocal Tics in Diagnosis and Treatment

A diagnosis of Tourette disorder versus persistent motor/vocal tic disorder depends solely on whether an individual has motor tics, vocal tics, or both. While these are listed as separate diagnoses in the DSM-5, the importance of the distinction between motor and vocal tics is unclear from either a conceptual or treatment perspective. On the one hand, many of the vocalizations that are typically considered vocal tics (e.g., grunting, sniffing) involve spontaneous contraction of the diaphragm, oropharynx, and associated musculature and thus might be better considered to be motor tics (Walkup et al., 2010). Further, motor and vocal tics respond to the same treatment approaches (Besag et al., 2021; McGuire et al., 2014). On the other hand, studies have shown that the presence of vocal tics is associated with higher rates of psychiatric comorbidity (Khalifa & von Knorring, 2005), and some studies suggest that motor and vocal tics differentially predict impairment and disability (Conelea et al., 2013).

19.1.1.5 The Semi-Volitional Nature of (Some) Tics

Although there is ample evidence showing that tics are involuntary, many individuals subjectively experience at least some of their tics as "semi-volitional" responses that are performed to alleviate aversive premonitory sensations, and most can temporarily suppress their tics with concentrated effort (Leckman et al., 1993). These two phenomena, suppressibility/controllability and the semi-volitional subjective experience, challenges how we traditionally conceptualize volition, can be a source of misunderstanding regarding the deliberate nature of tics (e.g., cause and intent), and can complicate diagnosis, especially when attempting to distinguish between complex tics and other repetitive behaviors (e.g., compulsions).

19.1.1.6 Swearing as a Hallmark Symptom

Although tics involving socially inappropriate vocalizations (i.e., coprolalia) or gestures (i.e., copropraxia) were once thought to be a hallmark symptom of tic disorders, these are relatively uncommon with lifetime prevalence ranging from approximately 15% to 20% for females and males, respectively, and are not the most representative symptoms (Freeman et al., 2009). Nevertheless, coprolalia continues to be portrayed in the media as a defining symptom of tic disorders, perpetuating stigma and misunderstanding (Calder-Sprackman et al., 2014).

19.1.1.7 How Often Do Tics Remit in Adulthood?

It is well established that for most individuals tics will improve in adulthood (Bloch & Leckman, 2009). Extant research findings regarding how often tics completely remit are somewhat contradictory, however, due in part to differing definitions of "remission." For example, one early study followed 42 patients with a tic disorder for an average of 7 years and found that, by 18 years of age, 50% of the cohort was "virtually tic free" (Leckman et al., 1998). A subsequent study by the same group followed a cohort of 82 children into adulthood and found that only 37% were tic-free with an additional 46% showing "minimal" or "mild" tic severity, and 19% showing "moderate or greater" tic severity (Bloch & Leckman, 2009). More recently, Rizzo and colleagues (2012) retrospectively analyzed the long-term clinical course of 100 patients with a tic disorder and found that none of the patients in their sample were tic free at follow-up, but 80% reported that their control over symptoms had improved since childhood. Collectively, these findings suggest that tics do improve to some extent for many individuals in the adult years. However, overconfidence in the extent to which tics remit after adolescence risks neglecting a sizeable cohort of patients with tic disorders whose symptoms will persist into adulthood and cause substantial impairment in functioning (Conelea et al., 2013).

19.1.1.8 Adult-Onset Tics

Although tic disorders are considered to be developmental disorders with childhood onset, there have been several cases of adult-onset tics reported in the literature. As noted by Robakis (2017), most are secondary to drug use, trauma, or neurodegenerative disease (i.e., acquired secondary tics) or, after careful history taking, have been determined to be a re-emergence of childhood-onset tics. While relatively rare, adult-onset primary (i.e., idiopathic) tics have also been reported. Unfortunately, there have been no studies to date examining the prevalence or incidence of adult-onset primary tics in the general population, and it remains unclear whether these cases are etiologically or phenomenologically similar to childhood-onset tic disorders or whether they respond to treatments that have been shown to be effective for childhood-onset tics.

19.1.1.9 Functional Tics

Functional neurological symptom disorder (FNSD, also referred to as conversion disorder) involves symptoms of altered motor and/or sensory functions that are not explained by neurological disease (APA, 2022). Although numerous reports of tic-like behaviors consistent with FNSD (i.e., functional tics) have been reported in the literature (see Ganos et al., 2019), it has historically been considered to be a relatively rare presentation. Recently, however, an increase in cases has emerged, seemingly corresponding to the onset of the COVID-19 pandemic in early 2020 (Heyman et al., 2021). In particular, several recent international reports have been published reporting a substantial increase in cases of adolescents and young adults, predominantly girls and women, presenting with rapid-onset, complex tic-like symptoms that in many cases cause substantial distress and functional impairment. Interestingly, in addition to the relatively late onset and female predominance, these cases appear to share several features that are atypical of "organic" tic disorders, including a lack of family history of tics, abrupt onset of complex movements and vocalizations (often involving coprolalia, self-abusive behavior, speaking with an accent, copro- and echo-phenomena, etc.), and absent history of simple motor and vocal tics, lack of premonitory urges, diminished ability to suppress the symptoms, and high rates of comorbid anxiety and depressive disorders (Pringsheim et al., 2021). In addition, the onset of these tic-like behaviors has been associated with significant psychosocial stressors and/or high levels of involvement with tic disorder-related social media in some cases (Pringsheim et al., 2021). Whether such cases will persist beyond the COVID-19 pandemic is unclear, but for now they remain a source of diagnostic controversy (atypical presentation/later onset of tic disorder versus FNSD), in large part due to the heterogeneity in the clinical course of a tic disorder and the lack of objective tests to confirm a diagnosis. Further, no established treatment guidelines exist for tic-like FNSD.

19.1.2 Questionable Claims about Treatments

19.1.2.1 Complementary and Alternative Medicines

Several surveys of patients with a tic disorder have shown that the use of complementary and alternative medicines, such as nutritional supplements, special diets, and homeopathy, are commonly used by individuals with tic disorders in an attempt to reduce or manage tics (Mantel et al., 2005). Although many alternative medicine users report some degree of subjective tic improvement (Kompoliti et al., 2009), there is currently little empirical evidence or plausible scientific justification supporting their use as an effective strategy. In addition, studies have shown that most people do not consult their doctor prior to taking complementary and alternative medicines and presume them to be safe (Kompoliti et al., 2009), which may be an erroneous and possibly dangerous assumption given that vitamins, supplements, and homeopathic remedies are not regulated by the Food and Drug Administration and thus their purity, potential side effects, and potential interactions with psychotropic medications remain largely unknown.

19.1.2.2 Chiropractic Treatments

Over the past several years, chiropractic treatments have increasingly been marketed as an effective way to alleviate tics based on the rationale that spinal misalignments (i.e., subluxations) can interfere with the transmission of nerve impulses throughout the body, thereby causing a variety of adverse health outcomes, including tics. To date, there is no empirical support for using chiropractic techniques as a means of reducing tics, aside from a few highly questionable case studies (e.g., Kuhn & Cambron, 2013), which are often cited in online marketing materials. Further, there is virtually no scientific evidence to suggest that spinal misalignments are etiologically related to tic disorders.

19.1.2.3 Biofeedback

The use of biofeedback in tic disorders is based on findings that tics are often exacerbated by physiological arousal (Nagai et al., 2009). The premise behind biofeedback training is to help an individual gain control over covert physiological responses (e.g., heart rate, galvanic skin response) by making the response visible real-time on a computer screen and teaching them to actively modify the targeted physiological process. Although there have been case reports of the successful use of biofeedback to reduce tics (Benvenuti et al., 2011), a small randomized controlled trial comparing electrodermal biofeedback to a sham condition found that while tics were modestly reduced in both groups, there were no significant between-group differences (Nagai et al., 2014). Furthermore, the active treatment group did not demonstrate increased ability to modify the targeted sympathetic response, suggesting that any reduction in tics resulting from biofeedback was likely due to nonspecific factors, not the intervention itself.

19.1.2.4 Repetitive Transcranial Magnetic Stimulation

Repetitive transcranial magnetic stimulation (rTMS), sometimes just referred to as TMS, is a noninvasive form of brain stimulation that involves the use of a changing magnetic field to provoke or inhibit neuronal firing in focal cortical areas of the brain, with the goal of inducing lasting modulation of neural network activity (e.g., oscillatory rhythms). Although several case studies and small open trials have reported promising results, especially in patients with comorbid OCD (see Grados et al., 2018), a recent randomized controlled trial failed to demonstrate the efficacy of rTMS relative to a sham stimulation control condition (Landeros-Weisenberer et al., 2015) and a recent meta-analysis of 18 studies examining rTMS for tic disorders concluded that although rTMS has been shown to improve tics relative to baseline, it has not been shown to be more effective than placebo (Hsu et al., 2018). Collectively, these findings suggest rTMS remains a questionable treatment for tic disorders.

19.1.2.5 Undermining Behavioral Treatments

Although behavioral approaches to treatment have recently gained recognition and acceptance as effective first-line interventions for reducing tics, early reports issued strong cautionary statements that behavioral therapies were potentially harmful (e.g., Burd & Kerbeshian, 1987). One of the most commonly raised concerns was that teaching tic suppression could result in a paradoxical worsening of tics following suppression (Woods et al., 2007). However, several empirical investigations evaluated tic severity before, during, and after successful tic suppression and failed to observe a resulting increase in tics above baseline levels (Müller-Vahl et al., 2014). Another common myth regarding behavior therapy is that efforts to suppress tics will result in the emergence of new tics. The idea of symptom substitution was central to early psychoanalytic models which posited that tics were expressions of unresolved unconscious conflicts or impulses that, if not properly addressed, would be expressed through other, possibly more problematic symptoms. Systematic studies have failed to find evidence of tic worsening or tic substitution during or following behavior therapy (Peterson et al., 2016). Finally, concerns have also been raised regarding the possibility that behavior therapy induces other aversive side effects that are not specific to tics, including somatic symptoms (e.g., headache, muscle pain), increased anxiety or irritability, concentration problems, or fatigue. Research has shown that such side effects are rarely reported (Wilhelm et al., 2012).

19.2 Research-Supported Approaches

Current best-practice guidelines recommend the use of behavior therapy as a first-line treatment option for tic disorders in adults, either before or in combination with medication (Pringsheim et al., 2019). The behavioral intervention with the strongest empirical support is CBIT (Woods et al., 2008; Wilhelm et al., 2012), which combines psychoeducation, habit reversal training, relaxation training, and individually tailored function-based strategies. Although the relative therapeutic benefit of the individual components of CBIT are unclear, habit reversal training (a primary component of CBIT) has also been shown to be effective without the additional components included in the CBIT package (see Himle et al., 2006). An adapted version of exposure and response prevention, which is an evidence-based behavioral therapy for OCD, has also shown to be effective in reducing tics, although it has been less rigorously studied (Verdellen et al., 2004).

Although a variety of medication options are recommended within best-practice guidelines and medical management remains a mainstay in the management of tics, there are relatively few rigorous placebo-controlled trials demonstrating the efficacy of the most prescribed medications (Besag et al., 2021). While neuroleptics are generally considered to be the most effective for suppressing tics, reaching an adequate therapeutic dose is often limited by intolerable side effects including drug-induced parkinsonism, sedation, and weight gain (Pringsheim et al., 2019). Alpha-2 agonists have also been shown to be modestly effective for reducing tics in children and adolescents, especially those with comorbid ADHD, and are typically better tolerated, but their efficacy has not been adequately studied in adults (Weisman et al., 2013). Although the additive benefit of combining medication with behavior therapy has not been explicitly studied, there is some evidence showing that medication status moderates treatment outcomes, suggesting that CBIT might be less effective for patients concurrently taking tic suppressing medication (Sukhodolsky et al., 2017).

For adults who do not respond to behavior therapy or more traditional medications, injection of botulinum toxin into specific tic-involved muscles can be effective for reducing targeted tics (Rath et al., 2010). Further, emerging research has implicated a possible role of the central cannabinoid receptor system in tic disorders, with delta-9-tetrahydrocannabinol (THC) demonstrating promising results suggesting that it is a potentially useful treatment for treatment refractory adults (Müller-Vahl et al., 2003). Finally, deep brain stimulation has been shown to be effective for managing tics in severe and life-threatening cases (Schrock et al., 2014).

19.3 Conclusion

Tic disorders are a class of childhood-onset neurodevelopmental disorders with considerable variability in clinical presentation and course. Although significant progress has been made in understanding tic disorders over the past several decades, several important clinical features are not fully understood. As a result, stubborn conceptual, diagnostic, and treatment controversies have persisted, and new disputes have emerged. While evidence-based treatments exist, many of the most prescribed medications have not been adequately studied in placebo-controlled trials, their efficacy has not been adequately studied in adults, their mechanisms of action are not adequately understood, and the most effective medications are limited by concerns over adverse side effects. Effective behavioral treatments have recently gained acceptance but remain underutilized in part due to a historical psychoanalytic hangover and lingering concerns over side effects that have been refuted by research. Perhaps most importantly, none of our existing treatments are effective for all patients and, among treatment responders, symptom reduction is often modest and incomplete. It is not surprising that a host of questionable treatments have emerged that are based on implausible conceptual models and that lack adequate evidence of safety and efficacy but are nonetheless marketed to patients desperate for symptom relief. Finally, although international patient organizations have launched admirable campaigns to increase awareness and understanding of tic disorders (see www.tourette.org and www.tourettes-action.org.uk), tics remain sensationalized and misrepresented in the media (Calder-Sprackman et al., 2014), perpetuating stigma and controversy. There in an urgent need for additional research to better understand tic disorders, resolve controversies, and to act as a safeguard against pseudoscientific treatments.

Kirsten Bootes, MA, **Brianna Wellen**, PhD, and **Emily Braley**, MA, are doctoral students at the University of Utah.

Michael B. Himle, PhD, is an Associate Professor of Psychology and the Director of Clinical Training at the University of Utah.

References

American Psychiatric Association. (1952). *Diagnostic and statistical manual of mental disorders* (1st ed.). American Psychiatric Association.
American Psychiatric Association. (1994). *Diagnostic and statistical manual of mental disorders* (4th ed). American Psychiatric Association.
American Psychiatric Association. (2013). *Diagnostic and statistical manual of mental disorders* (5th ed). American Psychiatric Association.
American Psychiatric Association. (2022). *Diagnostic and statistical manual of mental disorders, fifth edition, text revision* (DSM-5-TR). American Psychiatric Association.

Azrin, N. H., & Nunn, R. G. (1973). Habit-reversal: A method of eliminating nervous habits and tics. *Behaviour Research and Therapy, 11*, 619–628. https://doi.org/10.1016/0005-7967(73)90119-8.

Benvenuti, S. M., Buodo, G., Leone, V., & Palomba, D. (2011). Neurofeedback training for Tourette syndrome: An uncontrolled single case study. *Applied Psychophysiology and Biofeedback, 26*, 281–288. https://doi.org/10.1007/s10484-011-9169-7.

Besag, F., Vasey, M. J., Lao, K., Chowhury, U., & Stern, J. S. (2021). Pharmacological treatment for Tourette syndrome in children and adults: What is the quality of the evidence? A systematic review. *Journal of Psychopharmacology, 35*, 1037–1061. https://doi.org/10.1177/02698811211032445.

Bloch, M. H., & Leckman, J. F. (2009). Clinical course of Tourette syndrome. *Journal of Psychosomatic Research, 6*, 497–501. https://doi.org/10.1016/j.jpsychores.2009.09.002.

Burd, L., & Kerbeshian, J. (1987). Treatment-generated problems associated with behavior modification in Tourette disorder. *Developmental Medicine & Child Neruology, 29*, 831–833.

Calder-Sprackman, S., Sutherland, S., & Doja, A. (2014). The portrayal of Tourette syndrome in film and television. *Canadian Journal of Neurological Sciences, 41*, 226–232. https://doi.org/10.1017/S0317167100016620.

Chang, S. W., Piacentini, J., & Walkup, J. T. (2007). Behavioral treatment of Tourette syndrome: Past, present, and future. *Clinical Psychology: Science & Practice, 14*, 268–273. https://doi.org/10.1111/j.1468-2850.2007.00086.x.

Coffey, B. J., Biederman, J., Geller, D., Frazier, J., Spencer, T., Doyle, R., Gianini, L., Small, A., Frisone, D. F., Magovcevic, M., Stein, N., & Faraone, S. V. (2004). Reexamining tic persistence and tic-associated impairment in Tourette's disorder: Findings from a naturalistic follow-up study. *The Journal of Nervous and Mental Disease, 192*, 776–780. https://doi.org/10.1097/01.nmd.0000144696.14555.c4.

Conelea, C. A., Woods, D. W., Zinner, S. H., Budman, C. L., Murphy, T. K., Scahill, L. D., Compton, S. N., & Walkup, J. T. (2013). The impact of Tourette Syndrome in adults: results from the Tourette Syndrome impact survey. *Community Mental Health Journal, 49*, 110–120. https://doi.org/10.1007/s10597-011-9465-y.

Erenberg, G. (1988). Pharmacologic therapy of tics in childhood. *Pediatric Annals, 17*, 395–396, 398, 400–402, 404. https://doi.org/10.3928/0090-4481-19880601-07.

Ferenczi, S. (1921). Psycho-analytical observations on tic. *International Journal of Psychoanalysis, 2*, 1–30.

Freeman, R. D, Zinner, S. H., Müller-Vahl, K. R., Fast, D. K., Burd, L. J., Kano, Y., Rothenberger, A., Roessner, V., Kerbeshian, L., Stern, J. S., Jankovic, J., Loughlin, T., Janik, P., Shady, G., Robertson, M. M., Lang, A. E., Budman, C., Magor, A., Bruun, R., & Berlin Jr., C. M. (2009). Coprophenomena in Tourette syndrome. *Developmental Medicine & Child Neurology*, *51*, 218–227. https://doi.org/10.1111/j.1469-8749.2008.03135.x.

Ganos, C., Martino, D., Espay, A.J., Lang, A.E., Bhatia, K.P., & Edwards, M. J. (2019). Tics and functional tic-like movements. Can we tell them apart? *Neurology*, *93*, 750–758. https://doi.org/10.1212/WNL.0000000 000008372.

Grados, M., Huselid, R., & Duque-Serrano, L. (2018). Transcranial magnetic stimulation in Tourette syndrome: A historical perspective, its current use and the influence of comorbidities in treatment response. *Brain Science*, *8*, 129. https://doi.org/10.3390/brainsci8070129.

Heyman, I., Liang, H., & Hedderly, T. (2021). COVID-19 related increase in childhood tics and tic-like attacks. *Archives of Disease in Childhood*, *106*, 420–421. https://doi.org/10.1136/archdischild-2021-321748.

Himle, M. B., Woods, D. W., Piacentini, J., & Walkup, J. (2006). A brief review of habit reversal training for Tourette syndrome. *Journal of Child Neurology*, *21*, 719–725. https://doi.org/10.1177/08830738060210080101.

Hsu, C, Want, L., & Lin, P. (2018). Efficacy of repetitive transcranial magnetic stimulation for Tourette syndrome: A systematic review and meta-analysis. *Brain Stimulation*, *11*, 1110–1118. https://doi.org/10.1016/j.brs.2018.06.002.

Khalifa, N., & von Knorring, A.L. (2005). Tourette syndrome and other tic disorders in a total population of children: Clinical assessment and background. *Acta Paediatrica*, *94*, 1608–1614. https://doi.org/10.1111/j .1651-2227.2005.tb01837.x.

Kompoliti, M. D., Fan, W., & Leurgans, S. (2009). Complementary and alternative medicine use in Gilles de la Tourette syndrome. *Movement Disorders*, *24*, 1998–2019. https://doi.org/10.1002/mds.22724.

Kuhn, K. W., & Cambron, J. (2013). Chiropractic management using a brain-based model of care for a 15-year-old boy with migraine headaches and behavioral and learning difficulties: A case report. *Journal of Chiropractic Medicine*, *12*, 274–280. https://doi.org/10.1016/j.jcm.2013.10.005.

Kurlan, R. (2014). Hypothesis II: Tourette's syndrome is part of a clinical spectrum that includes normal brain development. *Archives of Neurology*, *51*, 1145–1150. https://doi.org/10.1001/archneur.1994.00540230083017.

Kushner, H. I. (1999). *A cursing brain? The histories of Tourette syndrome*. Harvard University Press.

Lajonchere, C., Nortz, M., & Finger, S. (1996). Gilles de la Tourette and the discovery of Tourette syndrome. *Archives of Neurology*, *53*, 567–574. https://doi.org/10.1001/archneur.1996.00550060111024.

Landeros-Weisenberger, A., Mantovani, A., Motlagh, M. G., de Alvarenga, P. G., Katsovich, L., Leckman, J. F., & Lisanby, S. H. (2015). Randomized sham controlled double-blind trial of repetitive transcranial magnetic stimulation for adults with severe Tourette syndrome. *Brain Stimulation*, *8*, 574–581. https://doi.org/10.1016/j.brs.2014.11.015.

Leckman, J. F., Walker, D. E., & Cohen, D. J. (1993). Premonitory urges in Tourette's syndrome. *American Journal of Psychiatry*, *150*, 98–102. https://doi.org/10.1176/ajp.150.1.98.

Leckman, J. F., Zhang, H., Vitale, A., Lahnin, F., Lynch, K., Bondi, C., Kim, Y. S., & Peterson, B. S. (1998). Course of tic severity in Tourette syndrome: The first two decades. *Pediatrics*, *102*, 14–19. https://doi.org/10.1542/peds.102.1.14.

Mantel, B. J., Meyers, A., Tran, Q., Rogers, S., & Jacobson, J. S. (2005). Nutritional supplements and complementary/alternative medicine in Tourette syndrome. *Journal of Child & Adolescent Psychopharmacology*, *14*, 582–589. https://doi.org/10.1089/cap.2004.14.582.

McGuire, J. F., Piacentini, J., Brennan, E. A., Lewin, A. B., Murphy, T. K., Small, B. J., & Storch, E. A. (2014). A meta-analysis of behavior therapy for Tourette syndrome. *Journal of Psychiatric Research*, *50*, 106–112. https://doi.org/10.1016/j.jpsychires.2013.12.009.

Müller-Vahl, K. R., Riemann, L., & Bokemeyer, S. (2014). Tourette patients' misbelief of a tic rebound is due to overall difficulties in reliable tic rating. *Journal of Psychosomatic Research*, *76*, 472–476. https://doi.org/10.1016/j.jpsychores.2014.03.003.

Müller-Vahl, K. R., Schneider, U., Prevedel, H., Theloe, K., Kolbe, H., Daldrup, T., & Emrich, H. M. (2003). Delta 9-tetrahydrocannabinol (THC) is effective in the treatment of tics in Tourette syndrome: A 6-week randomized trial. *Journal of Clinical Psychiatry*, *64*, 459–465. https://doi.org/10.4088/jcp.v64n0417.

Nagai, Y., Cavanna, A., & Critchley, H. D. (2009). Influence of sympathetic autonomic arousal on tics: Implications for a therapeutic behavioural intervention for Tourette syndrome. *Journal of Psychosomatic Research*, *67*, 599–605. https://doi.org/10.1016/j.jpsychores.2009.06.004.

Nagai, Y., Cavanna, A. E., Critchley, H. D., Stern, J. J., Robertson, M. M., & Joyce, E. M. (2014). Biofeedback treatment for Tourette syndrome: A preliminary randomized controlled trial. *Cognitive & Behavioral Neurology*, *27*, 17–24. https://doi.org/10.1097/WNN.0000000000000019.

O'Rourke, J. A., Scharf, J. M., Yu, D., & Pauls, D. L. (2009). The genetics of Tourette syndrome: A review. *Journal of Psychosomatic Research, 67,* 533–545. https://doi.org/10.1016/j.jpsychores.2009.06.006.

Peterson, A. L., McGuire, J. F., Wilhelm, S., Piacentini, J., Woods, D. W., Walkup, J. T., Hatch, J. P., Villarreal, R., & Scahill, L. (2016). An empirical examination of symptom substitution associated with behavior therapy for Tourette's disorder. *Behavior Therapy, 47,* 29–41.

Piacentini, J. C., Woods, D. W., Scahill, L. D., Wilhelm, S., Peterson, A., Chang, S., Ginsburg, G. S., Deckersbach, T., Dziura, J., Levi-Pearl, S., & Walkup, J. T. (2010). Behavior therapy for children with Tourette Syndrome: A randomized controlled trial. *Journal of the American Medical Association, 303,* 1929–1937. https://doi.org/10.1001/jama.2010.607.

Pringsheim, T., Ganos, C., McGuire, J.F., Hedderly, T., Woods, D., Gilbert, D.L., Piacentini, J., Dale, R. C., & Martino, D. (2021). Rapid onset functional tic-like behaviors in young females during the COVID-19 pandemic. *Movement Disorders, 36,* 2707–2713. https://doi.org/10.1002/mds.28778.

Pringsheim, T., Okun, M.S., Müller-Vahl, K., Martino, D., Jankovic, J., Cavanna, A.E., Woods, D. W., Robinson, M., Jarvie, E., Roessner, V., Oskoui, M., Holler-Managan, Y., & Piacentini, J. (2019). Practice guideline recommendations summary: Treatment of tics in people with Tourette syndrome and chronic tic disorders. *Neurology, 92,* 896–906. https://doi.org/10.1212/WNL.0000000000007466.

Rath, J. J., Tavy, D. L., Wertenbroek, A. A., van Woerkom, T. C., & de Bruijn, S. F. (2010). Botulinum toxin type A in simple motor tics: short-term and long-term treatment effects. *Parkinsonism & Related Disorders, 16,* 478–481. https://doi.org/10.1016/j.parkreldis.2009.11.011.

Rizzo, R., Gulisano, M., Cali, P. V., & Curatolo, P. (2012). Long term clinical course of Tourette syndrome. *Brain and Development, 34,* 667–673.

Robakis, D. (2017). How much do we know about adult-onset primary tics? Prevalence, epidemiology, and clinical features. *Tremor and Other Hyperkinetic Movements, 7,* 441. https://doi.org/10.7916/D8SQ95ND.

Robertson, M. M. (2008). The prevalence and epidemiology of Gilles de la Tourette syndrome: Part 1: The epidemiological and prevalence studies. *Journal of Psychosomatic Research, 65,* 461–472. https://doi.org/10.1016/j.jpsychores.2008.03.006.

Schrock, L. E., Mink, J. W., Woods, D. W., Porta, M., Servello, D., Visser-Vandewalle, V., Silburn, P. A., Foltynie, T., Walker, H. C., Shahed-Jimenez, J., Savica, R., Klassen, B. T., Machado, A. G., Foote, K. D., Zhang, J.-G., Hu, W., Ackermans, L., Temel, Y., Mari, Z., ... Okun, M. S. (2014). Tourette syndrome deep brain stimulation: A review and updated recommendations. *Movement Disorders, 30,* 448–471.

Shapiro, A. K., & Shapiro, E. (1968). Treatment of Gilles de la Tourette's syndrome with Haloperidol. *The British Journal of Psychiatry*, *114*, 345–350. https://doi.org/10.1192/bjp.114.508.345.

Storch, E. A., Lack, C. W., Simons, L. E., Goodman, W. K., Murphy, T. K., & Geffken, G. R. (2007). A measure of functional impairment in youth with Tourette syndrome. *Journal of Pediatric Psychology*, *32*, 950–959. https://doi.org/10.1093/jpepsy/jsm0034.

Sukhodolsky, D. G., Woods, D. W., Piacentini, J., Wilhelm, S., Peterson, A. L., Katsovich, L., Dziura, J., Walkup, J. T., & Scahill, L. (2017). Moderators and predictors of response to behavior therapy for tics in Tourette syndrome. *Neurology*, *14*, 1029–1036. https://doi.org/10.1212/WNL .0000000000003710.

Verdellen, C. W. J., Keijsers, G. P., Cath, D. C., & Hoogduin, C. A. L. (2004). Exposure and response prevention versus habit reversal in Tourette's syndrome: A controlled study. *Behaviour Research & Therapy*, *42*, 501–511. https://doi.org/10.1016/S0005-7967(03)00154-2.

Walkup, J. T., Ferrao, Y., Lackman, J. F., Stein, D. J., & Singer, H. (2010). Tic disorders: Some key issues for DSM-V. *Depression and Anxiety*, *27*, 600–610. https://doi.org/10.1002/da.20711.

Weisman, H., Qureshi, I. A., Leckman, J. F., Scahill, L., & Bloch, M. H. (2013). Systematic review: Pharmacological treatment of tic disorders – Efficacy of antipsychotic and alpha-2 adrenergic agonist agents. *Neuroscience and Biobehavioral Reviews*, *37*, 1162–1171. https://doi.org/10.1016/j .neubiorev.2012.09.008.

Wilhelm, S., Peterson, A. L., Piacentini, J., Woods, D. W., Deckersbach, T., Sukhodolsky, D. G., Chang, S., Liu, H., Dziura, J., Walkup, J. T., & Scahill, L. (2012). Randomized trial of behavior therapy for adults with Tourette syndrome. *Archives of General Psychiatry*, *69*, 795–803. https://doi.org/10.1001/archgenpsychiatry.2011.1528.

Woods, D. W., Conelea, C. A., & Walther, M. R. (2007). Barriers to dissemination: Exploring the criticisms of behavior therapy for tics. *Clinical Psychology: Science & Practice*, *14*, 279–282.

Woods, D. W., Piacentini, J. C., Chang, S. W., Deckersbach, T., Ginsburg, G. S., Peterson, A. L., Scahill, L. D., Walkup, J. T., & Wilhelm, S. (2008). *Managing Tourette Syndrome: A behavioral intervention for children and adults: Therapist guide*. Oxford University Press.

20

Couples Discord

Erin F. Alexander and Matthew D. Johnson

Couples therapy involves individuals in an intimate partnership meeting with a therapist together to change aspects of their relationship, including managing conflict, improving satisfaction, and coping with contextual stressors. The most commonly cited reasons for seeking couples therapy are poor communication and a lack of emotional affection, although the individual members of a couple often disagree as to why they attend (Doss et al., 2004). The centrality of intimate relationship quality in overall life satisfaction has led experts to predict an expansion in the demand and offerings of couples therapy (Norcross et al., 2013).

Couples therapy is most often associated with *relationship distress with spouse or intimate partner* in the Other Conditions That May Be a Focus of Clinical Attention section of the *Diagnostic and Statistical Manual of Mental Disorders* (DSM-5-TR; American Psychological Association, 2022). Although this intervention is not designed to treat a specific diagnosis, marital dissatisfaction is linked to many health problems, both physical (McShall & Johnson, 2015b) and mental (McShall & Johnson, 2015a). Additionally, couples therapy has demonstrated efficacy in reducing symptoms in individuals with various mental health disorders, including posttraumatic stress disorder, substance use, and depression, as well as several physical health concerns (Gurman et al., 2015).

20.1 Pseudoscience and Questionable Ideas

From its inception, the field of couples therapy has been no stranger to pseudoscience. Paul Popenoe, a therapist known by some as the father of marriage counseling, declared that part of the "promotion of successful family life" included eugenics (as cited by Lepore, 2010, para. 5). In modern times, pseudoscience in couples therapy primarily presents as marketed interventions with little to no research support. In this chapter, we demonstrate that many widely advertised, readily accessible therapies and self-help resources have few or no experimental studies supporting their use. Some therapies have demonstrated statistical *efficacy* in the context of research but not clinically significant change in the real world, which is referred to as *effectiveness* (Flay et al., 2005). In the following section, studies on the efficacy and effectiveness of various couples therapy approaches are discussed.

In reading treatment outcome studies, attention should be paid to the distinction between quasi-experimental and experimental designs. In a true experiment, participants are randomly assigned to treatment conditions. In typical quasi-experimental designs, couples self-select into either the treatment or control condition. This self-selection has meant that some outcome studies had less committed couples in the control group than in the treatment group (for a review, see Johnson & Bradbury, 2015). Ideally, a couples therapy approach should have demonstrated efficacy and effectiveness in experimental studies.

In preparation for writing this chapter, we did a standard Google search for couples therapy. All of the therapeutic approaches discussed below appeared on the first page of search results for "couples therapy" or "types of marriage counseling." The therapies discussed as "pseudoscientific" (or at least "questionable") in this chapter are not research-supported, as we conducted a systematic review of the scientific literature to find all existing published studies on each of these therapeutic approaches.

20.1.1 Myths about Relationships

Before describing dubious approaches to treating relationship problems, it is worth reviewing some of the myths about intimate partnerships that make dubious approaches to treatment more compelling. In 2016, the second author of this chapter (Johnson) published a book refuting 25 persistent myths about intimate relationships. Here is a sampling of some such myths that continue to lead couples and those who seek to help them astray.

20.1.1.1 Myth: Men Have a Stronger Libido Than Women

Most people overestimate gender differences in sex drive (Hyde, 2005). As we note later in this chapter, this myth has led to a proliferation of pseudoscience. One's gender is less determinative of libido than other factors. Furthermore, evidence exists that compared to men, women may be more likely to be sexually attracted to people other than their partner, and that this myth may persist because women are bored with their current sex life (see Johnson, 2016, Myth #1 for details).

20.1.1.2 Myth: Opposites Attract

They do not. Partner differences are far less frequent and intense than partner similarities. Couples perceive differences because they develop over time as the couple becomes more complementary. That is, couples condition one another into opposite, complementing roles (e.g., the quiet partner and the loud one; the logical partner and the emotional one) through their interactions with one another. Conflict is often avoided when partners are not competing for these roles, thus reinforcing the pattern of becoming more complementary. However, these differences develop over time as opposed to at the moment of initial attraction, and the notion that opposites attract has been consistently refuted by scientists (see Johnson, 2016, Myth #6 for details).

20.1.1.3 Myth: Couples Who Are "Matched" By Online Dating Services Are More Likely to Have Satisfying Relationships

Claims by online dating services that they provide more satisfying relationships using matching algorithms are dubious. Until these companies share their proprietary formulas and outcome data, we will not know for sure; however, they may simply be screening out people who are unlikely to have successful relationships (see Johnson, 2016, Myth #10 for details).

20.1.1.4 Myth: Children Raised by Other-Sex Couples Are Better Off Than Children Raised by Same-Sex Couples

As cases about the legality of same-sex marriage were making their way through the courts, a group of activists and professors claimed to test whether children raised by same-sex parents had worse outcomes than other children (Regnerus, 2012). Rather than scientifically studying this question, they engaged in scientific misconduct. In the views of many, this damaged their cause, their reputations, and the public's understanding of same-sex parenting (see Johnson, 2016, Myth #13 for details).

20.1.1.5 Myth: Living Together Before Marriage Is a Good Way to Determine Whether You're with the Right Person

For over 30 years, researchers have consistently generated evidence showing no benefit to living with a partner before marriage, including no positive impacts on personal wellbeing, relationship satisfaction, or likelihood of divorce (see Johnson, 2016, Myth #14 for details).

20.1.1.6 Myth: Men Are from Mars, Women Are from Venus

No, men are from Earth and women are from Earth – both metaphorically and literally. As we describe later, there is more empirical support for the gender similarity hypothesis than the gender difference hypothesis (Hyde, 2005). More importantly, people who display both stereotypically masculine and feminine traits tend to have better relationships (see Johnson, 2016, Myth #21 for details).

20.1.2 Dangerous Assessment Practices

Before treating relational problems, it is important that practitioners assess couples carefully. Properly screening for intimate partner violence prior to beginning conjoint therapy sessions with a couple is essential. Evidence suggests that couples experiencing a type of intimate partner violence in which one partner exhibits controlling, abusive behaviors over the other may not be suitable for treatment in a couples setting. In fact, it may be dangerous to engage in couples therapy with such couples due to the potential for retaliation against the victim for statements made in therapy (Stith & McCollum, 2012). Careful consideration should be given to the selection of intimate partner violence assessment instruments because many existing measures have not been properly validated (Alexander et al., 2021).

20.1.3 Implausible and Ineffective Treatments

All of the following treatment approaches are either untested or under-tested and some have studies suggesting a lack of utility. However, these therapies are still widely publicized, leading some couples to choose questionable treatments over evidence-based approaches.

20.1.3.1 Unhelpful Couples Self-Help

Couples therapy is an area with a vast self-help industry. Hundreds of books are written that promise to improve relationship functioning, help struggling single people understand the opposite sex, and form lasting relationships. However, the quality of many of these books is questionable.

A common premise of these books is that men and women are so different they cannot possibly understand each other. For example, *Act Like a Lady, Think Like a Man* by television personality Steve Harvey declares that "the women need a voice – someone to help get them through and decipher the muck" (Harvey & Millner, 2010, p. 6). Harvey goes on to give advice around the simplistic, stereotypic idea that men want sex, women do not, and in order to succeed in a relationship, women must trade sex for romance. Similar ideas are prevalent in the self-help industry. For example, one author promotes the idea that men and women are inherently different in *Love and Respect: The Love She Most Desires; The Respect He Desperately Needs*. He notes that "wives are made to love" and "husbands are made to be respected" (Eggerichs, 2004, p. 6).

Perhaps the most well-known self-help book promoting the idea that men and women are incapable of understanding each other is *Men Are from Mars, Women Are from Venus*. One clear signal of pseudoscience is the sensationalistic promises of an intervention's efficacy. The book declares that by using the Mars–Venus framework, the author has seen "relationships dramatically transform overnight" and "*miraculously* change[d]" (Gray, 1993, p. 3). In fact, the idea that men and women are so different as to be unable to understand each other has been disputed in many studies. A compilation of 46 meta-analyses provided evidence for what is called the "gender similarity hypothesis" (Hyde, 2005). This hypothesis, supported by hundreds of studies, declares that women and men are actually quite similar on most psychological constructs, including what they want in a relationship. Finally, some popular self-help books are based on the principles of the therapies described below. These books often make overblown promises, such as the ability to eliminate all negativity from couples' interactions. Often sold with a slew of other self-help resources including DVDs, webinars, card games, postcards, and workshops, these resources are based on therapies with limited empirical support.

20.1.3.2 Gottman Therapy

Gottman Therapy or Gottman Method Couples Therapy is a style of couples therapy developed to "help create and maintain greater love and health in relationships" (The Gottman Institute, 2020a, para. 1). The Gottman Method is described as beginning with thorough assessment and feedback, and then focusing on friendship, conflict management, and creating shared meaning. The therapy is based around the Sound Relational House Theory, which involves nine components of a healthy relationship (The Gottman Institute, 2020b).

In a systematic search for studies on Gottman Method couples therapy, no randomized controlled trials were located. The largest study on the Gottman Method focused on gay and lesbian couples (Garanzini et al., 2017), in which 88 gay and 18 lesbian couples who were seeking treatment for relationship distress were included. All couples received Gottman Method couples therapy by therapists trained in using the Gottman Method. There was no control group. Results showed significant differences in relationship satisfaction across time points. However, without a control group, it is unknown whether the Gottman Method was instrumental in leading to these changes over the course of treatment, if some other nonspecific factor was at play simply by virtue of being in treatment, or whether these couples would have naturally improved over time.

Three additional studies on the efficacy of Gottman Method couples therapy were located. All three studies were conducted in Iran, had sample sizes of fewer than 20 couples, and used quasi-experimental designs (Davoodvandi et al., 2018; Havaasi et al., 2017; Rajaei et al., 2019). In one study, Davoodvandi and colleagues (2018) showed that eight treatment couples had greater increases in satisfaction and intimacy than eight control couples; however, the small sample size and quasi-experimental design precludes the conclusion that the intervention was efficacious. Similarly, Havaasi and colleagues (2017) compared the efficacy of the Gottman Method and emotion-focused therapy in treating marital burnout and changing the way couples approach conflict resolution. Results showed that both treatments reduced burnout and increased constructive conflict resolution styles; however, emotion-focused therapy was found to be more effective than the Gottman Method. Finally, Rajaei and colleagues (2019) demonstrated that a treatment group receiving the Gottman Method was more likely to remain married and had better communication skills than controls. Yet once again, couples were not randomly assigned to conditions (i.e., the design was quasi-experimental), so inferences about the efficacy of the intervention cannot be made. Another important limitation of this study includes the fact that the therapist who conducted the sessions had not received training on the Gottman Method but self-trained by reading about it, so adherence to the formal intervention was unclear.

Overall, studies on Gottman Method couples therapy reveal positive results when comparing the Gottman Method to self-selected, no-treatment control conditions. However, when compared to an active treatment comparison group, the Gottman Method is less effective. Additionally, none of the studies had the methodological rigor required to make conclusive determinations of its efficacy or effectiveness. Most sample sizes were small, and the largest study was uncontrolled. Much more rigorous research would be needed before considering Gottman Method couples therapy an evidence-based treatment, as some popular media articles suggested. Given that preliminary evidence suggests other treatment alternatives to be more effective, the popularity and promotion of Gottman Method couples therapy is unwarranted.

20.1.3.3 Imago Therapy

Imago Therapy, first developed in 1980, is based on the idea that so-called childhood wounds lead to conflict in adult relationships (Imago Relationships Worldwide, 2020). Gehlert and colleagues (2017) describe several aspects of this approach. The therapy is based on the theory that unconscious drives from childhood impact the partners we select and the conflicts we have with those partners. The therapy aims to heal these childhood wounds through communication and understanding between partners. This process is intended to bring about growth and personality development. Core components of the therapy include dialogue between partners in which one plays the role of the childhood caregiver, making specific requests of one another, and identifying similarities between one's partner and childhood caregiver.

Two publications were located that described different outcome metrics from one randomized controlled trial in which 30 couples were randomized to Imago Therapy or a control (Gehlert et al., 2017; Schmidt & Gelhert, 2017). The researchers found that the treatment group showed an increase in relationship satisfaction, while the control group's satisfaction remained stable (Gehlert et al., 2017). However, the authors found that while the treatment group showed an increase in satisfaction, the change was *not clinically significant* because the satisfaction scores were still in the distressed range (Schmidt & Gelhert, 2017). The same study measured empathy levels as an outcome. The treatment group increased in empathy, while the control group decreased. However, the pretreatment empathy levels were already within the functional range, so it is questionable whether empathy was a useful treatment target.

One qualitative study on Imago therapy involved six couples who reported subjective effectiveness in improving communication skills and understanding of themselves and their partners (Martin & Bielawski, 2011). Two additional articles on Imago therapy using a pretest–posttest quasi-experimental design were located; however, these articles were from foreign language journals that were so poorly translated into English, they lost important methodological information (Cheraey et al., 2019; Farahani et al., 2018).

Overall, there was one objective, useable study on Imago therapy (Gehlert et al., 2017; Schmidt & Gelhert, 2017). While this study showed improvements in relationship satisfaction and empathy levels, the improvement in relationship satisfaction was deemed not clinically significant and the improvement in empathy not relevant. Additionally, a single study cannot be the basis to establish an evidence-based practice, and multiple lines of evidence are needed before such a claim can be made. Given these findings, the wide publicization of Imago therapy is unwarranted.

From a theoretical perspective, aspects of Imago seem to contradict empirical knowledge about healthy relationship development and functioning. A core element of Imago includes the directive that clients examine how the personality traits of their partner align with personality traits of their parents (Gehlert et al., 2017). Specifically, Imago involves one partner directing how they feel about their childhood caregiver toward their partner and requesting their partner perform a behavior to meet a childhood need. This is theoretically similar to the construct of displaced aggression, which is thought to be an unhealthy defense mechanism associated with narcissism (Martinez et al., 2008).

20.1.3.4 Narrative Couples Therapy

Narrative therapy is a therapeutic orientation not specific to couples therapy. It utilizes a narrative metaphor to help clients make sense of their lives (Freedman & Combs, 2015). Narrative couples therapy involves restructuring the way a couple views their joint story (Freedman & Combs, 2015). Only one experimental study endeavoring to test the efficacy of narrative couples therapy was located (Roozdar et al., 2019). Fifteen married couples in Iran received 8 weeks of treatment in conjoint narrative therapy, and 15 others were part of a waitlist control group. Unfortunately, the article included no descriptive statistics and limited inferential statistics, therefore we cannot draw any meaningful conclusions. It is clear that much more research is needed to determine whether the narrative couples therapy approach is effective. Proponents have said that "practice-based evidence" is preferred over "evidence-based practice," in that therapists ask patients in the room with them whether they are experiencing therapy as helpful (Freedman & Combs, 2015, p. 287). However, anecdotal evidence is insufficient for making determinations about treatment effectiveness. Therefore, we do not recommend the use of narrative couples therapy when well-tested couples therapy approaches exist (detailed below).

20.1.3.5 Relational Life Therapy

Relational Life Therapy (RLT) focuses on obtaining a power balance in the couple, as well as a balance between shame and grandiosity. RLT is different from other therapies in that the therapist takes sides, the therapist is extremely directive in telling the clients what to do, and there is sometimes intensive individual therapy work done with one member of the couple while the other observes in the room. An article written by the developer of RLT says that in this approach, the therapist is extremely honest with the client and says things that would normally not be said to a client directly but reserved for consulting with colleagues (Real, 2012).

A statement on a related website notes that the first study on RLT was completed in 2017 and returned a nonsignificant trend for the effectiveness of the therapy. The lack of significance was explained by noting the small sample size. No references to other studies on RLT were found. No empirical publications located mention RLT. From a theoretical perspective, aspects of RLT are contrary to empirical knowledge. For example, RLT suggests that the therapist should take sides. This is disputed by evidence suggesting the importance of couples therapists developing a balanced rapport that considers the broader systemic dynamic of the couple (Perkins et al., 2019). Additionally, some of its suggested techniques are in contrast to the common factors theory of efficacious psychotherapy (Norcross & Wampold, 2011) and at odds with empirical findings showing that a lack of perceived empathy leads to dissatisfaction with therapy and early termination (Khazaie et al., 2016).

20.2 Research-Supported Approaches

Several couples therapy approaches exist that are well-studied with demonstrated efficacy. Multiple reviews reveal that behavioral therapies (including cognitive-behavioral and integrative behavioral couples therapy), as well as emotion-focused couples therapy, have demonstrated efficacy and effectiveness (Bradbury & Bodenmann, 2020; Gurman & Fraenkel, 2002; Rathgeber et al., 2019; Snyder & Halford, 2012).

Behavioral therapies apply learning principles, especially those from social learning theory, to the relationship context. Typical components include teaching communication skills and changing how behaviors in the relationship are rewarded and punished. Goals of this type of couples therapy include teaching couples previously unlearned skills to resolve conflict and helping couples receive more rewards than costs from their relationship. Cognitive-behavioral couples therapy combines traditional behavioral couples therapy strategies with a focus on changing distorted cognitions about one's partner and relationship, ranging from attention biases to deeply rooted standards about what a relationship should be (Baucom et al., 2015). Integrative behavioral couples therapy adds a component of acceptance of what cannot be changed about one's partner and relationship (Jacobson et al., 2000).

Emotion-focused couples therapy is based upon experiential and family systems theoretical orientations, incorporating ideas from attachment theory to focus on emotion within couples' interactions (Johnson, 2015). Emotion-focused couples therapy aims to help couples reorganize their interactional patterns and experience their emotions in the present moment during interactions with their partner (Johnson, 2015).

A recent review described the core components of effective couples therapies as providing a contextualized, dyadic, objective conceptualization of problems; modifying emotion-driven, dysfunctional, and destructive interpersonal behavior; eliciting avoided, emotion-based private behavior; fostering productive communication; and emphasizing strengths and encouraging positive behavior (Bradbury & Bodenmann, 2020). Given that evidence suggests these core goals are conducive to positive couples outcomes, and that research-supported therapies are shown to be widely effective, the popularity and dogmatic marketing of nonscience-based couples interventions is unwarranted. Couples are advised to choose research-supported methods. They may not promise an overnight transformation into a negativity-free couple, but results suggest that these methods are far more effective than any of the questionable approaches described in this chapter.

20.3 Conclusion

In conclusion, there are many resources for couples that are widely marketed without the outcome research to ensure their efficacy or effectiveness. Many myths about relationships persist in our society that impact relationship expectations. These myths are publicized in self-help claims promising to provide magical cures for relationship problems and secrets to understanding the opposite sex. Readily available to the public, these books, videos, and seminars are often promoted as being research-based, transformative, and effective. Yet many popular therapy techniques lack research evidence of their effectiveness. Gottman Therapy, Imago Therapy, narrative therapy, and

Relational Life Therapy are all publicized without proper evidence to support their use. While some of these therapies have preliminary evidence that suggest potential efficacy, without trials that include adequate sample sizes, control groups, and outcome measures, it remains unclear whether these options are effective. Investing in these interventions can draw couples away from scientifically sound, well-established treatments. Rather than investing in magical cures or dubious interventions, we recommend that couples seek research-supported treatments such as behavioral (as well as cognitive-behavioral and integrative-behavioral) couples therapy or emotion-focused couples therapy.

Erin F. Alexander, MS, is a doctoral student of psychology at Binghamton University.

Matthew D. Johnson, PhD, is a Professor of Psychology at Binghamton University. He is author of the book *Great Myths of Intimate Relationships: Dating, Sex, and Marriage* (2016).

References

Alexander, E. F., Backes, B. L., & Johnson, M. D. (2021). Evaluating measures of intimate partner violence using consensus-based standards of validity. *Trauma, Violence, and Abuse, 23*(5), 1549–1567.

American Psychiatric Association. (2022). *Diagnostic and statistical manual of mental disorders, fifth edition, text revision* (DSM-5-TR). American Psychiatric Association.

Baucom, D. H., Epstein, N. B., Kirby, J. S., & LaTaillaide, J. J. (2015). Cognitive behavioral couple therapy. In A. S. Gurman, J. L. Lebow, & D. K. Snyder (Eds.), *Clinical handbook of couple therapy* (5th ed., pp. 23–60). Guilford.

Bradbury, T. N., & Bodenmann, G. (2020). Interventions for couples. *Annual Review of Clinical Psychology, 16*, 99–123. https://doi.org/10.1146/annurev-clinpsy-071519-020546.

Cheraey, L., Goudarzi, M., Akbari, M. (in press). Comparing the effectiveness of couple therapy with imago-therapy and Feldman's integrated approach on marital commitment of conflicting spouses. *Quarterly Journal of Women and Society, 10*(39), 239–254.

Davoodvandi, M., Nejad, S. N., & Farzad, V. (2018). Examining the effectiveness of Gottman couple therapy on improving marital adjustment and couples' intimacy. *Iranian Journal of Psychiatry, 13*(2), 135–141.

Doss, B. D., Simpson, L. E., & Christensen, A. (2004). Why do couples seek marital therapy? *Professional psychology: Research and practice, 35*(6), 608–614.

Eggerichs, E. (2005). *Love & respect: The love she most desires, the respect he desperately needs*. Christian Art.

Farahani, F., & Delavar, A. (2018). Comparison of the effectiveness of coupled communication imaging therapy (imago therapy) with acceptance and commitment therapy (ACT) on the mental health of couples. *Iranian Journal of Educational Sociology*, *1*(9), 91–103.

Flay, B. R., Biglan, A., Boruch, R. F., Castro, F. G. l., Gottfredson, D., Kellam, S., Moscicki, E. K., Schinke, S., Valentine, J. C., & Ji, P. (2005). Standards of evidence: Criteria for efficacy, effectiveness and dissemination. *Prevention Science*, *6*(3), 151–175. https://doi.org/10.1007/s11121-005-5553-y.

Freedman, J., & Combs, G. (2015). Narrative couple therapy. In A. S. Gurman, J. L. Lebow, & D. K. Snyder (Eds.), *Clinical handbook of couple therapy* (5th ed., pp. 271–299). Guilford.

Garanzini, S., Yee, A., Gottman, J., Gottman, J., Cole, C., Preciado, M., & Jasculca, C. (2017). Results of Gottman Method Couples Therapy with gay and lesbian couples. *Journal of Marital and Family Therapy*, *43*(4), 674–684. https://doi.org/10.1111/jmft.12276.

Gehlert, N. C., Schmidt, C. D., Giegerich, V., & Luquet, W. (2017). Randomized controlled trial of imago relationship therapy: Exploring statistical and clinical significance. *Journal of Couple & Relationship Therapy*, *16*(3), 188–209. https://doi.org/10.1080/15332691.2016.1253518.

Gray, J. (1992). *Men are from Mars, women are from Venus: A practical guide for improving communication and getting what you want in your relationships*. HarperCollins.

Gurman, A. S., & Fraenkel, P. (2002). The history of couple therapy: A millennial review. *Family Process*, *41*(2), 199–260.

Gurman, A. S., Lebow, J. L., & Snyder, D. K. (Eds.). (2015). *Clinical handbook of couple therapy*. Guilford.

Harvey, S., & Millner, D. (2009). *Act like a lady, think like a man: What men really think about love, relationships, intimacy, and commitment*. Amistad.

Havaasi, N., Zahra Kaar, K., & Mohsen Zadeh, F. (2017). Compare the efficacy of emotion focused couple therapy and Gottman couple therapy method in marital burnout and changing conflict resolution styles. *Journal of Fundamentals of Mental Health*, *20*(1), 15–25.

Hyde, J. (2005). The gender similarities hypothesis. *The American Psychologist*, *60*(6), 581–592.

Imago Relationships Worldwide. (2020, January 12). Imago relationships. https://imagorelationships.org/.

Jacobson, N. S., Christensen, A., Prince, S. E., Cordova, J., & Eldridge, K. (2000). Integrative behavioral couple therapy: An acceptance-based, promising new treatment for couple discord. *Journal of Consulting and Clinical Psychology*, *68*(2), 351–355.

Johnson, M. D. (2016). *Great myths of intimate relationships: Dating, sex, and marriage.* Wiley.

Johnson, M. D., & Bradbury, T. N. (2015). Contributions of social learning theory to the promotion of healthy relationships: Asset or liability? *Journal of Family Theory & Review, 7*(1), 13–27. https://doi.org/10.1111/jftr.12057

Johnson, S. M. (2015). Emotionally focused couples therapy. In A. S. Gurman, J. L. Lebow, & D. K. Snyder (Eds.), *Clinical handbook of couple therapy* (5th ed., pp. 97–128). Guilford.

Khazaie, H., Rezaie, L., Shahdipour, N., & Weaver, P. (2016). Exploration of the reasons for dropping out of psychotherapy: A qualitative study. *Evaluation and Program Planning, 56,* 23–30. https://doi.org/10.1016/j.evalprogplan.2016.03.002.

Lepore, J. (2010, March 29). The rise of marriage therapy, and other dreams of human betterment. *The New Yorker.*

Martin, T. L. & Bielawski, D. M. (2011). What is the African American's experience following imago education? *Journal of Humanistic Psychology, 51*(2), 216–228. https://doi.org/10.1177/0022167809352379.

Martinez, M. A., Zeichner, A., Reidy, D. E., & Miller, J. D. (2008). Narcissism and displaced aggression: Effects of positive, negative, and delayed feedback. *Personality and Individual Differences, 44*(1), 140–149.

McShall, J. R., & Johnson, M. D. (2015a). The association between relationship distress and psychopathology is consistent across racial and ethnic groups. *Journal of Abnormal Psychology, 124*(1), 226–231. https://doi.org/10.1037/a0038267.

McShall, J. R., & Johnson, M. D. (2015b). The association between relationship quality and physical health across racial and ethnic groups. *Journal of Cross-Cultural Psychology, 46*(6), 789–804. https://doi.org/10.1177/0022022115587026.

Norcross, J. C., Pfund, R. A., & Prochaska, J. O. (2013). Psychotherapy in 2022: A Delphi poll on its future. *Professional Psychology: Research and Practice, 44*(5), 363–370. https://doi.org/10.1037/a0034633.

Norcross, J. C., & Wampold, B. E. (2011). Evidence-based therapy relationships: Research conclusions and clinical practices. *Psychotherapy, 48*(1), 98–102. https://doi.org/10.1037/a0022161.

Perkins, S. N., Glass, V. Q., & D'Aniello, C. (2019). It's all about the balance: Therapists' experience of systemic alliance development. *Contemporary Family Therapy, 41*(4), 420–434. https://doi.org/10.1007/s10591-019-09500-1.

Rajaei, A., Daneshpour, M., & Robertson, J. (2019). The effectiveness of couples therapy based on the Gottman method among Iranian couples with conflicts: A quasi-experimental study. *Journal of Couple & Relationship Therapy, 18*(3), 223–240.

Rathgeber, M., Bürkner, P. C., Schiller, E. M., & Holling, H. (2019). The efficacy of emotionally focused couples therapy and behavioral couples therapy: A meta-analysis. *Journal of Marital and Family Therapy*, *45*(3), 447–463. https://doi.org/10.1111/jmft.12336.

Real, T. (2012, November/December). Joining through the truth: Therapeutic coaching tests our assumptions. *Psychotherapy Networker*, *36*(6), 36–43, 60–61.

Regnerus, M. (2012). How different are the adult children of parents who have same-sex relationships? Findings from the New Family Structures Study. *Social Science Research*, *41*(4), 752–770.

Roozdar, E., Hamid, N., Beshlideh, K., & Arshadi, N. (2019). The effectiveness of narrative couple therapy on improving the psychological well-being maladaptive couples. *Biannual Journal of Applied Counseling 9*(1), 67–86. https://doi.org/10.22055/jac.2020.31058.1703.

Schmidt, C. D. & Gehlert, N. C. (2017). Couples therapy and empathy: An evaluation of the impact of imago relationship therapy on partner empathy levels. *The Family Journal*, *25*, 23–30. https:/doi.org/10.1177/1066480716678621.

Snyder, D. K., & Halford, W. K. (2012). Evidence-based couple therapy: Current status and future directions. *Journal of Family Therapy*, *34*(3), 229–249.

Stith, S. M., McCollum, E. E., Amanor-Boadu, Y., & Smith, D. (2012). Systemic perspectives on intimate partner violence treatment. *Journal of Marital and Family Therapy*, *38*(1), 220–240.

The Gottman Institute. (2020a). Our mission. www.gottman.com/about/.

The Gottman Institute. (2020b). The Gottman method. www.gottman.com/about/the-gottman-method/.

Postscript: Scientific Skepticism Resources

Stephen Hupp

It can feel overwhelming to think about all of the pseudoscience in the world. But it can also be motivating. This book might have made you hungry for more information about skepticism. Or perhaps you may even want to get involved in the skeptical community. Resources are described in the last chapter of the book *Pseudoscience in Child and Adolescent Psychotherapy* (Hupp, 2019), and a few will be described here, as well.

The Committee for Skeptical Inquiry (CSI) is a great starting point for learning more about scientific skepticism. The organization's magazine, *Skeptical Inquirer*, has a large number of articles related to psychology and just about every other discipline (https://skepticalinquirer.org/). You can also get involved through the CSI conference – CSICon – typically held annually in Las Vegas and/or online. Many of the presentations are freely available by searching the Internet for "Skeptical Inquirer Presents." Some of the notable presentations by psychologists include: Carol Tavris on cognitive dissonance; Maria Konnikova on deception; and Richard Wiseman in conversation with David Copperfield about the relationship between magic and skepticism.

Another prominent conference is the Northeast Conferences on Science and Skepticism (NECSS), a joint effort of the New England Skeptical Society (NESS) and the New York City Skeptics. The NESS President, Neurologist Steven Novella, also runs the Science-Based Medicine website (https://sciencebasedmedicine.org/), which has a large collection of skeptical articles, many of which relate to psychological therapies. Novella also hosts *The Skeptic's Guide to the Universe* podcast along with a group of "skeptical rogues" including this book's co-editor, Cara L. Santa Maria. She also hosts another podcast, *Talk Nerdy with Cara Santa Maria*, in which she interviews scientists across many disciplines. Together Novella, Santa Maria, and their co-authors published a book which helps explain many of the cognitive biases and logical fallacies that influence the way people think about science and pseudoscience – *The Skeptics' Guide to the*

Universe: How to Know What's Really Real in a World Increasingly Full of Fake (Novella et al., 2018).

In the field of psychology specifically, Scott O. Lilienfeld has been the tip of the skeptical spear for decades. He published hundreds of articles about topics such as the scientific status of different types of therapy (Lilienfeld, 2014), treatments that cause harm (Lilienfeld, 2007), and the distinction between *evidence*-based practice and *science*-based practice (Lilienfeld et al., 2018). He also taught critical thinking skills through his books *50 Great Myths of Psychology* (Lilienfeld et al., 2010), *Science and Pseudoscience in Clinical Psychology* (Lilienfeld et al., 2015), and *Psychology: From Inquiry to Understanding* (Lilienfeld et al., 2022). Thanks to these and other works written by Lilienfeld and his long-time collaborator, Steven Jay Lynn, the scientific understanding of psychology has forever been elevated to a higher level. Lilienfeld's passion for the science of psychology is also described in the book *Toward a Science of Clinical Psychology: A Tribute to the Life and Works of Scott O. Lilienfeld* (Cobb et al., 2023).

If you're interested in promoting critical thinking by participating in scientific skepticism, Hupp and Santa Maria (2019) offer several suggestions for how to get engaged. Some relatively easy but impactful ways include: attending and presenting at skeptical conferences; submitting articles to journals, magazines, or blogs; and reviewing and/or rating skeptical books and podcasts to help increase their visibility. Lastly, an organization called Guerilla Skepticism works to increase the likelihood that topics on Wikipedia are described in a way that promotes science (Gerbic, 2019). Taking the initial step toward getting involved in any of these ways will help you gain access to a like-minded community of scientific thinkers.

Stephen Hupp, PhD, is a Professor of Psychology at Southern Illinois University Edwardsville. He is co-editor of the book *Investigating Pop Psychology: Pseudoscience, Fringe Science, and Controversies* (Hupp & Wiseman, 2023).

References

Cobb, C. L., Lynn, S. J., & O'Donohue, W. (2023). *Toward a science of clinical psychology: A tribute to the life and works of Scott O. Lilienfeld*. Springer.

Gerbic, S. (2019). What is guerrilla skepticism on Wikipedia? Sidebar in S. Hupp (Ed.), *Pseudoscience in child and adolescent psychotherapy: A skeptical field guide* (pp. 6–7). Cambridge University Press.

Hupp, S. (2019). *Pseudoscience in child and adolescent psychotherapy: A skeptical field guide*. Cambridge University Press.

Hupp, S. & Santa Maria, C. (2019). Scientific skepticism and critical thinking about therapy. *the Behavior Therapist, 42*(5), 158–162.

Lilienfeld, S. O. (2007). Psychological treatments that cause harm. *Perspectives on Psychological Science, 2*(1), 53–70.

Lilienfeld, S. O. (2014). The Dodo Bird verdict: Status in 2014. *the Behavior Therapist, 37*(4), 91–95.

Lilienfeld, S. O., Lynn, S. J., & Bowden, S. C. (2018). Why evidence-based practice isn't enough: A call for science-based practice. *the Behavior Therapist, 41*(1), 42–47.

Lilienfeld, S. O., Lynn, S. J., & Lohr, J. M. (2015). *Science and pseudoscience in clinical psychology*. Guilford.

Lilienfeld, S. O., Lynn, S. J., & Namy, L. L. (2022). *Psychology: From inquiry to understanding*. Pearson.

Lilienfeld, S. O., Lynn, S. J., Ruscio, J., & Beyerstein, B. L. (2010). *50 great myths of popular psychology: Shattering widespread misconceptions about human behavior*. John Wiley & Sons.

Novella, S., Novella, B., Santa Maria, C., Novella, J., & Bernstein, E. (2018). *The skeptics' guide to the universe: How to know what's really real in a world increasingly full of fake*. Grand Central Publishing.

Index

For EU product safety concerns, contact us at Calle de José Abascal, 56–1°,
28003 Madrid, Spain or eugpsr@cambridge.org.

www.ingramcontent.com/pod-product-compliance
Ingram Content Group UK Ltd.
Pitfield, Milton Keynes, MK11 3LW, UK
UKHW020402140625
459647UK00020B/2599